T0316828

YOU *CAN* MINIMIZE
THE HARMFUL EFFECTS OF STRESS WITH
THE STRESS SOLUTION

When stressful things happen to you, how effectively do you handle them? *THE STRESS SOLUTION* can help you to understand your personal STRESS PROFILE, and to put that knowledge to work in your STRESS ACTION PLAN.

Many activities can reduce your vulnerability to stress—*and safeguard your health and life.* You are protecting yourself from stress's damaging effects if you almost always:

* Eat at least one hot, balanced meal per day
* Get 7–8 hours of sleep at least 4 nights a week
* Give and receive affection regularly
* Exercise to the point of perspiration at least twice a week
* Regularly attend club or social activities
* Have one or more friends to confide in about personal matters
* Limit yourself to fewer than three cups of coffee (or tea or cola drinks) per day
* Take quiet time for yourself during the day
* Do something for fun at least once a week
* Have an optimistic outlook

Stress is a highly personal experience—different for everyone. The good news is that there are practical, specific tools *you* can use to control its effect on *your* life.

"Chock full of helpful information . . . *THE STRESS SOLUTION* . . . provides useful tools and strategies for dealing with [stress]."
—Paul F. Rosch, M.D., F.A.C.P.
President, The American Institute of Stress

For orders other than by individual consumers, Pocket Books grants a discount on the purchase of **10 or more** copies of single titles for special markets or premium use. For further details, please write to the Vice-President of Special Markets, Pocket Books, 1230 Avenue of the Americas, New York, NY 10020.

For information on how individual consumers can place orders, please write to Mail Order Department, Paramount Publishing, 200 Old Tappan Road, Old Tappan, NJ 07675.

THE STRESS SOLUTION

AN ACTION PLAN TO MANAGE THE STRESS IN YOUR LIFE

LYLE H. MILLER, Ph.D., and
ALMA DELL SMITH, Ph.D., ABPP,
with LARRY ROTHSTEIN, Ed.D.

POCKET BOOKS
New York   London   Toronto   Sydney   Tokyo   Singapore

The sale of this book without its cover is unauthorized. If you purchased this book without a cover, you should be aware that it was reported to the publisher as "unsold and destroyed." Neither the author nor the publisher has received payment for the sale of this "stripped book."

POCKET BOOKS, a division of Simon & Schuster Inc.
1230 Avenue of the Americas, New York, NY 10020

Copyright © 1993 by Lyle H. Miller, Ph.D.,
Alma Dell Smith, Ph.D., ABPP,
and Larry Rothstein, Ed.D.

All rights reserved, including the right to reproduce
this book or portions thereof in any form whatsoever.
For information address Pocket Books, 1230 Avenue
of the Americas, New York, NY 10020

ISBN: 978-1-5011-5240-5

First Pocket Books paperback printing April 1994

10 9 8 7 6 5 4 3 2 1

POCKET and colophon are registered trademarks of
Simon & Schuster Inc.

Printed in the U.S.A.

This book is dedicated to our students
and clients from whom we have
learned so much, and to Logan, for being
such a good sport.

LHM

ADS

And to Anthony C. Westerhof, Ph.D., who
taught me more than he'll ever know.

LHM

ACKNOWLEDGMENTS

We owe an incalculable debt of gratitude to those scholars, researchers, and clinicians upon whose shoulders we stand. We are particularly grateful to the giants among that throng, Claude Bernard, William James, Adolph Meyer, Walter B. Cannon, Hans Selye, Franz Alexander, John and Beatrice Lacey, Stewart Wolf, and Richard Lazarus. It is their thoughts and formulations on stress and the mind/body connection that have shown us the way in our research and clinical work and in writing this book. We owe a similar debt to our clients, whose personal stories have guided our research and formed the basis of the composite examples used throughout the book.

Our most special thanks to Joan Johnson. A key member of the Institute team, she has been truly invaluable. Without her intelligence, good humor, patience, and unstinting effort over the last ten years, the Institute would surely have collapsed in chaos and confusion.

Thanks to Bruce Mehler for his contributions to the development of the *Stress Audit* and to the programs at the Institute.

No book is written without help. We appreciate the ideas of the students and faculty of the Biobehavioral Institute who have contributed so much to the research and clinical findings on which we have based our comments, Jacqueline Buchin, John Davey, Susan Davidson, Elizabeth Handleman-Kling, Ira Rudolph, Saundra Schoicket, and A. Eugene Palchanis. We have also learned from the experience and advice of the Women's Health Group at The University Hospital at

Boston University Medical Center. The ongoing support of Joan Goldberg, Shirley Partoll, Carole Rubin, and Kathryn Kirshner of the writers' group kept us optimistic we would finish.

To Ron Finch, Susan Miller Houston, Linda Lesky, Pat Mehler, Paul Rosch, Curt Sandman, Derek and Priscilla Shows, Marilyn Smith, Mary Smith, Richard Turcotte, Anna Williams, and Stewart Wolf, who waded through initial drafts of the manuscript and gave us invaluable advice and criticism, thank you, thank you, thank you.

In the last stages of the manuscript, Kimberly Lucas joined us to offer astute comments and invaluable assistance in editing and typing. Thanks, Kim, for the long hours and your cheery good humor.

Thanks to Dan Jones for shooting promotional videotapes and to Richard "Dixie" Tourangeau for his photography.

We want to thank our agent and champion, Kris Dahl, for her knowledge of the publishing world and her steadfast support and encouragement throughout the project. We owe much to our editors at Pocket Books, Leslie Wells, who first recognized the book's merit, and Sally Peters, whose patience and hard work helped bring it in on time.

Finally, we owe our deepest debt to Larry Rothstein for his constant cheerful guidance, his knowledge of books, the clarity of his exposition, but most of all for his Boston Celtics tickets.

CONTENTS

III | SYMPTOMS: SOOTHING THE BODY, CALMING THE MIND

IV IF AT FIRST YOU DON'T SUCCEED, YOU'RE HUMAN

APPENDICES

THE
STRESS
SOLUTION

INTRODUCTION

This is a book about stress and how it affects your life. It is written from our personal, clinical, and research experience. This book teaches you how to use a set of powerful tools for measuring and identifying the stress in your life. Finally, this book helps you design personalized stress management plans and connects you to the resources and support systems needed to implement these plans.

We approach stress from the scientific perspective of behavioral medicine, which draws on a variety of disciplines, both traditional and nontraditional. We believe strongly that you are your own best health resource and that you can minimize the use of costly medication, extensive psychotherapy, and hospitalization. In fact, we are convinced you'll see results in a few months, even a few weeks, if you follow the system described in this book.

At the Biobehavioral Institute of Boston, we enable our clients to move beyond vague complaints and confusions—"I can't sleep"; "I'm fighting with people at work"; "I just can't seem to have fun anymore"; "I don't know what's happening to me, but it's not stress"—to a new understanding of what's really wrong and how to change it.

Our most important tools are the *Stress Audit, Stress Profiles*, and *Stress Action Plans*. More than 250,000 people have taken the *Stress Audit*. Hospitals, clinics, physicians, psychiatrists, psychologists, and corporate employee assistance programs use the *Audit* to diagnose stress and stress-related illness. The *Stress Audit* helps our clients quickly find out how susceptible they are to stress, where stress comes from, and how it manifests itself in physical and mental symptoms.

With this information, we construct *Stress Profiles* that show our clients the pattern of their stress problems and whether their stress levels are low, moderate, high, or critical compared to those of other people.

The *Audit* and the *Stress Profiles* increase and sharpen our clients' awareness of their specific problems and motivate them to act. After reviewing their *Stress Audit* and *Stress Profiles*, we work with our clients to design comprehensive *Stress Action Plans*. With these plans our clients increase their tolerance to stress, alter, avoid, or accept stressful situations, and reduce stress symptoms. *Stress Action Plans* also aid our clients in overcoming barriers to taking action and teach them how to locate sources of support for their plans.

We have seen thousands of clients over the last fifteen years. Each one has contributed to our thinking about stress and how to help others. We have incorporated their stories into this book. We hope that through their experience you'll gain a perspective of your own stress problems as you realize that millions of others suffer from similar complaints. We have also included our personal stories because our situations are probably not too different from yours.

LYLE'S STORY

It was a Friday afternoon in June 1970. I was speeding across the Lake Pontchartrain bridge returning to New Orleans when I thought I saw a large chunk of the roadway disappear. But I knew no hole existed in the road. Rather, a hole in my vision, what neurologists call a visual scotoma, made it look that way. I'd had scotomas before and understood their tricks too well.

That "hole in the road" was my first warning that a pounding migraine would soon surge through my head. I'd had a string of them over the previous six weeks. I knew this one was going to be especially bad. I was in the middle of a twenty-six-mile bridge, surrounded by traffic, with no place to pull over. I was nauseated. I worried about throwing up the red beans and rice I'd had for lunch. I desperately wanted to make it home.

Since I couldn't see anything in front of me, I used the bridge's guard rail as a guide. I managed to get home without running into anybody or anything—or throwing up in the car. I called my office to cancel my late afternoon appointments. By this time I was having trouble talking. My lips and tongue were numb. I couldn't find the words to express my thoughts. My secretary thought I was having a stroke and wanted to call an ambulance. Annoyed, I stumblingly told her to mind her own business, that I was just having a migraine. Then I crawled into bed and stayed there all evening and half the next day.

I was sick, I was miserable, and, worst of all, I couldn't think or talk coherently. But I knew there was no "quick fix" medication for my migraines. Only a cool cloth on my forehead, a dark quiet room, and sleep would help.

Migraines run in the Miller family. My father, an uncle, my sister Jane, and I have had incapacitating migraines. But I knew other factors besides genetics played a part. Red wine, cheese, caffeine, lack of sleep, and stress could, singly or in combination, trigger a migraine. But I'd been avoiding red wine and cheese, didn't drink much coffee, and, apart from occasional carousing in the French Quarter, I'd been getting enough sleep. Stress certainly couldn't have been the culprit. I was a national stress expert and my life was going great.

Married with three children, I had entered college at age 31 and graduated Phi Beta Kappa in three years while working full-time as a printing pressman on the graveyard shift. Six years later, I'd earned a Ph.D. in clinical psychology with a minor in neurophysiology, was Associate Professor and Head of Psychology at Louisiana State University Medical School, and was pursuing a career in behavioral medicine. I had brilliant graduate students and we published research papers at a dizzying pace. I was a sought-after speaker and consultant. Although I had started late, I had caught up with my age peers. I was proud of myself and determined to do even better.

But as I lay in the dark of my bedroom, I realized that the stress of the last six years had caught up with me. All the signs had been there, but somehow I had successfully ignored them. I was exhausted and unhappy. There had been too many changes in too short a time. I had gone from a dead-end blue collar job on the graveyard shift to the fast track in the academic world.

For an expert on stress, I was doing a lousy job. I was ignoring almost everything I knew. First of all, I hadn't been honest with myself. New Orleans is a party town and I partied my socks off. Because friends and relatives visited us regularly in New Orleans, late-night tours of the French Quarter had become obligatory. In reality, I was *always* having "a little" wine and cheese. I avoided coffee but drank gallons of tea. I was working sixty-plus hours per week, breaking only for a working lunch (they always included a couple of martinis or a Sazerac cocktail or two). I wasn't exercising and had gained twenty pounds.

But there were also demands and pressures I hadn't noticed. When I took a sobering look I was stunned. While I saw myself as a hard-driving, aggressive, selfless leader, many colleagues viewed me as "a tyrannical, self-seeking empire builder." I pictured myself as a good provider and father, yet my wife saw me as an "egotistical workaholic" who used work to escape family responsibilities.

I was grandiose and expansive. I enthusiastically promised too many people too much. And I got angry when they expected me to live up to my promises. Meaningful communication with colleagues and family was nonexistent, so nothing ever got resolved.

My realizations and insights in June of 1970, however, didn't alter my behavior. I kept doing the same things. But in 1979 I began to change, when we started developing the tools and techniques that form the core of this book. As I applied the findings of our stress research to the problems of my clients, I saw that much of what I was providing my clients applied to me as well. I became my own best patient.

One of the tools we used was the *Stress Audit*. When I first took the *Audit*, I was shocked at my scores. I was as stressed as many of my patients. Somehow, seeing my stress scores in black and white brought my problems into sharper focus. Another tool, the *Stress Profile*, forced me to take a hard, structured look at what it was I really wanted. I then designed *Stress Action Plans* for myself. Slowly but surely my life changed. Over time I altered the way I looked at career, competition, and "success." I ate and slept well, exercised regularly, avoided caffeine, nicotine, and alcohol, found time for myself each day, and talked on the telephone with my family more often. I practiced self-regulation techniques such as progressive muscle relaxation and meditation and used biofeedback regularly.

After many years, I finally realized that stress was what I had been telling my clients and patients all along—a complex, multifaceted, uniquely personal problem that responds only to a treatment program tailored to the individual.

ALMA DELL'S STORY

For most people, their lives are marked by a few incidents that alter the course they have set for themselves. At the time they occur such incidents may go unnoticed, be denied, or be seen as destructive. But as the years pass their importance becomes clear. Mine came nearly twenty years ago in a rathskeller in Charleston, South Carolina.

I had been drifting through my life up to that point. I had graduated from Smith College in 1968 with little idea of what I wanted to do. Married at 20, I was divorced at 24. I tried being a public school teacher but was temperamentally unsuited for the job. A series of temporary jobs followed—substitute teacher, research assistant on an education project, secretarial work. These were unhappy times. I cried a lot, felt blue, and withdrew from family and friends. On several occasions I sought the counsel of a psychiatrist. Our sessions were largely unproductive—I talked, he listened, I became more confused, and nothing changed.

In 1973 I found myself in Charleston. I had followed my boyfriend there, giving up my job to do so. I took menial work: filing, "gofer" for a construction company, "tender" on a deep-sea-diving rig. Again, I was periodically depressed, unhappy, adrift, and defining my life through my relationship with a man. Finally, I found a job as a psychophysiological research technician at the nearby Medical University of South Carolina. At the same time, at the urging of my sister and a co-worker at the medical center, I joined the National Organization for Women (NOW). These two events changed my life forever.

In consciousness-raising groups, with the support of other women, I started to reconsider my life, my relationships with men, and my upbringing. For the first time since Girl Scouts, I formed close bonds with a group of strong, independent women. This "informal" therapy worked for me. I became more and more aware of the tremendous pressures and restrictions women face, and how I had been underachieving in terms of my life and my career. In addition to personal growth, I began to push for political and community change.

Normally after meetings, a number of us would head to a nearby rathskeller for a few beers and further discussion. That's what happened on a warm spring evening in 1974. After sharing a round of beers, I excused myself and left for the ladies' room, which was at the end of a long, dark corridor. The ladies' room was empty when I entered it. I closed the stall door. I was still in the stall when I heard the door swing open. I flushed the toilet and opened the stall door. A large man, obviously drunk, stood in the doorway. I looked at him and said, "This is the ladies' room." He stared at me. He obviously knew that. It was instantly clear to me what his intentions were. I felt like a trapped wildcat. My heart pounded furiously. Just then I saw a sliver of space between him and the door frame. Like a charging fullback I bolted for the door. I crashed into him, knocking my glasses to the ground. I was free! I raced down the corridor to the dining area. I cried for help. As I reached the table where my companions sat, the bartender flew by me with a pistol in his hand. Moments later he returned, hustling the large man out of the bar.

For the next few weeks, whenever I thought of what had happened, I became upset. But along with those feelings came others—pride and regret. I had dealt with that threatening situation, taking action against a man intent on harming me; yet, I had been too confused to demand that he be held for questioning. Still what had happened to me was minor compared to a tragic event a few weeks later.

A 12-year-old girl had been raped in a local park by a college student. Little was being done for the girl—the law moved slowly, the police doubted her story, and school officials stonewalled the press. NOW members asked the girl's mother and physician to attend a meeting to tell us how we could help.

It was a highly emotional meeting, as her mother poured out her grief and anger. Afterward we decided to form a rape crisis center. At the center we did lay counseling, which meant we talked to victims brought to hospital emergency rooms. During those terrible initial moments, and in the weeks that followed an assault, we'd listen to women's feelings and help them place blame on the assailant, not themselves. Working with professionals from the Medical University of South Carolina, we developed an emergency room procedure for collecting evidence about rape. We also designed innovative, behaviorally oriented protocols for helping women to overcome the aftermath of rape, what is called post-traumatic stress disorder (PTSD).

As I saw more and more women with PTSD I became determined to go to graduate school to learn more about the disorder and the special challenges facing women. Because of the urging of my mentor at the medical school, I entered a doctoral program in clinical psychology at the University of Georgia. Within several years I graduated and headed north again to Boston University

Medical Center as a new faculty member in the Department of Biobehavioral Sciences. This is where I met Lyle and where we together developed the *Stress Audit*. Eventually we also found time to get married.

Lyle and I have complementary viewpoints on stress and psychology. He focuses more on the physiological aspects of health, due in part to his medical training in graduate school, and his research interests in physiology and neuropeptides, the hormones that affect brain function. He thinks more about the causes and treatment of the physical side of stress. His training also includes more traditional psychotherapy.

I think more about the cognitive and behavioral side of stress. I'm interested in what makes people vulnerable to stress, how coping skills and social networks buffer them, and the strategies available to counteract stress.

Over the years I've learned that I'm responsible for managing my own stress. When I'm stressed I become depressed, tending to withdraw and become passive. Now I use cognitive restructuring, which you'll read about later in the book, as a way of dealing with my negative thoughts. And I do common-sense things: I maintain my social network, the most essential part of my stress prevention plan; I call friends and family; I exercise; and I plan activities that make me feel good. In short, I work to keep myself happy by building positive events into my life.

Since that startling incident at the rathskeller in Charleston, my life turned around. I gained a deeper understanding of myself and the many demands and pressures women face. And it became my professional goal to develop new ways to help men and women face and manage stress.

TOOLS FOR CHANGE

Two people, two different stories of stress. Lyle's story is the all too common one of an ambitious, hard-driving man who loses sight of the important things in life in his blind pursuit of "success." Alma's stress problems involve searching for meaning in a confusing, rapidly changing world of conflicting demands and expectations.

While every person's story of stress is different, they are enough alike to tell us a lot about stress in general, to allow scientific analysis and research, and to enable us to create tools for managing stress.

We believe anyone can use the *Stress Audit* and *Stress Profiles* to gain a greater understanding of their lives and can then tailor comprehensive *Stress Action Plans* that work for them. Guided by this belief, we have tried to write a book that parallels in its structure the basic steps we help our clients follow: increasing *awareness* of the specific problem, taking appropriate *action*, overcoming *barriers to change*, and developing *supports for change*. In its content, this book replicates the information and methods we provide our clients at the Institute.

We have divided the book into four sections. The first section, "Getting in Touch with Stress," opens with the chapter "Stress Points," in which we describe the myths and truths about stress and argue for self-regulation as the key to managing stress. We mention many case studies throughout the book to illustrate these points. One woman you will encounter repeatedly as she struggles with stress is Anne. In chapter 2, you take the *Stress Audit* and plot your own *Stress Profile*. In chapter 3, "The Tougher You Are, The More You Can Take," we tell you how to design *Stress Action Plans* for your susceptibility to stress and locate your sources and symptoms of stress.

The book's second section, "Playing Hardball with Stress," its third section, "Soothing the Body, Calming the Mind," and its fourth section, "If at First You Don't Succeed, You're Human," focus on those personal factors that make altering our lives difficult, how to deal effectively with these factors, and how to get assistance for change from friends, family, self-help organizations, and professionals. Extensive appendices close the book, instructing where you can find detailed descriptions of self-regulation techniques, recommended readings, and scientific data on the *Stress Audit*, and directions on fax scoring the *Stress Audit*.

You can connect with us directly by removing the

FaxScore form from the back of the book and faxing it to us for scoring and interpretation. Just follow the directions. We'll return your personalized *Stress Audit* report to you on your own fax machine within eight minutes. You may also be interested in our Multi-Media Support Package of biofeedback devices and audio and videotapes. Our clients have found them to be profoundly helpful in promoting deep relaxation and counteracting the unwanted effects of stress.

We believe our book will help you deal with the most pervasive health problem of our time: Through the book we hope to do for you what we do for our clients—help set you on the road to a new way of living, one where you feel a sense of personal power, and the ability to manage your own stress problems. We know from experience that there is no more precious gift.

1

GETTING IN TOUCH WITH STRESS

1 STRESS POINTS

Not long ago, a young woman named Anne came to the Biobehavioral Institute after her cardiologist referred her to us for stress management and treatment of "heart attack" symptoms. Anne, 36, seemingly had the world by the tail. Marketing director for a local high-tech firm, she was in line for promotion to vice president. Anne drove a new sports car, traveled extensively, and was socially active.

Although on the surface everything seemed fine, Anne felt that, in her words, "the wheels on my tricycle are about to fall off. I'm a mess." Over the last several months she had attacks of shortness of breath, heart palpitations, chest pains, dizziness, and tingling sensations in her fingers and toes. Filled with a sense of impending doom, she would become anxious to the point of panic. Every day she awoke with a dreaded feeling that an attack might strike without reason or warning.

On two occasions, she rushed to a nearby hospital emergency room fearing she was having a heart attack. The first episode followed an argument with Mark, her boyfriend of three years, about the future of their relationship. After studying her electrocardiogram (ECG, a record of the electrical activity of the heart), the emergency room doctor told Anne she was "just hyperventilating" and showed her how to breathe into a paper bag to handle the situation in the future. Anne felt foolish and went home that night embarrassed, angry, and confused. She remained convinced that she had almost had a heart attack.

Anne's next severe attack occurred after a fight at work with her boss over a new marketing campaign. This time she insisted that she be hospitalized overnight for extensive diagnostic tests and that her internist be consulted. The results were the same—no heart attack. Her internist prescribed Xanax, a tranquilizer, to calm her down.

Convinced now that her own doctor was wrong, Anne sought the advice of a cardiologist, who conducted another battery of diagnostic tests, again with no physical findings. Her conclusion—stress was the primary cause of Anne's panic attacks and "heart attack" symptoms. The doctor referred Anne to the Institute. We will use her experience to illustrate our approach throughout the book.

During her first visit, we gave Anne the *Stress Audit* and explained how stress could cause her physical symptoms. At her next visit, utilizing her *Stress Audit* results, we described to her the sources and nature of her health problems. The *Stress Audit* revealed that Anne was highly susceptible to stress, that she was enduring enormous stress from her family, her personal life, and her job, and that she was experiencing a number of stress-related symptoms in her emotional, sympathetic nervous, muscular, and endocrine systems. Her *Stress Profiles* showed Anne's stress was at a critical level. She wasn't sleeping or eating well, didn't exercise, abused caffeine and alcohol, and lived on the edge financially.

The *Stress Audit* and the *Stress Profiles* crystallized for Anne how susceptible she was to stress, what was causing her stress, and how stress was expressing itself in her "heart attack" and other symptoms. This newly found knowledge eliminated a lot of her confusion and separated her concerns into simpler, more manageable problems.

She now realized that she was feeling tremendous pressure from her boyfriend, Mark, as well as her mother to settle down and get married; yet, she didn't feel ready. At the same time, work was overwhelming her as a new marketing campaign began. Any serious emotional incident—a quarrel with Mark or her boss—sent Anne over the edge. Her body's response was hyperventilation, palpitations, chest pain, dizziness, anxiety, and a dreadful sense of impending doom. Stress, in short, was destroying Anne's life.

She's not alone. Forty-three percent of all adults suffer adverse health effects from stress; 75 to 90 percent of all physician office visits are for stress-related ailments and complaints; stress is linked to the six leading causes of death—heart disease, cancer, lung ailments, accidents, cirrhosis of the liver, and suicide. The Occupational Safety and Health Administration has declared stress a hazard of the workplace.[1]

Stress is expensive. We all pay a stress tax whether we know it or not. As this book is written, health care costs account for 12 percent of our gross domestic product, escalating yearly at a dizzying rate.[2] In terms of lost hours due to absenteeism, reduced productivity, and workers' compensation benefits, stress costs American industry more than $300 billion annually, or $7,500 per worker per year.

Stress plays havoc with our health, our productivity, our pocketbooks, and our lives, but stress is necessary, even desirable. Exciting or challenging events such as the birth of a child, completion of a major project at work, or moving to a new city generate as much stress as does tragedy or disaster. Without it, life would be dull.

Stress is a confusing and mysterious problem for the clients who seek help at the Biobehavioral Institute, to many of the physicians who refer these people to us, and to our corporate clients, who pay ever mounting health insurance premiums. Six myths surround stress. Dispelling them enables our clients to understand their problems and then take action against them. Let's look at these myths.

Stress Myths

Myth 1: Stress is the same for everybody.

Completely wrong. Stress is *different* for each of us. What is stressful for one person may or may not be stressful for another; each of us responds to stress in an entirely different way.

Myth 2: Stress is always bad for you.

According to this view, zero stress makes us happy and healthy. Wrong. Stress is to the human condition what tension is to the violin string: too little and the music is dull and raspy; too much and the music is shrill or the string snaps. Stress can be the kiss of death or the spice of life. The issue, really, is how to manage it. Managed stress makes us productive and happy; mismanaged stress hurts and even kills us.

Myth 3: Stress is everywhere, so you can't do anything about it.

Not so. You can plan your life so that stress does not overwhelm you. Effective planning involves setting priorities and working on simple problems first, solving them, and then going on to the more complex difficulties. When you mismanage stress, it's difficult to prioritize. All your problems seem to be equal and stress seems to be everywhere.

Myth 4: The most popular techniques for reducing stress are the best ones.

Again, not so. No universally effective stress reduction technique exists. We are all different, our lives are different, our situations are different, and our reactions are different. Only a comprehensive program tailored to the individual works.

Myth 5: No symptoms, no stress.

Don't be fooled by this one. Absence of symptoms does not mean the absence of stress. In fact, camouflaging symptoms with medication may deprive you of the signals you need for reducing the strain on your physiological and psychological systems.

Myth 6: Only major symptoms of stress require attention.

This myth assumes that the "minor" symptoms, such as headaches or stomach acid, may be safely ignored. Wrong again. Minor symptoms of stress are the early warnings that your life is getting out of hand and that you need to do a better job of managing stress.

How Stress Works

Now that you know what stress isn't, what is it? We've thought a lot about stress over the years. The Biobehavioral Model of Stress, shown below, has helped us organize the thoughts and ideas that underlie the *Stress Audit*, the *Stress Profiles*, and the *Stress Action Plans*. It provides a comprehensive way of looking at stress.

A BIOBEHAVIORAL MODEL OF STRESS

We define stress as the state of dynamic tension created when you respond to perceived demands and pressures from outside and from within yourself. These demands and pressures build up, while you mobilize your resources to deal with them. In the illustration (page 18), the person peers out at the external demands and pressures, indicating the role played by subjective interpretation—how you feel about a situation determines whether it will cause stress, not the situation itself. Cold and snow are a burden when you're shoveling your car out; they're exhilarating when you're skiing.

Notice in the illustration that there are two kinds of external demands and pressures: physical and psychosocial. External physical demands and pressures—gravity, air pollution, noise pollution, extreme weather conditions, etc.—generally aren't acknowledged as stressful. But consider the time and effort that has gone into dealing with gravity—elevators, escalators, airplanes, automobiles, arch supports, support hose, face-lifts, and so on. Psychosocial pressures and demands include family, personal, social, environmental, financial, and work or school problems. This is what most of us think of when we talk about stress. (We'll discuss them extensively in the Sources section of the book.)

Demands and pressures compete with one another for attention. Psychological research has shown that we can pay attention only to seven items, plus or minus two, at a time.[3] We set our own, subjectively defined priorities as to what we'll pay attention to and when. Sometimes we do this poorly, overextend ourselves, and create stress.

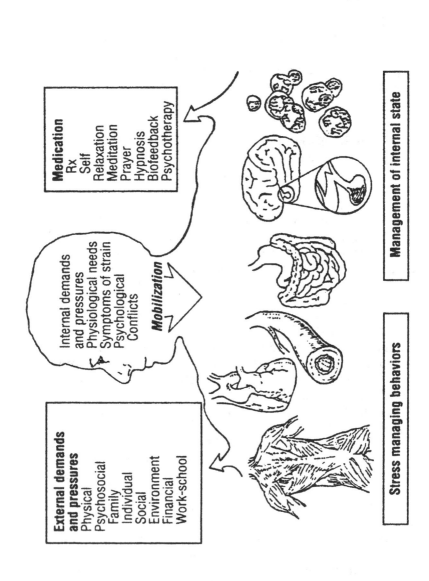

**External demands
and pressures**
Physical
Psychosocial
Family
Individual
Social
Environment
Financial
Work-school

Internal demands
and pressures
Physiological needs
Symptoms of strain
Psychological
Conflicts

Mobilization

Medication
Rx
Self
Relaxation
Meditation
Prayer
Hypnosis
Biofeedback
Psychotherapy

Management of internal state

Stress managing behaviors

Such decision-making is particularly problematic when the demands and pressures not only compete but conflict—work versus leisure time, for example. When this happens, stress escalates further. External competing and conflicting demands and pressures—a big lump of items we "have to do"—are combined with internal demands and pressures. In the illustration, the items within the person's head include:

- physiological demands and pressures such as hunger, thirst, fatigue, pain, sexual desire, needs for elimination, etc.
- psychological demands and pressures concerning your views of who and what you are, what your rights and privileges are, expectations of yourself and others, psychological baggage from the past, etc.

Your internal demands and pressures are thus added to your external demands and pressures to produce a *total* burden of demand and pressure composed of many competing and conflicting elements all clamoring for your attention.

Obviously, the solution to stress is to set priorities on this clamorous throng. But organization becomes another demand and pressure in and of itself. How many times have you said, "When I get time, I'm going to get organized." But you never do.

Under these circumstances, stress now becomes overwhelming. In response, your body automatically and unconsciously mobilizes. Energy reserves are tapped. The electrical activity of the skin, respiration, heart rate, and blood pressure increase. Muscles tense, blood vessels constrict, blood flow shifts from skin and gut to muscle and brain. Your temperature rises, your metabolism speeds up, and your immune system prepares for battle—platelets become sticky so that blood will coagulate faster, the kidneys conserve sodium, etc. The process of mobilization is orchestrated by the autonomic nervous system and the endocrine glands, powered by adrenaline and similar biochemical substances, and assisted by a variety of hormones.

When you're angry or afraid, this mobilization is sudden and intense. The great physiologist Walter B. Cannon called this the "fight or flight response." This response is proportional. The greater the demand or threat from your viewpoint, the greater your mobilization. The more sudden and intense the demand or threat, the more sudden and intense the mobilization. The longer the demand or threat continues, the longer you stay mobilized. The more frequently you experience demand and pressure, the more frequently you mobilize. The more overwhelming your demands and pressures, the more serious the health consequences of your mobilizations.

You can only push yourself so hard for so long. When you exceed your physical limits of responding, something in your mind and/or body breaks down. Like Anne, you develop stress-related symptoms. Sometimes they're physical, sometimes they're mental. They occur within seven discrete physiological systems:

- the neuromuscular system
- the parasympathetic nervous system (stomach, gut, and bowel)
- the sympathetic nervous system (heart, blood vessels, and sweat glands)
- the limbic system (the emotional part of the brain)
- the neocortical system (the thinking part of the brain)
- the endocrine system (glands and hormones)
- the immune system

(We'll discuss these systems and how they indicate strain and breakdown with symptoms in more detail in section 3, "Soothing the Body, Calming the Mind.")

The particular symptoms you develop depend on a complex interaction between the physical constitution you inherited and the intensity, frequency, and duration of your mobilizations in response to your perceived demands and pressures.

THE DIFFERENT KINDS OF STRESS

Stress management is complicated and confusing because there are different types of stress—acute stress, episodic acute stress, chronic stress, and traumatic stress—each with its own characteristics, symptoms, duration, and treatment approaches. Let's look at each one.

Acute Stress

Acute stress is the most common form of stress. It comes from demands and pressures of the recent past and anticipated demands and pressures of the near future. Acute stress is thrilling and exciting in small doses, but too much is exhausting. A fast run down a challenging ski slope, for example, is exhilarating early in the day. That same ski run late in the day is taxing and wearing. Skiing beyond your limits can lead to falls and broken bones. By the same token, overdoing on short-term stress can lead to psychological distress, tension headaches, upset stomach, and other symptoms.

Fortunately, acute stress symptoms are recognized by most people. It's the laundry list of what has gone awry in their lives: the auto accident that crumpled the car fender, the loss of an important contract, a deadline they're rushing to meet, their child's occasional problems at school, and so on.

Because it is short term, acute stress doesn't have enough time to do the extensive damage associated with long-term stress. The most common symptoms of acute stress are:

- Emotional distress—some combination of anger or irritability, anxiety, and depression, the three stress emotions.
- Muscular problems including tension headache, back pain (upper and lower), jaw pain (TMJ, temporomandibular jaw), and the muscular tensions that lead to pulled muscles and tendon and ligament problems.
- Stomach, gut, and bowel problems such as heart-

burn, acid stomach, ulcers, flatulence, diarrhea, constipation, and irritable bowel syndrome.
- Transient overarousal leads to elevation in blood pressure, rapid heartbeat, sweaty palms, heart palpitations, dizziness, migraine headaches, cold hands or feet, shortness of breath, and chest pain.

Acute stress can crop up in anyone's life. But it is highly treatable and manageable, in eight to twelve weeks, through the self-regulation techniques we describe in chapter 19 and appendix I.

Episodic Acute Stress

There are those, however, who suffer acute stress frequently, whose lives are so disordered that they are studies in chaos and crisis. They're always in a rush, but always late. If something can go wrong, it does. They take on too much, have too many irons in the fire, and can't organize the slew of self-inflicted demands and pressures clamoring for their attention.

One of our clients, Ralph, 43, a salesman, exemplified this problem. Recently he ran out of gas on the way to an important meeting. Ralph didn't have a car phone and couldn't call from a pay phone because he had left his money on his dresser as he hurried out of the house to make sure he got to his meeting on time. Ralph hadn't had time to get gas the night before because he had to go to a dinner party. The party ran late. When he left at two in the morning, Ralph couldn't find a station open and was in too much of a hurry to stop for gas that morning.

Although appearance is important in his line of work, Ralph had difficulty finding time to get a haircut or get to the dry cleaners. His checkbook was always out of balance and he frequently bounced checks. He described his wife as being even more disordered than he and their expensive home in an exclusive suburb as "really messy."

Like so many of our clients who seem perpetually in the clutches of acute stress, Ralph didn't think he had the time to step back, see what had to be done, set priorities, and take care of problems in their order of importance. His perception was, "I'm so busy doing the things I need to do to live the way I want to live, I don't have the *time* to live the way I want to live."

It is common for people with acute stress reactions to be overaroused, short-tempered, irritable, anxious, and tense. Often, they describe themselves as having "a lot of nervous energy." Always in a hurry, they tend to be abrupt, and sometimes their irritability comes across as hostility. Interpersonal relationships deteriorate rapidly when others respond with real hostility. The world becomes a very stressful place for them.

The cardiac prone, "Type A" personality described by cardiologists Meyer Friedman and Ray Rosenman is similar to an extreme case of episodic acute stress. Type A's have an "excessive competitive drive, aggressiveness, impatience, and a harrying sense of time urgency." In addition there is a "free-floating, but well-rationalized form of hostility, and almost always a deep-seated insecurity." Such personality characteristics would seem to create frequent episodes of acute stress for the Type A individual. Friedman and Rosenman found Type A's to be much more likely to develop coronary heart disease than Type B's, who showed an opposite pattern of behavior.[4]

Another form of episodic acute stress comes from ceaseless worry. "Worry warts" see disaster around every corner and pessimistically forecast catastrophe in every situation. The world is a dangerous, unrewarding, punitive place where something awful is always about to happen. These "awfulizers" also tend to be overaroused and tense, but are more anxious and depressed than angry and hostile.

The symptoms of episodic acute stress are the symptoms of extended overarousal: persistent tension headaches, migraines, hypertension, chest pain, and heart disease. Treating episodic acute stress requires intervention on a number of levels, generally requires professional help, and may take many months.

Often, lifestyle and personality issues are so ingrained and habitual with these individuals that they see nothing wrong with the way they conduct their lives. They blame their woes on other people and external events. Frequently they see their lifestyle, their patterns of interacting with others, and their ways of perceiving the world as part and parcel of who and what they are. Sufferers can be fiercely resistant to change. Only the promise of relief from the pain and discomfort of their symptoms can keep them in treatment and on track in their recovery program. Anne's symptoms, for instance, were symptoms of the extended overarousal created by chronic acute stress. They motivated her to turn her life around.

Chronic Stress

While acute stress can be thrilling and exciting, chronic stress is not. This is the grinding stress that wears people away day after day, year after year. Chronic stress destroys bodies, minds, and lives. It wreaks havoc through long-term attrition. It's the stress of poverty, of dysfunctional families, of being trapped in an unhappy marriage or in a despised job or career. It's the stress that the never-ending "troubles" have brought to the people of Northern Ireland, that the tensions of the Middle East have brought to Arab and Jew, and the endless ethnic rivalries that have been brought to the people of Eastern Europe and the former Soviet Union.

Chronic stress comes when a person never sees a way out of a miserable situation. It's the stress of unrelenting demands and pressures for seemingly interminable periods of time. With no hope, the individual gives up searching for solutions.

Some chronic stresses stem from traumatic, early childhood experiences that become internalized and remain forever painful and present. Such experiences profoundly affect personality. A view of the world, or a belief system, is created that causes unending stress for the individual (e.g., the world is a threatening place, people will find out you are a pretender, you must be perfect at all times). When personality or deep-seated convictions and beliefs must be reformulated, recovery requires active self-examination, often with professional help.

The worst aspect of chronic stress is that people get used to it. They forget it's there. People are immediately aware of acute stress because it's new; they ignore chronic stress because it's old, familiar, and, sometimes, almost comfortable. One patient whose long-term anger and rage at her dead father served as a chronic source of potentially life-threatening stress for her believed that she couldn't give it up because she wouldn't be herself anymore. "And besides," she said, "I like being mad."

Chronic stress kills through suicide, violence, heart attack, stroke, and, perhaps, even cancer. People wear down to a final, fatal breakdown. Because physical and mental resources are depleted through long-term attrition, the symptoms of chronic stress are difficult to treat and may require extended medical as well as behavioral treatment, therapy, and stress management. Many chronic stress situations can only be addressed through group or community efforts where individuals must act together to create alternatives.

The good news is that recovery from the ravages of chronic stress is possible. Dr. Dean Ornish at the University of San Francisco Medical School, for instance, has demonstrated that coronary heart disease can be reversed with a program of diet, exercise, and stress management.[5] Norman Cousins insisted that hope was key in the remission of his progressive illness.[6]

The popular literature is replete with stories of "miracle" cures of terminal illness through a variety of means, including prayer, laughter, diet, exercise, and love. Regardless of how these reversals, cures, or remissions come about, we believe it's the stress reduction and stress management inherent in them all that makes it possible.

Traumatic Stress

If not handled properly at the outset, overpowering trauma—accidents, rape, verbal, physical, psychological, or sexual abuse, being in the presence of extreme violence, a brush with death, natural disasters (hurricanes, earthquakes, floods, landslides), death of a loved one, imprisonment—can cause a special kind of chronic stress known as post-traumatic stress disorder (PTSD).

PTSD brings with it intrusive memories of events associated with the trauma (flashbacks), symptoms of overarousal, emotional numbness or loss of feeling, along with extreme emotional outbursts to minor events. Problems with concentration, controlling impulses, decision making, and memory become chronic and unremitting.

Several factors increase the stress of an acute traumatic event. For instance, if the trauma occurred because of a deliberate act of aggression as opposed to an accident (having a leg broken by someone versus breaking a leg in a skiing accident), stress is much more severe and overpowering. If the trauma results in ongoing stress, such as a lawsuit or an injury that does not heal and requires modification of activities (e.g., auto accident resulting in chronic, debilitating back pain), it contains the worst features of both PTSD and chronic stress. Stress is greater in cases where the trauma is repeated and there is little hope of escape (e.g., prisoners of war, soldiers in war, child abuse victims, hostages in a criminal activity or international politics, or a kidnapping). Where the trauma was inflicted by a supposedly protective person or loved one (intrafamilial battering or verbal or sexual abuse, abuse by teacher, counselor, pastor, police officer, or other person with public responsibilities), the stress can be overwhelming. Long-term psychological consequences such as depression, anxiety, behavioral disorders, multiple personality disorder, and suicide are not unusual. The more exacerbating factors present, the worse the stress.

The case of Joanie and Kim, her 14-year-old daughter, shows how traumatic stress problems can interact to compound the stress of an initial trauma. Kim's accident happened in an instant, but the repercussions lasted more than two years.

Kim was at a birthday party for Susan, a friend from school. Food and drinks were being served on the patio. Along the edge of the patio were what appeared to be boards, covered with a cloth, resting on a pair of saw horses. As Kim spoke to Susan, she leaned back and sat on the boards. Instantly, she crashed to the floor. The "boards" were actually panes of glass.

In her surprise, Kim barely felt the pain in her back and was unaware that she was bleeding badly. Someone shouted to get an ambulance. But Susan said, "Don't call, it's not that serious." Unassisted, Kim started to walk back to the house to clean herself. But she became weak with pain, saw the blood on the back of her dress, and fainted. Several minutes passed before anyone called for help. More than a half-hour went by before the ambulance arrived.

At the hospital Kim was taken immediately into surgery. The doctors labored for hours, slowly removing each piece of glass. The glass had narrowly missed her lungs and other vital organs.

Joanie rushed to the hospital and was told Kim was in surgery. She sat in the waiting room alone, terrified that Kim might die. Numbly she thought how empty her life would be. No one from the party came to the hospital. Joanie sat alone with her fearful thoughts until the surgeon told her that Kim was all right.

What happened in the weeks following was as unexpected as the accident. Susan's family blamed Kim for the incident. Susan, in fact, remarked to her friends that Kim had ruined her party. No one acknowledged that storing glass in such a way was hazardous. No one came to visit.

When Joanie approached Susan's parents about household insurance to cover part of Kim's medical expenses, they said they were not at fault and would not file a claim. Joanie, a single mother with a limited income, couldn't pay the medical bills and sued Susan's parents.

To Kim, the shock of being treated this way by her "friend," Susan, was more distressing than the surgery. To make matters worse, when she returned to school, Kim was in the same class with Susan, who would not speak to her because "she is suing my parents." Kim's other friends dared not take sides against the popular Susan, and Kim became a social outcast.

Kim's initial trauma was compounded because her accident was the result of negligence. It shouldn't have happened. In the initial moments after the injury, doubt and confusion delayed treatment and support. The very people Kim expected help from turned away because of fear of litigation. Blame was directed at Kim, the victim. Responsibility was shifted to her and her mother. Kim had little social support because her friends were afraid of being caught in the middle. As a consequence of all this stress, Kim withdrew socially and eventually changed schools. She continued to have unexplained pains in her back and feared there was still glass in her body. Such thoughts brought back the old panicky feelings. Her mother became anxious and depressed and worried constantly about the future.

A number of things could have lessened Joanie and Kim's trauma, minimized their stress, and eliminated their consequent reactions. Perhaps the most important would have been discussing the accident soon after it happened. Just talking about trauma to someone lessens its impact. Victims of trauma may need to tell their stories time and time again to a trauma team, other survivors, family, friends, reporters, or anyone who will listen. With each repeated telling, the victim puts the experience a little more in perspective. By reliving the experience, bit by bit, the impact of the trauma decreases proportionally.

Traumatic stress can also be reduced by community support. Hostages, for instance, need to feel they have not been forgotten, that somebody cares and is loyal. Community support provides hope and a feeling that help is available or on the way. Family "hostages" of abusive families, for instance, need to know about the presence of shelters and self-help groups even if they are not yet ready to leave the situation.

A personal, political, or religious belief system that justifies the trauma also helps. If one dies for one's country or God, is injured severely in doing something one loves, or finds a sense of meaning in the experience, the trauma is somehow lessened. Victims reveal their belief systems with comments like, "It wasn't my time to die. God wasn't ready for me yet. There is something more for me to do in this life. I have another chance." Victims injured for a cause in which they deeply believe, such as political or religious freedom, do not suffer the same psychological trauma as victims for whom an event is meaningless.

Had Joanie and Kim had more of these resources available to them, they wouldn't have ended up in our clinic. They would have been upset over the accident and Kim's injuries, but they would have coped. As it was, their stress kept feeding on itself until it became a monster.

WHERE YOU START

Overcoming stress and getting control of your life can be a tough and complicated proposition. Not only are there different types of stress each with its own patterns of cause, duration, symptoms, and treatment, but in many instances they have to be dealt with all at once. Chronic stress can be aggravated by acute and episodic acute stress. You may have to struggle with all three simultaneously. If so, start with the easiest to control— acute stress. For instance, this is what Janine had to do to manage her stress.

Abandoned and abused as a teenager, Janine struggled with PTSD compounded by the grinding, chronic stress of a miserable marriage, an acrimonious divorce, and raising three young children as a single parent. Small wonder that she was devastated by even the slightest disappointment or additional demand or pressure.

It was not unusual for Janine to fall apart and require psychiatric hospitalization around the first of the year. Christmas, New Year's, and child-care problems during school vacation would compound all the normal stress in her life. An incapacitating depression would settle over her like a thick fog. At the hospital, where she could rest and be relieved of her immediate demands and pressures, Janine's natural restorative processes took over. As her energy came back, she would talk about her early traumas and the misery of her life. Her depression would slowly lift. In about six weeks or so, on heavy antidepressant medication, she would be back at home. Luckily, Janine received health and disability insurance as part of her divorce settlement.

Janine came to us following her last hospitalization. She was unhappy with the side effects of her medication and had heard we worked with people like her. Her case was difficult, but we started a long-term program for her depression and her stress problems. That was five years ago and Janine hasn't seen the inside of a hospital since.

She still checks in with us from time to time, but she's doing well. Most of what we did was to help Janine develop ways of handling her acute stress. Our intervention focused on the nuts and bolts of working and managing a home and three children. We worked on setting up schedules for the children's household chores, disciplining the children, getting everyone out of the house on time in the morning, putting more responsibility on the children, and taking her husband back to court for an increase in child support. These concerns were more immediately important for her than her traumatic and chronic stress problems. We also provided her with psychotherapy, relaxation and imagery techniques, and biofeedback.

As with most complex stress problems, the key was to help Janine handle her acute stress first. Why? First, you can do something about acute stress; it's going on at the moment, and it's the easiest kind of stress to handle. Second, you reduce your total burden of stress every time you eliminate something, giving you more time to heal or take care of other stress issues. Most important, though, you learn how to handle stress by starting with the easiest problems. This makes you feel you are not helpless against a mysterious and omnipotent enemy.

The same approach worked for Anne. Based on her new understanding of herself and what her problems really were, we helped Anne create a comprehensive set of *Stress Action Plans* for doing something about her stress complaints. First, we developed a *Stress Action Plan* to reduce her susceptibility, focused initially on improving her sleeping habits. Later, she designed new *Action Plans* for improved nutrition, exercise, money management, and cutting back on alcohol and caffeine. Together, we created an *Action Plan* for reducing pressures on the job. Most important, we introduced her to a set of self-regulatory techniques that reduced her symptoms by soothing her body and calming her mind. These became Anne's basic *Action Plans* for dealing with her symptoms of stress.

Finding out what the problems are and setting up *Action Plans*, however, was only a beginning. Anne had to actually do it. She had to follow through. That was the hard part. Changing your life is difficult under the best of circumstances. It's even harder when you're under enormous stress as Anne was. In the tragedy of *Pudd'nhead Wilson* Mark Twain said, "Habit is habit, not to be flung out of the window by any man, but coaxed downstairs a step at a time." He was right.

Anne had to make time to do her prescribed self-regulatory exercises and be courageous about facing her fears about her future. There were setbacks due to her own resistances and there were barriers she had to overcome in carrying out her first set of *Stress Action Plans*. Once she got the hang of it, though, she generated new *Action Plans* to deal with the rest of her stress problems.

Within a couple of months, Anne was in control again. Her attacks had subsided. Her relationship with Mark, her mother, and her boss had improved. She felt a new sense of self-efficacy and was determined to manage the demands and pressures placed on her, rather than letting them manage her.

Now that you have the basic ideas about what stress isn't, what it is, the different kinds of stress, and different approaches on how to handle it, it's time for you to start tailoring your own program. We start by identifying what your problems are through the *Stress Audit*.

N O T E S

1. *Healthy People: 2000 National Health Promotion and Disease Preventive Objectives*, U.S. Publication No. (PHS) 91-50213, 1990, p. 99. Department of Health and Human Services Public Health Service.

2. Ibid., p. 5.

3. Wittenborn, J. R. (1943), "Factorial equations for the test of attention," *Psychometrika* 8, 19–35.

Miller, G. A. (1956), The magical number seven, plus or minus two: Some limits on our capacity for processing information, *Psychological Review* 63, 81–97.

4. Friedman, M., and Rosenman, R. H. (1974), *Type A Behavior and Your Heart*, Greenwich, CT, Fawcett.

5. Ornish, D. (1990), *Dr. Dean Ornish's Program for Reversing Heart Disease*, New York, Ballantine.

6. Cousins, N. (1981), *Anatomy of an Illness as Perceived by the Patient*, New York, Bantam.

2 YOUR STRESS PROFILE

The *Stress Audit* is one of the most important tests you'll ever take. It shows you how susceptible you are to stress and why. You learn what parts of your life are most and least stressful and your particular pattern of stress symptoms. Filling out the *Stress Audit* is your first step in managing the stress in your life.

Our research indicates that just taking the *Stress Audit* reduces stress. If you're like most people, some problems will be solved almost as soon as you recognize them. Even if the problems are difficult to deal with, identifying them helps to eliminate confusion.

After you've defined the nature of your stress problems by taking the *Stress Audit*, you'll plot your *Stress Profile*. If you score in the high or critical zones, read those chapters designated for you. In them you'll find out specifically what to do to reduce your susceptibility to stress, deal more effectively with your sources, and manage your symptoms.

After you have absorbed this information, you'll be set to design your *Stress Action Plans* to fit your unique needs.

The *Stress Audit* is broken down into three major sections: Susceptibility, Sources, and Symptoms. Take one section at a time if you like, but you should complete each section without stopping. The entire *Audit* can be finished in about a half-hour.

You may make one photocopy of the *Stress Audit* for your own use. The *Stress Audit* is protected by international copyright laws and may not be reproduced by any means without specific written permission from the authors.

Turn to the back of the book to see how you can get a professional computerized interpretation of your *Stress Audit* over your own fax machine.

THE *STRESS AUDIT*

SUSCEPTIBILITY TO STRESS SECTION

This part of the *Audit* helps you look at some of the lifestyle, health behaviors, and coping resources that make you more or less susceptible to stress. Read each of the items below and decide whether it is true of you ALMOST ALWAYS, NEVER, or somewhere in between. Then, circle the appropriate number—1 for ALMOST ALWAYS, 5 for NEVER, 2, 3, or 4 for in-between levels.

SUSCEPTIBILITY SECTION

1 = ALMOST ALWAYS   5 = NEVER

1 2 3 4 5	**1.** I eat at least one hot balanced meal per day.
1 2 3 4 5	**2.** I get seven to eight hours of sleep at least four nights per week.
1 2 3 4 5	**3.** I give and receive affection regularly.
1 2 3 4 5	**4.** I have at least one relative within 50 miles on whom I can rely.
1 2 3 4 5	**5.** I exercise to the point of perspiration at least three times a week.
1 2 3 4 5	**6.** I limit myself to half a pack of cigarettes per day.
1 2 3 4 5	**7.** I limit myself to fewer than five alcoholic drinks per week.
1 2 3 4 5	**8.** I am the appropriate weight for my height.
1 2 3 4 5	**9.** I have an income adequate to meet basic expenses.
1 2 3 4 5	**10.** I get strength from my religious beliefs.
1 2 3 4 5	**11.** I regularly attend club or social activities.
1 2 3 4 5	**12.** I have a network of friends and acquaintances.
1 2 3 4 5	**13.** I have one or more friends to confide in about personal matters.
1 2 3 4 5	**14.** I am in good health (including eyesight, hearing, teeth).
1 2 3 4 5	**15.** I am able to speak openly about my feelings when angry or worried.
1 2 3 4 5	**16.** I have regular conversations with the people I live with about domestic problems (e.g., chores, money, and daily living issues).
1 2 3 4 5	**17.** I do something for fun at least once a week.
1 2 3 4 5	**18.** I am able to organize my time effectively.
1 2 3 4 5	**19.** I limit myself to fewer than three cups of coffee (or tea or cola drinks) a day.
1 2 3 4 5	**20.** I take quiet time for myself during the day.
1 2 3 4 5	**21.** I have an optimistic outlook on life.

SUSCEPTIBILITY TO
STRESS SCORE

Add the circled numbers to get your TOTAL SUSCEPTIBILITY TO STRESS SCORE.
Mark your TOTAL SUSCEPTIBILITY TO STRESS SCORE on the graph below. If you
score in the High or Serious range, be sure to read chapter 3 to see what to do about it.

Your Susceptibility to Stress Profile

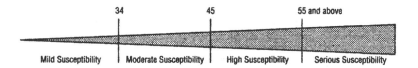

34	45	55 and above
Mild Susceptibility	Moderate Susceptibility	High Susceptibility	Serious Susceptibility

---

SOURCES OF STRESS

This next section of the *Audit* is somewhat longer than the Susceptibility section,
but it, too, should be completed in one session. Here you gain a perspective on the
sources of the demands and pressures that create the stress in your life—job, family,
personal, social, environmental, financial.

Read each of the potential sources of demand and pressure below. If an item
happened or was a problem, but was NOT STRESSFUL, in the last six months circle
the number 1 in the PAST COLUMN; if it was VERY STRESSFUL, circle the number
5; if it was somewhere in between a 1 and a 5, circle 2, 3, or 4. Now do the same
for the next six months.

SKIP ITEMS THAT DO NOT APPLY TO YOU!

Job Stress

PAST		FUTURE
1 = NOT STRESSFUL		*1 = NOT STRESSFUL*
5 = VERY STRESSFUL		*5 = VERY STRESSFUL*

PAST		FUTURE
1 2 3 4 5	1. Beginning new work or school	1 2 3 4 5
1 2 3 4 5	2. Poor job description	1 2 3 4 5
1 2 3 4 5	3. Ambiguous lines of authority	1 2 3 4 5
1 2 3 4 5	4. Poorly defined responsibilities at work or school	1 2 3 4 5

PAST		FUTURE	
1 = NOT STRESSFUL **5 = VERY STRESSFUL**		**1 = NOT STRESSFUL** **5 = VERY STRESSFUL**	
1 2 3 4 5	**5.** Setting work or school goals	1 2 3 4 5
1 2 3 4 5	**6.** Meeting work or school goals	1 2 3 4 5
1 2 3 4 5	**7.** Failure to understand or accomplish assignments	1 2 3 4 5
1 2 3 4 5	**8.** Lack of necessary skills and abilities to perform adequately at work or school	1 2 3 4 5
1 2 3 4 5	**9.** Too tired to get work done	1 2 3 4 5
1 2 3 4 5	**10.** Difficulties with career decisions	1 2 3 4 5
1 2 3 4 5	**11.** Overwork	1 2 3 4 5
1 2 3 4 5	**12.** Pressured deadlines	1 2 3 4 5
1 2 3 4 5	**13.** Many emergencies at work	1 2 3 4 5
1 2 3 4 5	**14.** Uncooperative co-workers or students	1 2 3 4 5
1 2 3 4 5	**15.** Language problems with co-workers or other students	1 2 3 4 5
1 2 3 4 5	**16.** Too much responsibility at work	1 2 3 4 5
1 2 3 4 5	**17.** Fear of error	1 2 3 4 5
1 2 3 4 5	**18.** Fired from job/expelled from school	1 2 3 4 5
1 2 3 4 5	**19.** Laid off	1 2 3 4 5
1 2 3 4 5	**20.** Work hours too long	1. 2 3 4 5
1 2 3 4 5	**21.** Family members interfering with work or school	1 2 3 4 5
1 2 3 4 5	**22.** Pressure to do well at work or school	1 2 3 4 5
1 2 3 4 5	**23.** Lack of company/school concern about workers/students	1 2 3 4 5
1 2 3 4 5	**24.** Labor-management/student-school conflict	1 2 3 4 5
1 2 3 4 5	**25.** Quit job or school	1 2 3 4 5
1 2 3 4 5	**26.** Promotion	1 2 3 4 5
1 2 3 4 5	**27.** Outstanding personal achievement at work or school	1 2 3 4 5
1 2 3 4 5	**28.** Change to a different line of work or study	1 2 3 4 5
1 2 3 4 5	**29.** Picking a school, college, or course of study	1 2 3 4 5
1 2 3 4 5	**30.** Equipment malfunctions at work	1 2 3 4 5
1 2 3 4 5	**31.** Company/school interference in personal life	1 2 3 4 5
1 2 3 4 5	**32.** Insufficient in-service training or supervision	1 2 3 4 5
1 2 3 4 5	**33.** Boredom with work or school	1 2 3 4 5
1 2 3 4 5	**34.** Little opportunity for advancement	1 2 3 4 5
1 2 3 4 5	**35.** Responsibility without authority	1 2 3 4 5
1 2 3 4 5	**36.** Lack of privacy at work	1 2 3 4 5
1 2 3 4 5	**37.** Irregular work hours	1 2 3 4 5
1 2 3 4 5	**38.** Retirement	1 2 3 4 5
1 2 3 4 5	**39.** Change in responsibilities at work or school	1 2 3 4 5
1 2 3 4 5	**40.** Trouble with boss	1 2 3 4 5

PAST						FUTURE				
1 = NOT STRESSFUL						**1 = NOT STRESSFUL**				
5 = VERY STRESSFUL						**5 = VERY STRESSFUL**				

1	2	3	4	5	**41.** Change in work hours or conditions	1	2	3	4	5
1	2	3	4	5	**42.** Work-related travel	1	2	3	4	5
1	2	3	4	5	**43.** Dangerous working conditions	1	2	3	4	5
1	2	3	4	5	**44.** Death or injury of coworker	1	2	3	4	5
1	2	3	4	5	**45.** Toxic working conditions	1	2	3	4	5

PAST   FUTURE

TOTAL JOB
STRESS SCORE

Add the circled numbers in the past columns to get your PAST score. Add the circled numbers in the future columns to get your FUTURE score. Add your PAST and your FUTURE scores to get your TOTAL JOB STRESS SCORE. Mark your TOTAL JOB STRESS SCORE on the graph below. If you score in the High or Serious range, be sure to read the work/school section of chapter 4, "Planning a Winning Strategy," and chapter 5, "Getting the Upper Hand on Job Stress," for suggestions on what to do about it.

Your Job Stress Profile

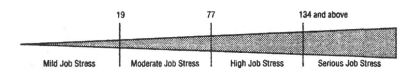

19	77	134 and above
Mild Job Stress	Moderate Job Stress	High Job Stress	Serious Job Stress

SKIP ITEMS THAT DO NOT APPLY TO YOU!

Family Stress

PAST						FUTURE				
1 = NOT STRESSFUL						**1 = NOT STRESSFUL**				
5 = VERY STRESSFUL						**5 = VERY STRESSFUL**				

1	2	3	4	5	**1.** Holidays, family celebrations, family vacations	1	2	3	4	5
1	2	3	4	5	**2.** Marriage or starting a significant relationship	1	2	3	4	5

		PAST						FUTURE		
		1 = NOT STRESSFUL						**1 = NOT STRESSFUL**		
		5 = VERY STRESSFUL						**5 = VERY STRESSFUL**		

1	2	3	4	5		1	2	3	4	5
1	2	3	4	5	**3.** Marital difficulties	1	2	3	4	5
1	2	3	4	5	**4.** Marital separation	1	2	3	4	5
1	2	3	4	5	**5.** Marital reconciliation	1	2	3	4	5
1	2	3	4	5	**6.** Divorce	1	2	3	4	5
1	2	3	4	5	**7.** Death of a spouse	1	2	3	4	5
1	2	3	4	5	**8.** Death of a close relative	1	2	3	4	5
1	2	3	4	5	**9.** Death of a distant relative	1	2	3	4	5
1	2	3	4	5	**10.** Disciplinary problems with children	1	2	3	4	5
1	2	3	4	5	**11.** Alcoholism or drug problems in family	1	2	3	4	5
1	2	3	4	5	**12.** Pregnancy in family	1	2	3	4	5
1	2	3	4	5	**13.** Son or daughter leaving home	1	2	3	4	5
1	2	3	4	5	**14.** Adult son or daughter returning home	1	2	3	4	5
1	2	3	4	5	**15.** Sex difficulties	1	2	3	4	5
1	2	3	4	5	**16.** Difficulties with other family members	1	2	3	4	5
1	2	3	4	5	**17.** Serious illness in family	1	2	3	4	5
1	2	3	4	5	**18.** Divorce or remarriage of parents	1	2	3	4	5
1	2	3	4	5	**19.** Family conflict around household chores	1	2	3	4	5
1	2	3	4	5	**20.** Divorce or remarriage of children	1	2	3	4	5
1	2	3	4	5	**21.** Difficulty in meeting obligations to family	1	2	3	4	5
1	2	3	4	5	**22.** Family conflict over money	1	2	3	4	5
1	2	3	4	5	**23.** Child care responsibilities	1	2	3	4	5
1	2	3	4	5	**24.** Birth of a child or adoption	1	2	3	4	5
1	2	3	4	5	**25.** Abortion, miscarriage, or stillbirth	1	2	3	4	5
1	2	3	4	5	**26.** Inability to have children	1	2	3	4	5
1	2	3	4	5	**27.** Change in number of arguments with spouse	1	2	3	4	5
1	2	3	4	5	**28.** Family violence	1	2	3	4	5
1	2	3	4	5	**29.** Troubles with in-laws	1	2	3	4	5
1	2	3	4	5	**30.** Wife or husband begins or stops work	1	2	3	4	5
1	2	3	4	5	**31.** Change in number of family get-togethers	1	2	3	4	5
1	2	3	4	5	**32.** Child with special needs	1	2	3	4	5
1	2	3	4	5	**33.** Responsibility for aging relative(s)	1	2	3	4	5
1	2	3	4	5	**34.** Difficulties with stepparents or step-children	1	2	3	4	5
1	2	3	4	5	**35.** Sibling rivalry or conflict	1	2	3	4	5

PAST   **FUTURE**

**TOTAL FAMILY
STRESS SCORE**

Add the circled numbers in the past columns to get your PAST score. Add the circled numbers in the future columns to get your FUTURE score. Add your PAST and your FUTURE scores to get your TOTAL FAMILY STRESS SCORE. Mark your TOTAL FAMILY STRESS SCORE on the graph below. If you score in the High or Serious range, be sure to read chapter 6, "Managing Family Stress," to see what to do about it.

Your Family Stress Profile

10	39	68 and above

| Mild FAM Stress | Moderate FAM Stress | High FAM Stress | Serious FAM Stress |

SKIP ITEMS THAT DO NOT APPLY TO YOU!

Personal Stress

PAST	**FUTURE**
1 = NOT STRESSFUL	1 = NOT STRESSFUL
5 = VERY STRESSFUL	5 = VERY STRESSFUL

PAST		Item	FUTURE	
1 2 3 4 5		1. Vacations or travel	1 2 3 4 5	
1 2 3 4 5		2. Feeling unattractive	1 2 3 4 5	
1 2 3 4 5		3. Personal injury or illness	1 2 3 4 5	
1 2 3 4 5		4. Pregnancy	1 2 3 4 5	
1 2 3 4 5		5. Noticeable aging	1 2 3 4 5	
1 2 3 4 5		6. Started menopause	1 2 3 4 5	
1 2 3 4 5		7. Outstanding personal achievement	1 2 3 4 5	
1 2 3 4 5		8. Change in personal habits or schedule (smoking, bedtime, mealtimes, etc.)	1 2 3 4 5	
1 2 3 4 5		9. Problems from being too successful	1 2 3 4 5	
1 2 3 4 5		10. Lack of personal privacy	1 2 3 4 5	
1 2 3 4 5		11. Difficulty in meeting obligations to yourself	1 2 3 4 5	
1 2 3 4 5		12. Failure to meet personal goals	1 2 3 4 5	
1 2 3 4 5		13. Not enough time for yourself	1 2 3 4 5	
1 2 3 4 5		14. Problems with drug or alcohol dependence	1 2 3 4 5	
1 2 3 4 5		15. Problems with weight	1 2 3 4 5	
1 2 3 4 5		16. Not enough time to get things done	1 2 3 4 5	
1 2 3 4 5		17. Philosophical or religious preoccupations	1 2 3 4 5	
1 2 3 4 5		18. Assaulted or robbed	1 2 3 4 5	

PAST							FUTURE				
1 = NOT STRESSFUL							**1 = NOT STRESSFUL**				
5 = VERY STRESSFUL							**5 = VERY STRESSFUL**				
1	2	3	4	5		**19.** Involved in lawsuit or other court procedure	1	2	3	4	5
1	2	3	4	5		**20.** Minor violations of the law	1	2	3	4	5
1	2	3	4	5		**21.** Jail term	1	2	3	4	5
1	2	3	4	5		**22.** Change in living conditions	1	2	3	4	5
1	2	3	4	5		**23.** Change in residence	1	2	3	4	5
1	2	3	4	5		**24.** Change in recreation	1	2	3	4	5
1	2	3	4	5		**25.** Change in religious activities	1	2	3	4	5

_____

PAST   FUTURE

_____

TOTAL PERSONAL
STRESS SCORE

Add the circled numbers in the past columns to get your PAST score. Add the circled numbers in the future columns to get your FUTURE score. Add your PAST and your FUTURE scores to get your TOTAL PERSONAL STRESS SCORE. Mark your TOTAL PERSONAL STRESS SCORE on the graph below. If you score in the High or Serious range, be sure to read chapter 7, "Overcoming Personal Stress," for suggestions on what to do about it.

Your Personal Stress Profile

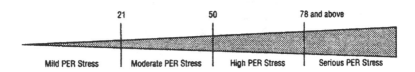

21	50	78 and above
Mild PER Stress	Moderate PER Stress	High PER Stress	Serious PER Stress

SKIP ITEMS THAT DO NOT APPLY TO YOU!

Social Stress

PAST						FUTURE				
1 = NOT STRESSFUL						*1 = NOT STRESSFUL*				
5 = VERY STRESSFUL						*5 = VERY STRESSFUL*				

1	2	3	4	5		1	2	3	4	5
1	2	3	4	5	**1.** Leading a group	1	2	3	4	5
1	2	3	4	5	**2.** Identification as a group leader	1	2	3	4	5
1	2	3	4	5	**3.** Following along with a group	1	2	3	4	5
1	2	3	4	5	**4.** Major responsibility for or to a social group	1	2	3	4	5
1	2	3	4	5	**5.** Feeling excluded from a group	1	2	3	4	5
1	2	3	4	5	**6.** Starting new relationship(s)	1	2	3	4	5
1	2	3	4	5	**7.** Ending old relationship(s)	1	2	3	4	5
1	2	3	4	5	**8.** Special care in maintaining relationship(s)	1	2	3	4	5
1	2	3	4	5	**9.** Not having freedoms and privileges acquaintances enjoy					
1	2	3	4	5	**10.** High popularity	1	2	3	4	5
1	2	3	4	5	**11.** Feelings of superiority toward friends and acquaintances	1	2	3	4	5
1	2	3	4	5	**12.** Feeling inferior to friends and acquaintances	1	2	3	4	5
1	2	3	4	5	**13.** Feeling unwanted and alone	1	2	3	4	5
1	2	3	4	5	**14.** Lack of social stimulation	1	2	3	4	5
1	2	3	4	5	**15.** Death of a close friend	1	2	3	4	5
1	2	3	4	5	**16.** Close friend moves away	1	2	3	4	5
1	2	3	4	5	**17.** Problems with social discrimination	1	2	3	4	5
1	2	3	4	5	**18.** Feeling victim of ethnic, racial, religious, or sexual prejudice	1	2	3	4	5
1	2	3	4	5	**19.** Change in social activities	1	2	3	4	5
1	2	3	4	5	**20.** Feeling self-conscious in social situations	1	2	3	4	5
1	2	3	4	5	**21.** Feelings of competition and comparison	1	2	3	4	5

_____   _____

PAST   FUTURE

_____

TOTAL SOCIAL
STRESS SCORE

Add the circled numbers in the past columns to get your PAST score. Add the circled numbers in the future columns to get your FUTURE score. Add your PAST and your FUTURE scores to get your TOTAL SOCIAL STRESS SCORE. Mark your TOTAL SOCIAL STRESS SCORE on the graph below. If you score in the High or Serious range, be sure to read chapter 8, "Dealing with Social Stress," for suggestions on what to do about it.

Your Social Stress Profile

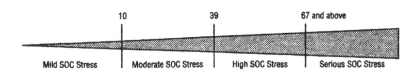

	10		39		67 and above
Mild SOC Stress		Moderate SOC Stress		High SOC Stress	Serious SOC Stress

SKIP ITEMS THAT DO NOT APPLY TO YOU!

Environmental Stress

PAST		**FUTURE**
1 = NOT STRESSFUL		*1 = NOT STRESSFUL*
5 = VERY STRESSFUL		*5 = VERY STRESSFUL*

PAST		FUTURE
1 2 3 4 5	**1.** Problems with zoning issues/local government	1 2 3 4 5
1 2 3 4 5	**2.** Noisy or unfriendly neighbors	1 2 3 4 5
1 2 3 4 5	**3.** Construction work in neighborhood or community	1 2 3 4 5
1 2 3 4 5	**4.** Problems with traffic, parking, transportation	1 2 3 4 5
1 2 3 4 5	**5.** Problems with shifts in population	1 2 3 4 5
1 2 3 4 5	**6.** Problems with schools	1 2 3 4 5
1 2 3 4 5	**7.** Local politics or election results	1 2 3 4 5
1 2 3 4 5	**8.** Adjustments to new neighborhood	1 2 3 4 5
1 2 3 4 5	**9.** Neighbors failing to maintain property	1 2 3 4 5
1 2 3 4 5	**10.** Problems with municipal services or utilities	1 2 3 4 5
1 2 3 4 5	**11.** Vandalism or other minor crime in neighborhood	1 2 3 4 5
1 2 3 4 5	**12.** Violent crime in neighborhood	1 2 3 4 5
1 2 3 4 5	**13.** Ethnic or racial conflict	1 2 3 4 5
1 2 3 4 5	**14.** Lack of recreational facilities	1 2 3 4 5

PAST						FUTURE				
1 = NOT STRESSFUL						**1 = NOT STRESSFUL**				
5 = VERY STRESSFUL						**5 = VERY STRESSFUL**				
1	2	3	4	5	**15.** Crowding	1	2	3	4	5
1	2	3	4	5	**16.** Remodeling in home	1	2	3	4	5
1	2	3	4	5	**17.** Major renovation or construction of home	1	2	3	4	5
1	2	3	4	5	**18.** Problems with landlord, tenant, roommate, condo association	1	2	3	4	5
1	2	3	4	5	**19.** Concern about toxic substances	1	2	3	4	5
1	2	3	4	5	**20.** Environmental pollution (air, noise, water, earth)	1	2	3	4	5
1	2	3	4	5	**21.** Environmental deterioration or destruction	1	2	3	4	5

PAST _____   FUTURE _____

TOTAL ENVIRONMENTAL STRESS SCORE

Add the circled numbers in the past columns to get your PAST score. Add the circled numbers in the future columns to get your FUTURE score. Add your PAST and your FUTURE scores to get your TOTAL ENVIRONMENTAL STRESS SCORE. Mark your TOTAL ENVIRONMENTAL STRESS SCORE on the graph below. If you score in the High or Serious range, be sure to read chapter 9, "Beating Environmental Stress," for suggestions of what to do about it.

Your Environmental Stress Profile

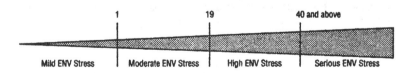

| 1 | 19 | 40 and above |

| Mild ENV Stress | Moderate ENV Stress | High ENV Stress | Serious ENV Stress |

SKIP ITEMS THAT DO NOT APPLY TO YOU!

Financial Stress

PAST						FUTURE				
1 = NOT STRESSFUL						*1 = NOT STRESSFUL*				
5 = VERY STRESSFUL						*5 = VERY STRESSFUL*				

1	2	3	4	5		1	2	3	4	5
1	2	3	4	5	**1.** Not enough money to pay bills	1	2	3	4	5
1	2	3	4	5	**2.** Loss of income	1	2	3	4	5
1	2	3	4	5	**3.** Increased expenditures	1	2	3	4	5
1	2	3	4	5	**4.** Declining net worth	1	2	3	4	5
1	2	3	4	5	**5.** Lack of funds for recreation	1	2	3	4	5
1	2	3	4	5	**6.** Major purchase	1	2	3	4	5
1	2	3	4	5	**7.** Financial loss	1	2	3	4	5
1	2	3	4	5	**8.** Cash-flow problems	1	2	3	4	5
1	2	3	4	5	**9.** Loss of credit	1	2	3	4	5
1	2	3	4	5	**10.** Dramatic increase in net worth	1	2	3	4	5
1	2	3	4	5	**11.** Inheritance	1	2	3	4	5
1	2	3	4	5	**12.** Major financial gain	1	2	3	4	5
1	2	3	4	5	**13.** Went on or off welfare	1	2	3	4	5
1	2	3	4	5	**14.** Business readjustment	1	2	3	4	5
1	2	3	4	5	**15.** New mortgage or loan	1	2	3	4	5
1	2	3	4	5	**16.** Foreclosure of mortgage	1	2	3	4	5

PAST _____   FUTURE _____

_____
TOTAL FINANCIAL
STRESS SCORE

Add the circled numbers in the past columns to get your PAST score. Add the circled numbers in the future columns to get your FUTURE score. Add your PAST and your FUTURE scores to get your TOTAL FINANCIAL STRESS SCORE. Mark your TOTAL FINANCIAL STRESS SCORE on the graph below. If you score in the High or Serious range, be sure to read chapter 10, "Conquering Financial Stress," for suggestions on what to do about it.

Your Financial Stress Profile

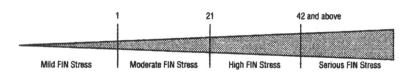

1	21		42 and above
Mild FIN Stress	Moderate FIN Stress	High FIN Stress	Serious FIN Stress

SYMPTOMS OF STRESS

This part of the *Audit* measures the symptoms of stress you experience as a result of too much demand and pressure and/or too much susceptibility to stress. The following items are symptoms of stress that you may have experienced or anticipate experiencing. The symptoms of stress can be stressful themselves. If you have had one or more of the symptoms below, rate the amount of stress it has caused you in the past six months and the amount of stress you anticipate it will cause you in the next six months.

SKIP ITEMS THAT DO NOT APPLY TO YOU!

Muscular (MS) Stress Symptoms

PAST 1 = NOT STRESSFUL 5 = VERY STRESSFUL						FUTURE 1 = NOT STRESSFUL 5 = VERY STRESSFUL				
1	2	3	4	5	**1.** Tight muscles or muscular aches	1	2	3	4	5
1	2	3	4	5	**2.** Nervous tics	1	2	3	4	5
1	2	3	4	5	**3.** Stuttering, voice shaky or strained	1	2	3	4	5
1	2	3	4	5	**4.** Frowning, wrinkling forehead	1	2	3	4	5
1	2	3	4	5	**5.** Tension headaches	1	2	3	4	5
1	2	3	4	5	**6.** Bruxism (grinding or clenching teeth)	1	2	3	4	5
1	2	3	4	5	**7.** Jaw pain or ache	1	2	3	4	5
1	2	3	4	5	**8.** Pacing finger or foot tapping, difficulty sitting still	1	2	3	4	5
1	2	3	4	5	**9.** Trembling or shaking	1	2	3	4	5
1	2	3	4	5	**10.** Back pain	1	2	3	4	5

PAST   FUTURE

TOTAL MUSCULAR SYMPTOMS SCORE

Add the circled numbers in the past columns to get your PAST score. Add the circled numbers in the future columns to get your FUTURE score. Add your PAST and your FUTURE scores to get your TOTAL MUSCULAR SYMPTOMS SCORE. Mark your TOTAL MUSCULAR SYMPTOMS SCORE on the graph below. If you score in the High or Serious range, be sure to read chapter 12, "Your Aching Back, Head, Jaw, Etc.," for suggestions on what to do about it.

Your Muscular Stress Symptoms Profile

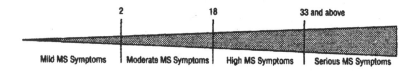

	2	18	33 and above

Mild MS Symptoms | Moderate MS Symptoms | High MS Symptoms | Serious MS Symptoms

SKIP ITEMS THAT DO NOT APPLY TO YOU!

Parasympathetic Nervous System (PNS) Stress Symptoms

PAST		**FUTURE**
1 = NOT STRESSFUL		*1 = NOT STRESSFUL*
5 = VERY STRESSFUL		*5 = VERY STRESSFUL*

PAST							FUTURE				
1	2	3	4	5	**1.** Change in appetite		1	2	3	4	5
1	2	3	4	5	**2.** Nausea		1	2	3	4	5
1	2	3	4	5	**3.** Gas pains or cramping		1	2	3	4	5
1	2	3	4	5	**4.** Acid stomach, heartburn		1	2	3	4	5
1	2	3	4	5	**5.** Problems with urination		1	2	3	4	5
1	2	3	4	5	**6.** Constipation		1	2	3	4	5
1	2	3	4	5	**7.** Diarrhea		1	2	3	4	5
1	2	3	4	5	**8.** Frigidity or impotence		1	2	3	4	5
1	2	3	4	5	**9.** Dry mouth or throat		1	2	3	4	5
1	2	3	4	5	**10.** Difficulty swallowing		1	2	3	4	5

PAST	FUTURE
_____	_____

**TOTAL PNS
SYMPTOMS SCORE**

Add the circled numbers in the past columns to get your PAST score. Add the circled numbers in the future columns to get your FUTURE score. Add your PAST and your FUTURE scores to get your TOTAL PNS SYMPTOMS SCORE. Mark your TOTAL PNS SYMPTOMS SCORE on the graph below. If you score in the High or Serious range, be sure to read chapter 13, "When It Gets You in the Gut," for suggestions on what to do about it.

Your PNS Stress Symptoms Profile

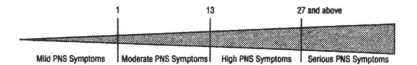

1	13	27 and above

Mild PNS Symptoms | Moderate PNS Symptoms | High PNS Symptoms | Serious PNS Symptoms

SKIP ITEMS THAT DO NOT APPLY TO YOU!

Sympathetic Nervous System (SNS) Stress Symptoms

PAST		**FUTURE**	
1 = NOT STRESSFUL		*1 = NOT STRESSFUL*	
5 = VERY STRESSFUL		*5 = VERY STRESSFUL*	

PAST				Item	FUTURE				
1 2 3 4 5				**1.** High blood pressure	1 2 3 4 5				
1 2 3 4 5				**2.** Dizziness	1 2 3 4 5				
1 2 3 4 5				**3.** Palpitations	1 2 3 4 5				
1 2 3 4 5				**4.** Sweaty palms, increased perspiration	1 2 3 4 5				
1 2 3 4 5				**5.** Cold hands or feet	1 2 3 4 5				
1 2 3 4 5				**6.** Rapid heartbeat	1 2 3 4 5				
1 2 3 4 5				**7.** Sudden bursts of energy	1 2 3 4 5				
1 2 3 4 5				**8.** Migraine headaches	1 2 3 4 5				
1 2 3 4 5				**9.** Chest pain	1 2 3 4 5				
1 2 3 4 5				**10.** Shortness of breath	1 2 3 4 5				

_____   _____
PAST   FUTURE

_____
TOTAL SNS
SYMPTOMS SCORE

Add the circled numbers in the past columns to get your PAST score. Add the circled numbers in the future columns to get your FUTURE score. Add your PAST and your FUTURE scores to get your TOTAL SNS SYMPTOMS SCORE. Mark your TOTAL SNS SYMPTOMS SCORE on the graph below. If you score in the High or Serious range, be sure to read the SNS section of chapter 14, "If Your Heart Runs Hot or Cold," for suggestions on what to do about it.

THE STRESS SOLUTION

Your SNS Stress Symptoms Profile

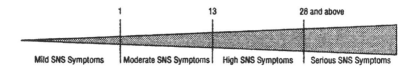

Mild SNS Symptoms	Moderate SNS Symptoms	High SNS Symptoms	Serious SNS Symptoms

SKIP ITEMS THAT DO NOT APPLY TO YOU!

Emotional (EM) Stress Symptoms

PAST		**FUTURE**
1 = NOT STRESSFUL		1 = NOT STRESSFUL
5 = VERY STRESSFUL		5 = VERY STRESSFUL

PAST		FUTURE
1 2 3 4 5	1. Feeling that things are getting out of control	1 2 3 4 5
1 2 3 4 5	2. Anxiety or panic	1 2 3 4 5
1 2 3 4 5	3. Frustration	1 2 3 4 5
1 2 3 4 5	4. Anger and irritation	1 2 3 4 5
1 2 3 4 5	5. Feeling desperate, hopeless	1 2 3 4 5
1 2 3 4 5	6. Feeling trapped, helpless	1 2 3 4 5
1 2 3 4 5	7. Feeling blue or depressed	1 2 3 4 5
1 2 3 4 5	8. Feeling guilty	1 2 3 4 5
1 2 3 4 5	9. Feeling self-conscious	1 2 3 4 5
1 2 3 4 5	10. Feeling restless	1 2 3 4 5

PAST _____   FUTURE _____

**TOTAL EMOTIONAL
SYMPTOMS SCORE** _____

Add the circled numbers in the past columns to get your PAST score. Add the circled numbers in the future columns to get your FUTURE score. Add your PAST and your FUTURE scores to get your TOTAL EMOTIONAL SYMPTOMS SCORE. Mark your TOTAL EMOTIONAL SYMPTOMS SCORE on the graph below. If you score in the High or Serious range, be sure to read chapter 15, "Angry, Depressed, and Anxious," for suggestions on what to do about it.

Your Emotional Stress Symptoms Profile

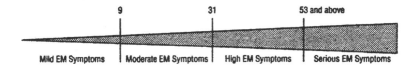

SKIP ITEMS THAT DO NOT APPLY TO YOU!

Cognitive (COG) Stress Symptoms

PAST						FUTURE				
1 = NOT STRESSFUL						*1 = NOT STRESSFUL*				
5 = VERY STRESSFUL						*5 = VERY STRESSFUL*				

PAST						FUTURE				
1	2	3	4	5	**1.** Poor memory	1	2	3	4	5
1	2	3	4	5	**2.** Daydreaming	1	2	3	4	5
1	2	3	4	5	**3.** Indecisiveness	1	2	3	4	5
1	2	3	4	5	**4.** Mental confusion	1	2	3	4	5
1	2	3	4	5	**5.** Racing thoughts	1	2	3	4	5
1	2	3	4	5	**6.** Conviction that everything turns out for the worst	1	2	3	4	5
1	2	3	4	5	**7.** Difficulty falling asleep	1	2	3	4	5
1	2	3	4	5	**8.** Poor judgment	1	2	3	4	5
1	2	3	4	5	**9.** Difficulty concentrating	1	2	3	4	5
1	2	3	4	5	**10.** Preoccupation	1	2	3	4	5

PAST   FUTURE

TOTAL COGNITIVE
SYMPTOMS SCORE

Add the circled numbers in the past columns to get your PAST score. Add the circled numbers in the future columns to get your FUTURE score. Add your PAST and your FUTURE scores to get your TOTAL COGNITIVE SYMPTOMS SCORE. Mark your TOTAL COGNITIVE SYMPTOMS SCORE on the graph below. If you score in the High or Serious range, be sure to read chapter 16, "Too Stressed to Think Straight," for suggestions on what to do about it.

Your Cognitive Stress Symptoms Profile

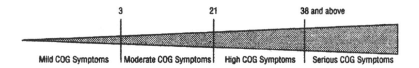

| 3 | 21 | 38 and above |

| Mild COG Symptoms | Moderate COG Symptoms | High COG Symptoms | Serious COG Symptoms |

SKIP ITEMS THAT DO NOT APPLY TO YOU!

Endocrine (END) Stress Symptoms

PAST		**FUTURE**
1 = NOT STRESSFUL		1 = NOT STRESSFUL
5 = VERY STRESSFUL		5 = VERY STRESSFUL

PAST		FUTURE
1 2 3 4 5	1. Arthritic joint pain	1 2 3 4 5
1 2 3 4 5	2. Menstrual difficulties	1 2 3 4 5
1 2 3 4 5	3. Unusual changes in body temperature	1 2 3 4 5
1 2 3 4 5	4. Diabetes	1 2 3 4 5
1 2 3 4 5	5. Skin rashes or pimples	1 2 3 4 5
1 2 3 4 5	6. Fatigue, feeling tired	1 2 3 4 5
1 2 3 4 5	7. Infertility	1 2 3 4 5
1 2 3 4 5	8. Bloating, water retention	1 2 3 4 5
1 2 3 4 5	9. Excessive thirst	1 2 3 4 5
1 2 3 4 5	10. Changes in skin color (e.g., gray pallor)	1 2 3 4 5

PAST _____   FUTURE _____

_____
TOTAL ENDOCRINE
SYMPTOMS SCORE

Add the circled numbers in the past columns to get your PAST score. Add the circled numbers in the future columns to get your FUTURE score. Add your PAST and your FUTURE scores to get your TOTAL ENDOCRINE SYMPTOMS SCORE. Mark your TOTAL ENDOCRINE SYMPTOMS SCORE on the graph below. If you score in the High or Serious range, be sure to read chapter 17, "Hormones in Disarray," for suggestions on what to do about it.

Your Endocrine Stress Symptoms Profile

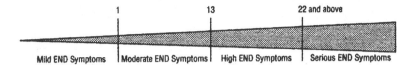

| 1 | 13 | 22 and above |

Mild END Symptoms | Moderate END Symptoms | High END Symptoms | Serious END Symptoms

SKIP ITEMS THAT DO NOT APPLY TO YOU!

Immune (IM) Stress Symptoms

PAST		**FUTURE**
1 = *NOT STRESSFUL*		1 = *NOT STRESSFUL*
5 = *VERY STRESSFUL*		5 = *VERY STRESSFUL*

PAST	Item	FUTURE
1 2 3 4 5	1. Many colds	1 2 3 4 5
1 2 3 4 5	2. Frequent bouts of flu	1 2 3 4 5
1 2 3 4 5	3. Allergies	1 2 3 4 5
1 2 3 4 5	4. Many low-grade infections	1 2 3 4 5
1 2 3 4 5	5. Hives	1 2 3 4 5
1 2 3 4 5	6. Feeling generally unwell or sick	1 2 3 4 5
1 2 3 4 5	7. Sores in mouth	1 2 3 4 5
1 2 3 4 5	8. Strep throat	1 2 3 4 5
1 2 3 4 5	9. Mononucleosis	1 2 3 4 5
1 2 3 4 5	10. Herpes	1 2 3 4 5

PAST   FUTURE

TOTAL IMMUNE
SYMPTOMS SCORE

Add the circled numbers in the past columns to get your PAST score. Add the circled numbers in the future columns to get your FUTURE score. Add your PAST and your FUTURE scores to get your TOTAL IMMUNE SYMPTOMS SCORE. Mark your TOTAL IMMUNE SYMPTOMS SCORE on the graph below. If your score in the High or Serious range, be sure to read chapter 18, "Sick of Stress," for suggestions on what to do about it.

Your Immune Stress Symptoms Profile

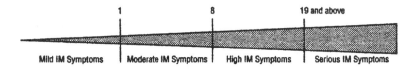

You've now taken the *Stress Audit* and discovered your individual *Stress Profiles*. We hope it was informative and that you learned some interesting aspects about yourself. If you are like most of our clients, you now have a much clearer picture of what stress means to you. You can use this information in the next section to construct your *Stress Action Plans*.

But stress, as we pointed out earlier, is additive, so you need some idea of what stress means to you overall. To do that, just add together the TOTAL scores from the Sources of Stress sections to get your TOTAL SOURCES OF STRESS score. Then add the TOTAL scores from the Symptoms of Stress sections to get your TOTAL SYMPTOMS OF STRESS score. Your SUSCEPTIBILITY TO STRESS score is already a total score. Write your scores below.

SOURCES

_____ JOB
_____ FAM
_____ PER
_____ SOC
_____ ENV
_____ FIN

_____
TOTAL SOURCES

SYMPTOMS

_____ MS
_____ PNS
_____ SNS
_____ EM
_____ COG
_____ END
_____ IM

_____
TOTAL SYMPTOMS

_____
SUSCEPTIBILITY

Find and mark your scores on the graphs below.

Your Total Sources of Stress Profile

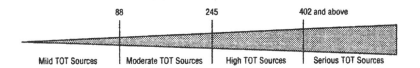

Your Total Symptoms of Stress Profile

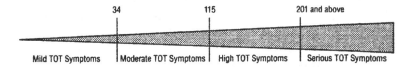

Your Susceptibility to Stress Profile

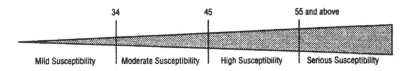

3 SUSCEPTIBILITY: THE TOUGHER YOU ARE, THE MORE YOU CAN TAKE

People are quite different from one another in their susceptibility to stress. Some are like horses, and some are like butterflies. The horses tolerate great amounts of stress without faltering or breaking stride; the butterflies fall apart under the slightest demand or pressure. Whether you're a horse or a butterfly depends on several ingredients: your physical constitution, how well you take care of yourself, and your resources for coping with stress. The tougher you are, the more you can take. If you have a stress-prone constitution, are lazy about exercise, eat poorly, abuse stimulants, don't get enough sleep, or don't use your coping resources, you don't stand much chance against stress.

Your physical constitution is a question of biology so there's not much you can do about that. But there is a lot you can do, whether you're a horse or a butterfly, to maximize your resistance to stress. You can develop good health habits, get rid of bad health habits, and use your familial, financial, social, spiritual, and personal resources for coping with stress more effectively. You can be stress tough even if you're a butterfly.

Dealing with your susceptibility to stress can be the quickest route to handling it effectively. A California State Department of Health Services study following seven thousand people over several years found that 45-year-old women whose health and living habits made them less susceptible to stress had seven years greater life expectancy than did controls. Forty-five-year-old men with good health and living habits had eleven years greater life expectancy.[1]

The health habits, lifestyle, and coping resources that make you stress tough are not new ideas. They're the kinds of things your grandmother may have told you when you were a child. They're part and parcel of the folk wisdom that served as the basis of ancient medicine. The writings of Huang Ti,[2] the "Yellow Emperor" (circa 2697–2597 B.C.), the foundation of Chinese medicine, are filled with admonitions on how one should take care of oneself to enjoy good health, happiness, and a long life.

Corporate wellness programs have taken grandmother's advice to heart and are fighting stress by helping their employees become stress tough. The better wellness programs include exercise, nutrition, weight management, employee assistance, smoking cessation, and alcohol and drug abuse elements. These are the topics addressed in the *Susceptibility* section of the *Stress Audit*.

Making yourself stress tough pays off in a number of ways. You'll feel better mentally and physically. You'll have fewer problems with stress. Our research indicates that about 14 percent of all stress-related symptoms are attributable to your susceptibility to stress.[3]

If you want to make yourself tougher and more stress resistant, it's going to take a little work. It's worth it, but it means making changes. As we tell our clients, "If you always do what you've always done, you'll always get what you've always got."

Many of the changes you need to make to get stress tough and less susceptible to stress can begin today. Start by going over the *Susceptibility* section of your *Stress Audit* and picking out an item—a good habit you want to emphasize, a bad habit you want to eliminate, or a coping resource you want to use more effectively.

Choose one you can change easily. Success breeds success. Once you get the hang of it, you can go on to design and carry out *Stress Action Plans* for your more difficult susceptibility items. Write down this item on your *Stress Action Plan: Susceptibility* form at the end of this chapter and then describe how that item affects your life and makes you more susceptible to stress.

You might want to take a look at Anne's sample *Stress Action Plan: Susceptibility* at the end of this chapter to see how she filled hers out. Anne didn't think she was getting enough sleep (item number 2 of the *Susceptibility* section). Poor sleep is a big problem for lots of people but it affects each person differently. Read Anne's behavioral description of why not getting enough sleep was a problem for her, then write a behavioral description of how the susceptibility item you've chosen affects your life.

Read the section of this chapter that discusses the item you've chosen to work on for tips on what you can do. Then decide which ideas have the most relevance to what you want to achieve. Finally, use those ideas to tailor a plan of action that best fits you and your situation. Write that plan down on your *Stress Action Plan: Sources* form at the end of chapter 4.

You might want to photocopy the form for reference in keeping you on track as you implement your plan. If all you get out of this book is some information and ideas that help you become more stress resistant, it will have been worth the time and effort for you.

As we said earlier, the key to effective stress management is self-regulation. But you can't just do it. Self-regulation is a five-step process:

- becoming aware of your problems
- deciding what you need to do about them
- breaking free of the pitfalls and obstacles that keep you from doing what you need to do
- using your resources, friends, and allies to help
- *doing it*

You've already taken your first step in reading chapter 1 and taking the *Stress Audit*. You know what stress points are and have discovered your own. Now you're ready to take your second step—deciding what to do about them and what actions you need to take. In this chapter you'll design a *Stress Action Plan: Susceptibility* to reduce your susceptibility to stress.

Your *Stress Action Plan* form has five sections:

- a specific item from the *Stress Audit: Susceptibility, Sources* or *Symptoms* sections that speaks to a particular problem you need to work on
- a behavioral description of the situation and problem
- a choice among possible courses of action
- obstacles to taking action
- supports for taking action

For now, concentrate on the first three elements of your plan: the item, a behavioral description of how it's a problem, and a chosen course of action—what you think you need to do to eliminate the problem. In this chapter you'll take the first three steps in developing an *Action Plan* to reduce your susceptibility to stress. In section II, you'll do the same for conquering a source of stress, and then you'll repeat the process by developing an *Action Plan* for conquering a symptom of stress in section III.

Each of these chapters contains stories illustrating how other people have dealt with particular problems and sample *Stress Action Plans* as examples to follow as you fill yours out. You'll also find information and suggestions on how to deal with specific issues and problems.

A good *Stress Action Plan* has particular characteristics:

- It makes your life better.
- You can execute a good *Stress Action Plan* in six to twelve weeks.
- The first step of a good *Stress Action Plan* doesn't have to solve the entire problem.
- The outcome of a good *Stress Action Plan* is described in behavioral terms.

- A good *Stress Action Plan* is leveraged. It gives you the "biggest bang for your buck."

You'll be able to complete your three *Stress Action Plans* after you read about barriers to action and supports for action in the last section of the book. But for now, just concentrate on filling out *Stress Action Plans* to decide what you need to do about your susceptibility to stress. The twenty-one items of the *Susceptibility Scale* were derived from research in health psychology that has linked certain behaviors with improved resistance to stress. These health behaviors and resources are your first line of defense against stress. Do what you can to increase the frequency of these items in your daily life.

1 | **I eat at least one hot balanced meal per day.**

You are what you eat. Sound nutrition is essential for lasting health and resistance to the ravages of stress. A good nutritional plan includes a variety of food such as dairy products, cereals and other grains, fruits, vegetables, and protein, and minimizes refined white flour, refined sugar, salt, saturated fats, alcohol, artificial preservatives and additives, and caffeine. You also need plenty of fluids, as much as eight to ten glasses of water and other beverages per day. Improving your nutritional habits makes you much less susceptible to stress.

Many people tend to overlook the importance of the vitamins contained in an adequate diet. The B and C vitamins, for instance, ensure the health of your nervous and immune systems. Stress burns them up quickly (so do alcohol, nicotine, processed sugar, and caffeine). The A, D, E, and K vitamins can be stored in our body fat so we can build up a supply to use as needed. The B and C vitamins, however, can't be stockpiled because they're water soluble and are excreted in perspiration and urine.

When you're under a lot of stress, you need to be more careful about proper nutrition to replenish your stores of B and C vitamins.

People eat poorly because they don't know any better, because sugary and fatty foods may taste better to them, or because they feel they don't have time to prepare or sit down to eat a balanced, nutritious meal. We are a nation on the go, and prepared or fast foods are quicker and less trouble.

However, they often contain more sugar, fat, and salt than is good for us. Our annual per capita consumption of refined sugar is more than 125 pounds and it increases every year. Most of it (about two-thirds) is added by food manufacturers. The average canned soft drink, for instance, contains ten to eleven teaspoons of sugar. Refined sugar not only adds unwanted calories, it increases our risk of cardiovascular problems by raising triglyceride levels. If you rely on sugar-laden foods as a primary source of energy, you have to eat something containing sugar every two or three hours just to keep your energy up.[4]

Sodium can also cause a problem. It is vital to the biological economy of our bodies, but we tend to consume too much. Most of our sodium is taken in as sodium chloride, or table salt. Excess is combed out of the bloodstream by our kidneys. Under stress, the kidneys conserve sodium. Since most of us eat five to ten times more salt than we need, our sodium blood levels increase dramatically under stress. Increased concentrations of blood sodium draw water from other tissues by osmosis, increasing the volume of blood and thereby raising blood pressure. This is a medical condition known as hypervolumia and is one way of developing stress-related hypertension.

But a hot, well-balanced meal at least once a day involves more than just nutrition. It usually means sitting down, relaxing, and focusing on enjoying your food. Meals shared with others also mean human contact, which fends off stress. Mealtime rituals, like saying grace, are calming, create a bond with others, and tell the body to prepare to receive and digest food.

> **2** | I get seven to eight hours of sleep at least four nights per week.

If you're like Anne, chronic lack of sleep leads to a state of exhaustion that not only harms the quality of your life but erodes health, lowers productivity, and, most of all, seriously decreases your ability to handle stress.

In *Macbeth*, almost four hundred years ago, Shakespeare wrote "The sleep that knits up the raveled sleeve of care." Modern research bears out his wisdom by showing that the mind and body require regular sleep to repair the wear and tear of everyday living. Mood, alertness, and work performance deteriorate progressively with sleep loss but return to normal with regular sleep.[5] The previously mentioned California study on health habits and longevity found proper sleep added years to life expectancy.

Not everyone has the same sleep requirements. Elderly people, for example, tend to sleep less. Some people require amazingly little sleep. Most of us, though, need at least seven to eight hours of sleep per night at least four nights a week. You can get by on less sleep for a while, but eventually you run into sleep debt. When you do, you become tired, tense, irritable, and on edge until you get caught up again. It may take several weeks of good sleep to feel truly rested.

Regular sleep means keeping regular hours. Go to bed and get up at the same time every day. Avoid alcohol, nicotine, and caffeine, especially for at least three hours before retiring. (Some over-the-counter medications have caffeine in them. Check the bottle for caffeine content or refer to the caffeine chart under item 19.) Never engage in stimulating activities such as physical exercise or heated discussions for at least an hour before bedtime. Turn off the TV before you get entranced into yet another program. Go to bed an hour earlier once a week and notice if you feel more rested in the morning. Develop bedtime routines such as taking a warm bath, listening to the radio, a gentle stretching routine, reading a book, or having a glass of milk. When you finally lie in bed, relax for a few moments before you turn out the light.

When our daily (or circadian) rhythms get out of sync, proper sleep becomes particularly difficult. Night-shift work and jet lag are two examples. For instance, night-shift workers who revert to normal nighttime sleeping patterns during weekends become sleepy when they're at work and wide awake when they should be sleeping. Shift workers who are rotated every three weeks have even more difficulty adjusting. If possible, keep your schedule consistent.

Some international business travelers have severe problems with jet lag because their circadian rhythms are out of sync with their new time zone. It's particularly bad for them flying east to west because their day is so much longer. They tend to wake up the next morning at their usual time, hours earlier than other people. The farther they go, the worse it is. Your circadian rhythms adjust to a new time zone, but it takes a little while. If your stay in the foreign time zone is short, your rhythms get disrupted again upon returning home. Gradually adjusting your sleep schedule in the days preceding your trip can lessen the disruption.

A word about naps. They should be limited to about thirty minutes. Much more and it can disrupt your regular sleep schedule. However, a nap during the day can leave you refreshed, with a renewed feeling of energy and alertness. An after-lunch siesta or a brief lie-down when you come home from work can make a big difference in both tension and fatigue levels.

There are times for all of us when sleep just won't come. Some people have difficulty sleeping under the best of circumstances. If you can't fall asleep, take a few minutes to notice what is interfering with your falling asleep. Racing or upsetting thoughts are common inhibitors of sleep. The most effective prescription for sleep-onset difficulties is progressive muscle relaxation (PMR) exercises (appendix I) combined with deep breathing and mental images of peace and quiet. Counting backward from one hundred, thinking of a special vacation spot, or counting your breaths can be helpful in slowing or eliminating worrisome thoughts.

Often people worry even more when they don't fall asleep right away, especially if they anticipate a big day ahead. Instead of becoming more agitated, tell yourself that your body is resting and direct your thoughts to the physical sensations of muscle relaxation. You'll get more sleep than you think, even if you wake up periodically. If you still can't fall asleep, get up, go into another room, and do something relaxing, such as reading, until you feel sleepy. Associate lying in bed with sleeping, not with insomnia. If you fall asleep easily but wake up in the middle of the night, don't panic. Gently talk yourself back to sleep.

Persistent insomnia is a sign of anxiety and may be a signal that you could benefit from counseling or consultation with a sleep specialist. If you persistently wake in the night and are unable to return to sleep, you may be suffering from depression and should consult a professional.

Unless you have been diagnosed with clinical depression, avoid sleep medications. Many have unwanted side effects and are helpful only for a few weeks at best. You will do better to find natural ways to regulate your sleeping and waking patterns.

Let's return again to Anne's story and her sleeping problems. They were fueled by her lifestyle, irregular hours, agitations about her job, anxieties over her future with Mark, and worries about her health. She had fallen into a pattern of chronic insomnia that sapped her ability to deal with the stresses in her life and became a source of stress in and of itself.

Her sleep debt was considerable. She not only had to make her hours more regular and modify her lifestyle, she had to deal with her worries and anxieties in a realistic fashion before she could get the quality of sleep she needed. She decided on a regular bedtime hour and stuck to it. She practiced saying, "I'll think about that tomorrow. There's nothing I can do about it tonight." She wrote down any particularly persistent thought as a way to get it out of her head and on paper instead. She practiced the progressive muscle relaxation exercises every night just before sleep. Some nights she never even heard the end of the tape.

It took her about six weeks to regain the sleep she needed to restore her energy reserves and feel rested and refreshed in the morning. Once Anne caught up, her productivity and efficiency increased dramatically at work. At one point, late in treatment, she told us, "I can't believe I had so much trouble with such simple problems."

---

3 | I give and receive affection regularly.

Research has shown that people who regularly give and receive affection live longer, are healthier, and report a higher quality of life than those who do not. Married people, for instance, have less stress, are healthier, and live longer than do single people. Affection does not necessarily mean sex. Widows and widowers with pets live longer than do those without pets.[6] Studies also indicate that single people with pets were shown to be happier, healthier, and to live longer than single people without pets.[7] Even having a plant to take care of has been shown to improve health.

Touch changes physiology. Animal researchers have found that a horse's heart rate goes down when touched by his trainer. Pigs who had been gentled and tamed with touch and calm words in the week prior to cardiac surgery had a 100 percent survival rate. This is compared to unadjusted pigs, who had a 100 percent death rate with identical surgery.[8]

Be generous with your warmth and affection. What goes around comes around. A warm smile and handshake, a gentle hug, and saying, "I'm glad to see you," are simple tokens but mean a lot. Affection costs you nothing and improves everyone's mental state. Make a practice of always greeting your loved ones with a hug or kiss or five minutes of undivided attention when meeting again at the end of the day.

Be willing also to ask for affection when you need it. Make requests such as, "I need a hug," or "Can I have a little sugar?" You must respect others in seeking affection and be sensitive to their moods. At the same time, don't be so sensitive to rejection that you are afraid to ask.

If you are in a relationship where there is little affectionate give and take, talk with your partner and see what can be done about this mutual concern. Ask about his or her needs and what you can do to fulfill them. Discuss your styles of expressing affection and learn how you might be more affectionate with your partner. If necessary, get professional marital or couple counseling.

If you don't have a partner, initiate contacts with people you think might make good friends for you. Get involved with other people in an activity you genuinely like. Volunteering in charitable activities may offer an outlet for your need to give to others.

4 | I have at least one relative within 50 miles upon whom I can rely.

Family gives you an unconditional charter membership in an emotional support group that really knows you for who you are and likes you anyway. Families provide emotional and practical help in times of crisis. Family teamwork is one of the best means of reducing stress.

Family members are often our oldest, closest, and most trusted friends. Brothers, sisters, mothers, fathers, aunts, uncles, and cousins are often the people with whom we share treasured childhood memories—schools, teachers, neighbors, pets, Wednesday night spaghetti dinners. Family is more than just a resource in reducing susceptibility to stress. A study by researchers at the Massachusetts General Hospital in Boston found that patients with relatives living within 50 miles had more successful hospital stays and fewer deaths than did patients without family.[9]

If you have family nearby that you're not close to, strengthen the bonds of kinship. Visit them, call them on the phone, invite them to dinner, have them over for the holidays. If you are not near to family, call or write. Be willing to draw on one another for emotional support and practical counseling and advice.

If you have no family, or if your family relationships are not healthy, attach yourself to one where you can become an honorary member. Strengthen bonds with neighbors through mutual assistance and social activities. Cultivate close friendships that include celebrating holidays and birthdays as well as assistance during times of need. In her book *Single Blessedness*, Margaret Adams has described the many ways that single people have created family-like relationships and traditions.[10]

5 | **I exercise to the point of perspiration at least three times a week.**

Exercise leads to fitness and fit people handle stress better. In a study at the University of Kansas, 112 people listed the stressful events they had experienced in the preceding year. They were then sorted into physically "fit" and "unfit" groups based on their measured aerobic capacity. For the next two months participants kept daily records of their physical health, mood, and level of psychological distress. Of those reporting the most "stressful" events in the previous year, the physically fit group reported fewer physical symptoms and less depression.[11]

Consistent moderate exercise improves almost every system of the body. It strengthens the heart, reduces the chance of a heart attack, improves overall circulation, and lowers cholesterol. It also helps control weight, decreases the need for insulin in diabetics and reduces conditions associated with hypertension. As you exercise, your muscle strength and flexibility increases, improving your posture and balance, and reducing the risk of muscle or joint injuries. Healthy muscles have fewer cramps and release tension more readily.

Exercise also has mental benefits. Forty minutes of fast-paced walking decreases anxiety for up to four hours. Exercise creates a sense of peace and well-being, probably by the release of a set of hormones called endorphins (endogenous morphine-like substances).[12]

How often should you exercise? At what pace? And for how long each time? You should exercise a minimum of three times a week to maintain fitness. Generally, the slower the pace, the longer you need to sustain exercise. Jog for twenty minutes, walk or swim for forty minutes. Try to keep a pace that increases your breathing and heart rate, but does not make you out of breath. If you can talk comfortably as you exercise you're not overdoing it.

If you begin an exercise program in your twenties or early thirties, your fitness will improve in a matter of days. If you're over forty, a month or so may pass before you feel the full impact.

The effects of stress are best counteracted by continuous, rhythmic, aerobic exercise such as walking, cycling, running, or swimming. But it can be any activity you enjoy, since you're more likely to stick with it. Alternating activities or cross training helps maintain your interest and exercises different groups of muscles. Join an exercise group or find someone to go jogging regularly with you. Check out a health, swim, or racquet club. If exercising becomes a social activity, all the better. You'll push yourself a little harder if you have company. Search your local newspapers and magazines for recreational opportunities such as biking, hiking, softball, basketball, etc. Or, call your municipal recreation department for information on recreational facilities and activities.

Remember, start your exercise program slowly, be consistent, and don't overdo. Periods of inactivity followed by bursts of effort can be harmful. Injuries from overexertion will be stressful in and of themselves. Be sensible. If you're out of condition, seek professional advice from an exercise physiologist, fitness coach, physical therapist, or your physician.

---

6 | **I limit myself to less than half a pack of cigarettes per day.**

Were it not for the cancer and cardiovascular risks, the fact that some of us crumble up dried weeds, roll them up in a paper tube, insert the paper tube into our mouths, and set it on fire would be little more than a curious aspect of our culture. You probably already know all about the health risks of cigarette smoking. If you're still smoking, you need to quit. But it's not easy. Nicotine is physically, behaviorally, and psychologically addictive. A successful smoking-cessation action plan takes all three aspects into account.

You may smoke because you think it relaxes you and reduces stress. Nothing could be further from the truth. Nicotine is a deadly poison that produces an artificial stress response involving lungs, heart, and the immune system. Like caffeine, it depletes your scarce stores of vitamins B and C.

Don't try to quit cigarettes all at once. Deal with each of the addictive components separately and give yourself time. First, keep a record of when and how much you smoke each day of the week. Fold your paper small enough to fit into your cigarette pack so it will be handy. Every time you light up, record the time of day. At the end of the week, review the total number of cigarettes. Notice the time of day you smoke the most cigarettes. Become aware of the times, locations, circumstances, and situations where you're most likely to light up.

Keep on smoking your usual daily number of cigarettes, still compiling those little charts, for the week, but switch to brands with lower nicotine and tar levels. If you like, you can record your daily nicotine intake and watch your nicotine levels go down. This gradual reduction in nicotine level takes care of your physiological dependence, lessening the probability of withdrawal symptoms.

Next, tackle the behavioral elements of the addiction. Start cutting down on the number of cigarettes smoked by *not smoking at all* in those places and situations where you don't smoke much anyway. Keep cutting back, and recording, for the next two weeks. Now, set time periods for yourself in which you are going to stop smoking. Start with an hour or two and gradually lengthen the time between cigarettes until you can comfortably go several hours without smoking. These are quitting-smoking practice sessions.

Finally, set a cessation date for yourself. Announce the date to friends and family. They'll be delighted to tease you if you don't make it. The social pressure is an added inducement not to start up again. Learn to tolerate the urge to light up. If you wait five minutes, and concentrate on taking long breaths of clean air, the urge usually passes. For the most difficult times, substitute other behaviors, such as drinking water, that are incompatible with smoking.

If you don't make it the first time, quit again right away. Look on your effort as a trial run that makes it easier next time. The best predictor for successful quitting is the number of prior attempts to quit. If you quit often enough, you're bound to quit for good.

Most important, reward yourself. When you quit, for example, each day put the money you would have spent on cigarettes in a jar. At the end of the month, buy yourself a present for having done something nice for yourself. Notice the advantages of not smoking: cleaner clothes, better stamina, the return of forgotten smells and tastes. Change your identity from a smoker to a nonsmoker. Allow yourself to let go of the rituals of smoking forever.

Psychological issues often complicate smoking cessation. One of our clients, Debby, had tremendous difficulty with withdrawal because she associated smoking with her deceased father, with whom she had had a turbulent and ambivalent relationship. She started smoking as a teenager, taking puffs off her father's cigarettes. Later, most of their positive interactions revolved around smoking and "bumming" cigarettes from each other since they smoked the same brand. She continued smoking after his death from heart disease complicated by emphysema. For Debby, even the smell of cigarette smoke reminded her of her father and, somehow, kept him with her. The last time she saw him she smuggled cigarettes to him in the hospital following his third heart attack.

We postponed our routine program for smoking cessation until we had dealt with Debby's unresolved grief and anger at a physically and verbally abusive father whom she still loved very much. After the psychological issues were out of the way, Debby moved through the program with less difficulty.

When you stop smoking, you'll probably do it on your own. The American Cancer Society estimates that 95 percent of the 30 million people who quit smoking between 1964 and 1980 did so on their own. One structured do-it-yourself program that we like is called Life Signs.[13] It centers around a device, much like a pocket calculator, that does all the record keeping of the withdrawal method we outlined. It designs your withdrawal schedule and then keeps you on it by beeping when it's time for you to smoke another cigarette. The kit also includes a manual and an instructional videotape. It's worked well for a number of our clients.

If you need outside help, the Yellow Pages lists many formal smoking-cessation programs such as Smoke Enders, or call your local chapter of the American Cancer Society or the American Heart Association for a referral. You can take part in the Great American Smokeout held by the American Cancer Society the third week of each November. Formal programs have about a 30 percent success rate after one year. If all else fails, check in with professionals who specialize in helping people get off nicotine. Your physician may prescribe a nicotine gum or skin patch that slowly reduces the nicotine addiction while you work on the habit or psychological addiction.

7 | I limit myself to fewer than five alcoholic drinks per week.

Many people drink to unwind after a busy day, to shift gears from the high energy, intense activity of the workday to a slower pace, a more relaxed, easier mood of evening. Yet, such relief from stress and tension is quite brief. Even in the short run, alcohol chews up your body's stores of vitamins B and C. For example, a blood alcohol level for intoxication is around 0.10. More than one drink (12 ounces of beer, 4 ounces of wine, 1.5 ounces of liquor) creates a blood alcohol level of 0.05. Just this amount inhibits activity in a part of the brain known as the locus coereleus, resulting in a state of overarousal. What starts as an effort at relaxation quickly backfires and creates more stress and tension. Alcohol also releases stress hormones such as hydrocortisone and adrenaline and creates a chemical imbalance leading to even higher levels of arousal, tension, and anxiety.

People tend to drink the most during periods of high stress, just when they need their wits about them to deal with their problems. They self-medicate themselves with alcohol to calm their physical reactions to stress. Yet, alcohol makes it difficult to think straight and respond appropriately. Five or more alcoholic drinks a week increases your susceptibility to stress and may even create an artificial, chemically induced stress state by releasing an oversupply of adrenaline.

There are many factors that contribute to the overuse of alcohol and other drugs: biological, chemical, psychological, and socioeconomic. Stress is only one factor that we can address here.

Cutting back on alcohol will increase your resistance to stress, and managing your stress will help you cut back on alcohol. Begin by asking yourself if you use alcohol as self-medication for your physical reactions to stress. Reread your *Stress Audit Profile* to determine your sources of stress. Then examine the pertinent chapters of section II to see what you can do about it and look at section III for alternative ways of handling your physiological reactions to stress. Begin to change your habits of drinking. Have a nonalcoholic drink first to quench your thirst. Use a one-ounce jigger to measure your liquor, and mix in more tonic to dilute the alcohol. Increase the number of your alcohol-free days. Substitute other ways of relaxing in social or tense times.

A client of ours, Jeff, age 45, provides a good example of how substituting another way of relaxing and unwinding after a hard day can short-circuit a daily alcohol routine. Jeff realized that alcohol was a problem for him and wanted us to hypnotize him to help him "get off the bottle." He was drinking at least two and sometimes three martinis in the early evening before dinner and "a cognac or two" after dinner every night. He wasn't an aggressive drunk. He just fell asleep in his chair most evenings until it was time to move to the bed. He came in for therapy because his wife was "talking separation" and his 16-year-old son had called him a "damned drunk."

We didn't hypnotize him. Instead, we went over his *Stress Audit* and suggested how he could reduce the stress in his life. We sent Jeff home with a business-size "stress card," which has a temperature-sensitive patch that changes color as hand temperature rises. We told him to sit, relax, and hold the card when he got home from work. He was not to take a drink until the card indicated that he was relaxed.

A month passed. One day Jeff called to ask if we had hypnotized him without his knowing it. He had been using the stress card and found that after it turned the "relaxed" color he didn't need or even want a drink. The time he took to relax allowed him to reach the good feeling that he thought only alcohol could give him.

Jeff's case was simple because his alcoholic use was not complicated by other psychological dependency. Chronic alcohol or substance abuse has many causes and may require intensive intervention, including support from family and friends, medical detoxification, and group support such as Alcoholics Anonymous. A key element in any substance abuse recovery program is to stop using alcohol or drugs as self-medication for the ravages of stress. If you need to decrease your alcohol intake and have trouble doing it on your own, get help. Drug and alcohol abuse counseling is a good place to start. Check with your local hospital for programs, or look in the Yellow Pages.

| 8 | **I am the appropriate weight for my height.** |

To be stress resistant, you need to get to, and stay at, a weight that makes you feel good about yourself and gives you a sense of physical well-being. A positive self-image is a key factor in developing resistance to stress. Being extremely overweight, or underweight, also threatens your physical health. At the same time, preoccupation with weight, hatred of your body, and yo-yo dieting can be more stressful than carrying a few extra pounds.

Eat sensibly several times a day. Don't get neurotic about eating. Don't play around with food fads and quick-weight-loss centers. Make positive changes slowly and stick to them. There are only four rules of diet that really matter: eat less fat, less sugar, more fiber, and a variety of healthful foods.

Any weight management plan should be a combination of eating awareness and exercise. Eating awareness means being consciously aware of your eating, noticing each mouthful, and eating only when hungry, not when bored, upset, for entertainment, or to relax from your stressed-out day. Mindful eating means that when you eat, just eat. Don't eat while watching television or otherwise occupied. Don't "graze"—that is, eat out of containers, while standing up, or while cooking. Eat only while sitting at a table and from a plate. Learn to notice and gauge your hunger. When you're partially full, stop eating.

You can probably lose about 10 percent of your standing body weight simply by reducing the fat content of your diet and increasing your level of physical activity. For larger weight gains or losses, look for a structured weight control program. Consult your physician about what program is best for you. The most sensible books we've found for weight management are *Fit or Fat*,[14] a humorous and informative book on nutrition and exercise physiology, and *E.A.T.: Eating Awareness Training*,[15] a twelve-week program that includes work on body image, eating habits, appetite awareness, and the connection between emotions and food.

---

9 | **I have an income or allowance adequate to meet basic expenses.**

Money can be a powerful resource in coping with stress and the demands and pressures of life and living. Our research with the *Stress Audit* indicates that if your income has been stable for two years, the higher your income, the lower your stress levels. Money can buy you assistance with your household chores, enabling you to hire nannies, nurses, and baby-sitters to help take care of the kids. It enables you to hire lawyers and accountants to look after your affairs, and gives you time to rest and recover from life's wear and tear. It buys food and shelter and pays for vacations. Having money can bolster your self-esteem and eliminate many of your worries about tomorrow. Money won't buy happiness, but poverty can buy misery.

Establishing financial security takes long-term planning, including career planning, budgeting, and regulation of impulse spending. In today's economy people are working longer and harder. Even two-income families have difficulty getting ahead of housing, medical, and education costs. A period of unemployment can be devastating. Stability and predictability of income and expenses is the most important aspect of financial security.

When things are predictable, we adjust accordingly. Senior citizens on fixed incomes are particularly threatened by changes beyond their control. If you are in a fluctuating economic situation, it is harder to plan.

If possible, don't let spending exceed your income. Not having money for basic needs leads to chronic worry about the future and limits your ability to handle even small financial emergencies. If you can, develop a long-term plan for increasing your income. If you must, adjust your standard of living to fit the realities of your finances. It is difficult to limit your spending in the face of advertising, credit cards, and the visible wealth of others around you. But the anguish of mounting debt with no plan for payment can be a chronic source of strain. If you lower your desire for material things, you are repaid with greater peace of mind.

One woman came to her session wearing a T-shirt with the slogan, WHEN THE GOING GETS TOUGH, THE TOUGH GO SHOPPING. For many people, it's no joke. Buying nice things is a way to cope with feeling down or to treat themselves. Be careful not to reduce your stress through shopping unless you can afford it. Playing the lottery is another way some people attempt to cope with stress, always hoping for the big hit, and not wanting to look at the actual amounts they've spent each week on tickets.

It is also important that the whole family unit shares the sense of responsibility for financial stability. Major purchases should be made jointly, and children can learn financial responsibility by budgeting their allowances and helping limit expenditures.

10 | I get strength from my religious beliefs.

If you scored 1, or "almost always," on this item, you have a powerful resource available to you during times of duress. The Twenty-third Psalm of the Bible sums it up, "Yea, though I walk through the valley of the shadow of death, I shall fear no evil, for Thou art with me." Trust in a Higher Power or a feeling of unity with a universal spirit decreases feelings of isolation and abandonment during times of loss or personal struggle. Spiritual beliefs provide guidelines for decision and comfort at times of despair, and give life a sense of meaning and purpose. Active participation in a spiritual community provides opportunity to discuss doubts and questions and to clarify values about what is truly important in life. Your spiritual community will also celebrate with you the important life transitions of births, adolescent maturation, marriages, and deaths.

If you scored 4 or 5 (Never) on this item, you may feel estranged from traditional or organized religion. You may feel that such approaches have not suited your philosophical view of the world. You may instead get strength from other beliefs—a deep respect for law or science, an admiration of the human community or an appreciation of the beauty and miraculous complexity of the natural world.

In any case, developing a source of meaning and guidance that is greater than yourself puts stressful events in perspective. Whatever your beliefs, allow yourself time for reading, discussion, and meditation on the themes of love, life and death, and the meaning of your existence and your place in the universe.

One of the oldest and most powerful forms of meditation is prayer. Prayer is not only calming and relaxing, it changes the way you think about life, lets you delegate "upstairs" your worries over situations out of your control, and permits you to unburden yourself without guilt or shame. Often religion creates a sense of "connectedness" or continuity that is comforting in a scattered, fragmented, or socially isolated life.

An elderly Jewish lady named Ruth, a refugee from communist Eastern Europe, was referred to us by her son. Ruth had been experiencing panic attacks and had been unable to sleep. In her early seventies, she was afraid of dying and was in the throes of a deep philosophical and religious crisis.

An Auschwitz survivor, she lived in Poland after World War II. To continue her education through college and graduate school, Ruth was forced to become communist and renounce her religious beliefs. Ruth and her husband, Morris, both scientists, defected to America with their children during the 1960s. After several years in this country, Morris and the children returned wholeheartedly to Judaism. But Ruth had difficulty resuming her faith.

Ruth had been convinced by her communist mentors that atheism was the only rational and intelligent view one could take on religion.

With the end of her life drawing nearer, Ruth felt a deep need to take her place in "the generations that have gone before and will come after," but had difficulty accepting her religion on "blind faith." "I am a scientist, you know," she said.

We had many discussions about Auschwitz and its brutality. Ruth's mother and father, along with thousands of others, were exterminated to prevent the spread of typhus after one case had been discovered. As we talked, her anger would mount and she would ask, "Why did this happen? We were good people. My father was a professor, my mother a doctor. Why did God hate us so?" Ruth was unaware that she was still angry at God for not having prevented her parents' deaths. She had embraced atheism out of her anger and disillusionment and now felt "empty." She felt a strong need to return to "the faith of my people," but couldn't forgive what the Holocaust had done to her.

We taught Ruth some relaxation and diaphragmatic breathing techniques, but mostly we listened as she relived her experiences *im lager* ("in the camp") and expressed her anger.

She joined an organization of Holocaust survivors where she found a comforting commonality of experience and interest. In sharing her memories with other survivors, Ruth cleansed the "Auschwitz poison from my mind," and made her peace with the God of her fathers.

She began going to synagogue with her family. She eventually regained her faith along with her "peace of mind" and finally faced her mortality with an equanimity she had never thought possible.

11 | **I regularly attend club or social activities.**

Clubs and social activities provide an organized and structured vehicle for socializing with like-minded people who share your interests and goals. Such activities can also provide opportunities for you to contribute to the larger community through special projects. Belonging to and regularly attending group or social activities contributes to a sense of identity in the community through relationships with others. In our mobile and largely urbanized society, organizations centered around common interests have partially replaced the sense of community formerly found in small towns. Friends you make through such organizations can provide a support network for enjoyable activities as well as in times of need.

There are clubs and organizations of every imaginable sort and description. Recreational organizations run the gamut from the local Y, bowling leagues, softball teams, and hiking and biking clubs, to urban athletic clubs and suburban golf clubs. Hobby organizations include those for people interested in history, computers, stamps, bird watching, and ballroom dancing. One friend of ours has had many meaningful experiences and relationships through his interest in mushrooms. His passion for fungi has led him to make friends from all over the world. He attends the annual meeting of amateur mycologists and avidly hunts specimens on hikes through the woods.

Professional, political, charitable, and volunteer organizations can be found in almost any community. Some are specifically organized as mutual aid societies and often have a commitment to assist members as well as people in need in the larger community. When Alma's father suffered a stroke, his physician recommended that we visit another stroke victim to see how the family managed his long-term care. This man's stroke had been far more debilitating, leaving him without speech, unable to stand or care for himself, or even to make meaningful signals with his hands. He had to be lifted into and out of bed each day. However, you could still see the spark of personality in his eyes. His wife had cared for him for more than ten years. As she spoke of her experience she said, "I never could have made it without the Kiwanis Club." Her husband had been a member years before. After the stroke, they organized a rotating volunteer list. Someone came each morning to help her bathe and dress him. Once a week, someone stayed for several hours so that she could go out to visit friends as a respite. This man's willingness to care for others years before had come back around to him in others' willingness to care for him.

If you rarely attend group activities, visit a few to see which ones might fit you best. Get information from friends who belong to clubs. Most communities have a community calendar in the local newspaper listing events. Be willing to attend an event even if you're not sure you'd like it. You can always leave if it's not what you had hoped for. If you don't see yourself as a "group" person, experiment with cognitive flexibility about your self-image. Imagine doing something a little bit out of character and give this form of long-term stress management a chance.

12 | I have a network of friends and acquaintances.

The Beatles sang, "I get by with a little help from my friends." They knew what they were singing about. A strong social network helps fight off feelings of loneliness, isolation, and despair. Supportive human relationships have been shown to protect stressed individuals against depression, ill health following job loss, feelings of dissatisfaction, anxiety or depression caused by on-the-job stress, pregnancy complications, and a recurrence of heart attack. Social support prevents feelings of demoralization, increases options, and facilitates active problem solving. Should you lose your job, sympathetic co-workers and friends can be of invaluable emotional support—even if they can't help with your unemployment problem.[16] Your network of friends is a smaller network within the larger community. These are people you visit more often, invite to your home, or see on a regular basis. A friend may share in only one part of your life or may share in almost everything you do. You may see your running buddy only for exercise and never get together for the movies. There may be another circle of friends with whom you always get together on the weekends.

Do your part to maintain this social network. Reciprocate invitations, return telephone calls, answer letters. If work makes you temporarily unavailable for socializing, let people know you haven't forgotten them and set a time to get together in the future. Let your friends know how important they are to you. As you keep in touch with old friends, allow new friends to enter your life. Your life changes over the course of time, and friends change as well.

There are limits to how large a social network you can maintain without being drained by its demands. As with any relationship, there are reciprocal obligations. Even the positive exchanges can be time consuming, and when a friend is in trouble, his or her stress can be contagious. If friends betray confidences, fail to fulfill expectations, or express disapproval, they in turn become sources of stress (see chapter 8). Find the right balance for you.

13	**I have one or more friends to confide in about personal matters.**

Having a network of acquaintances is a vital resource in coping with stress, but having one or more close friends is even more important. One study showed that women who experienced severe stress and did not have a close friend to confide in were twice as likely to be depressed than equally stressed women who did have a close, confiding relationship. Heart attack patients with no one to talk to were three times more likely to die than were those who had a confidant.[17] Women tend to maintain more emotionally intimate relationships than men do and report close relationships with siblings, children, and friends, while men tend to rely on their spouses or partners exclusively. This lack of alternative support leaves them particularly vulnerable upon the death of a spouse and may account for the higher mortality rates of widowers versus widows in the months following their loss. In contrast, it has been found that high-quality work relationships were more strongly related to well-being for men than for women.

A close friend shores up your morale and boosts your mental health just by being there. Close, confiding personal relationships buffer the stress connected not only to life's major changes such as deaths, births, marriages, divorces, geographic relocations, etc., but daily hassles as well. In *Just Friends*, Lillian Rubin describes the many varieties of friendships and the importance of friendship in our lives.[18]

When we were building the *Stress Audit*, one of our students, Carole, was particularly pleased that we had included the friendship item and told us why. She had stayed in an abusive relationship with a man named Ray for several years out of fear of being alone. Ashamed of the relationship, she hid her bruises from friends and family and told no one, becoming even more alone. One day, however, Carole went to work with a black eye and swollen lip. A co-worker, Mary, confronted Carole, who broke down and tearfully told her about her miserable marriage. A deep and confiding friendship began that day. Mary helped Carole face her fears of being without a man and referred her to a group for battered women. When Carole finally left Ray, Mary gave her a poster with the slogan, A WOMAN WITHOUT A MAN IS LIKE A FISH WITHOUT A BICYCLE.

After several years, with the continuing support of Mary and other new friends, Carole went to graduate school to study clinical psychology. Now a psychotherapist, she works with battered women and lectures on the importance of close, confiding friendships. The poster still hangs in Carole's office, reminding her of the power of a close friend.

14 | I am in good health (including eyesight, hearing, teeth).

Your health is your first line of defense against stress. If it isn't what it should be, your defenses are not only weakened, they may work against you. Health maintenance includes such mundane aspects as dental, hearing, and visual problems. A nagging dental problem can interrupt sleep, make concentration difficult, or be a source of uncertainty and anxiety. If you have an uncorrected hearing problem, you'll have difficulty communicating with other people, which leads to feelings of alienation and isolation. Uncorrected visual problems can create confusion, disorientation, and frustration. In addition, chronic feelings of being unwell or fatigued may indicate some kind of systemic disease. Make sure you get periodic physical and dental checkups, and if you need a hearing aid or glasses, buy them.

If you have a chronic medical condition such as hypertension, cardiovascular disease, diabetes, or back pain, be consistent in following your physician or other health care provider's advice on medication, diet, and exercise. Your health care providers can make recommendations and prescribe a treatment regimen, but they can't make you follow through at home. Just because life gets hectic is no excuse for shortcuts on health maintenance. Don't let an exacerbation of health symptoms due to neglect add to all your other pressures.

---

15 | **I am able to speak openly about my feelings when angry or worried.**

Anger, anxiety, and depression are the predominant stress emotions. "Bottling" them inside is mentally and physically damaging and decreases your resistance to stress. Expressing your emotions in an appropriate way is important. Be assertive and communicate your feelings to people in a direct, honest, and nonmanipulative way. Stand up for your rights while at the same time being sensitive to the rights and feelings of others. When you are angry at someone, tell him or her rationally what it is about the aggravating *behavior* that makes you angry rather than mount an emotional personal attack. Use "I" statements in explaining how you feel and why. Usually, expressing your feelings in a nonharmful way makes them subside more quickly. A nonattacking approach allows others to speak up about their feelings as well. An assertive approach allows both parties to better understand each other. Take your fair share of responsibility in addressing emotional concerns. If communicating your emotional feelings remains a problem for you, seek professional assistance in this area.

---

16 | **I have regular conversations with the people I live with about domestic problems (e.g., chores, money, and daily living issues).**

Teamwork makes life go smoothly and easily, whether it's on the basketball court or handling domestic chores and problems. Teams and teamwork don't just happen, though. It takes good communication. When the home team is working smoothly, home becomes a safe harbor in a stressful world. When it's not, home itself can become a source of stress. You have to talk with teammates openly, honestly, respectfully, and assertively—they have to talk with you in the same way. If you don't talk about problems, they don't get solved.

In the absence of regular communication, daily hassles become chronic sources of resentment. Roommates have particular difficulty with this one. If a roommate fails to do his or her share of household cleaning, is late paying his or her share of the electric bill, or borrows tools or clothing without asking, household tension can develop into icy silence, with no one wanting to confront the offender. What started out as friendship turns into animosity. A regular monthly "house meeting" is an opportunity to address such issues without personal attacks. Similarly, families need a regular forum to discuss assignment of chores, schedules, and the allocation of money. Some couples meet together each month to quickly go over the finances to see how they stand. Friday-night or Sunday-afternoon dinners that everyone is expected to attend provide another opportunity to bring up routine family organizational topics. Such meetings do not preclude on-the-spot problem solving but can prevent the accumulation of inequities that could blow up later.

17 | **I do something for fun at least once a week.**

Recreation is just what it says it is—re-creation. Doing something just for fun is not only enjoyable, it's a potent way to improve your stress resistance and recover from the effects of stress on mind and body. Our research indicates that people who report they "always" do something for fun at least once a week experience less stress from the demands and pressures of family, feel better about themselves, have less marital turmoil, and have fewer physical and mental symptoms of stress than those who report they "never" do. A half-smile relaxes muscle tension in the face; a good laugh relaxes the whole body and brings fresh air into the lungs.

Fun doesn't have to cost a lot of money or be anything fancy. Miah, a working mother with three children, had tension headaches and felt depressed and tired much of the time. She didn't have time to do anything "just for fun"—there were too many "important" things occupying her time.

When we asked her what she used to do for enjoyment, Miah recalled loving Laurel and Hardy movies. She smiled and laughed out loud as she described her favorites. Miah particularly liked when Oliver Hardy would get exasperated and call Stan Laurel a "blockhead." As part of her treatment we asked her husband, Bob, to start a Friday night "Blockheads" club. They would rent a Laurel and Hardy video, cook popcorn, and watch the movie with their kids. After the movie, they would take turns doing or saying something stupid. The stupidest stunt earned the perpetrator the title of "Blockhead of the Week."

We used other techniques with Miah to reduce her stress, but she thought "Blockheads" helped her the most. Her mood lifted, her energy returned, and her headaches went away. "Blockheads" has been expanded to include in-laws and neighbors, and Bob and Miah have made some "Blockheads" videos of their own.

Make a list of fun activities you like to do (include some activities you've never done but would like to try) and then include a few as a part of your weekly schedule. Read your local paper for fun activities. If you have difficulty having enjoyment at least once a week, think about what's holding you back and consider getting support for changing your mind. For example, do you think having fun is frivolous or sinful? Do you think you don't deserve to have fun? Explore these questions with family, friends, or a counselor.

18 | I am able to organize my time effectively.

Too much to do in too little time is a surefire recipe for stress. You can't make more time, but you can make better use of what time you have. Those who manage their time effectively have far less stress and fewer symptoms of stress. The three Ps central to effective time management are *Prioritize, Plan,* and *Protect.* Spend time on things that are important to you—set priorities on how to use your time through goal setting and project planning. Next, plan your time to handle your priorities. Decide on a schedule, know the times of day you function best, set realistic deadlines, and take time each day to think, relax, and exercise. Most of all, protect your time—say no to unwanted demands and avoid time wasters. Be willing to delegate certain tasks, utilize teamwork, and enlist support.

Watch out for the biggest time waster of all: *procrastination.* Procrastination is a mix of perfectionism, overestimation of the difficulty of the task, and undervaluing the rewards. Fear of failure and criticism, low frustration tolerance, guilt, and helplessness also contribute. Don't wait until you feel motivated. First comes action. Motivation follows when you see the results of your actions, and that leads you to further action.

Since starting a task is the most difficult stage, use the fifteen-minute rule we recommend to our clients. Do not think you will work for two hours on your project. Decide to do only fifteen-minute segments at a time. At the end of fifteen minutes, if you are working well, you can decide to continue for another fifteen minutes. If, however, you want to stop, you may. A lot more can be accomplished in a short time than you think. Murphy's Law states: "The task expands to fill the time allotted to it." In any case, after fifteen minutes you will know what needs to be done next. When you decide to quit for the time being, reward yourself for what you did accomplish, rather than berate yourself for what you left undone. Driving yourself with anxiety only increases your avoidance of the task the next time.

---

19 | **I limit myself to fewer than three cups of coffee (or tea or cola drinks) per day.**

The caffeine in one or two cups of coffee improves performance and efficiency and reduces fatigue. Too much caffeine, though, damages your health and increases your susceptibility to stress. It makes you irritable and nervous and disrupts your sleep and digestion. Very high doses of caffeine produce a condition indistinguishable from an anxiety neurosis. It can also increase blood pressure.

Caffeine is a highly addictive drug. Habitual users develop a tolerance for it. They need more and more caffeine for the same effect, resulting in a physical and psychological dependence. Abrupt caffeine withdrawal can create a state of lethargy, irritability, headache, depression, and anxiety.

Caffeine is a powerful stimulant because it releases large amounts of the major stress hormone, adrenaline, from the adrenal glands. Your body responds to caffeine in the same way it reacts to stress. A large mug of strong coffee releases enough adrenaline to triple the amount circulating in your bloodstream. Caffeine can stay in your system generating adrenaline release for hours, creating an artificial stress response that can keep you "wired" and tense for hours and interfering with sleep. It also destroys those vitamins B and C so vital to the functioning of your nervous and immune systems.

Coffee is only one source of caffeine. Caffeine is present in tea, certain soft drinks, many prescription and over-the-counter medications, and chocolate, just to name a few.

Fifty to 200 mg. of caffeine produces pharmacological actions, with 250 mg. considered to be a "large" pharma-

SOME COMMON SOURCES OF CAFFEINE

Source	Approximate Amounts of Caffeine per Unit
BEVERAGES	
Brewed coffee	100–150 mg. per cup
Instant coffee	86–99 mg. per cup
Tea	60–75 mg. per cup
Decaffeinated coffee	2–4 mg. per cup
Cola drinks	40–60 mg. per glass
PRESCRIPTION MEDICATIONS	
APCs (aspirin, phenacetin, caffeine)	32 mg. per tablet
Cafergot	100 mg. per tablet
Darvon compound	32 mg. per tablet
Fiorinal	40 mg. per tablet
Migral	50 mg. per tablet
OVER-THE-COUNTER ANALGESICS	
Anacin, Bromo-Seltzer	32 mg. per tablet
Cope, Easy-Mens, Empirin Compound, Midol	32 mg. per tablet
Vanquish	32 mg. per tablet
Excedrin	60 mg. per tablet
Pre-Mens	66 mg. per tablet
Many over-the-counter cold preparations	30 mg. per tablet
Many over-the-counter stimulants	100 mg. per tablet

Source: *American Journal of Psychiatry*, 131(10), pp. 1089–92, 1974, The American Psychiatric Association. Reprinted by permission.

cological dose. This dosage is easily exceeded by many people in the course of a day. For example, three cups of coffee, two over-the-counter headache tablets, and one caffeinated cola drink consumed in one morning equals approximately 500 mg. of caffeine.

Don't try to quit caffeine "cold turkey." Like smoking, put yourself on a gradual withdrawal schedule, taking about a month to "kick the habit." Over the years we've seen a lot of "stress" clients where caffeine, not stress, was the problem. George, a 46-year-old office manager, was referred to us by his family doctor for behavioral treatment of his insomnia after sleeping pills had been ineffective. George described himself as a "wreck." He was on the verge of being fired because he was "too tired and upset" to complete his work, and he was so irritable at home that his wife was sleeping in the spare bedroom. George claimed he had not slept at all for at least a month. When we suggested that he must be mistaken, he threw a temper tantrum in our office.

Based on our experience in treating insomnia, we immediately suspected caffeine abuse. As part of our interview we asked him for a detailed account of his daily consumption of caffeine.

Upon rising at 7:00 A.M. he had a large mug of coffee. "I have to have it to get started. I'm so exhausted," he told us. This first mug was followed by another with breakfast and yet a third cup that he drank while driving to work. At 8:30 A.M. he consumed a fourth cup of coffee as he entered the office, had a fifth one at his desk, and a sixth (with sugar doughnut) on his coffee break at 10:00 A.M. Lunch and his afternoon coffee break saw his seventh and eighth cups. Dinner was always followed by at least one cup, his ninth, and just before going to bed at ten or eleven, he routinely had a cup of coffee and a piece of pie. No wonder he would lie wide-eyed and fitful until the wee hours and rise exhausted and strung out, craving a caffeine "fix" to calm his jangled nerves and get him ready for another demanding day.

George had become addicted to caffeine. He had developed a tolerance and had to consume more and more caffeine not only to stay awake but to keep from going into withdrawal.

Caffeine abuse, like all substance abuse habits, involves one or more of three components: physical, behavioral, and psychological dependency. Where all three components are present, it's difficult to quit without professional help. In most cases of caffeine addiction, however, behavioral and physical dependency elements keep the process going. Separate behavior and dependency and you'll have a better chance of kicking caffeine.

We talked to George about his caffeine dependence and put him on a withdrawal schedule that had him completely off caffeine within six weeks. How? We used a simple principle of behavioral medicine—gradually change behavior. He continued to drink the same number of cups of coffee each day but he gradually substituted decaffeinated coffee for his late afternoon and evening cups, then for his midmorning cups, and finally for his early-morning drinks. As a result, his insomnia diminished and he was sleeping seven to eight hours most nights within two weeks. Once able to sleep, George got his work done easily and he and his wife resumed their normal life. His leveraged *Stress Action Plan: Susceptibility* paid big dividends.

---

20 | **I take quiet time for myself during the day.**

The ability to slow down during the day indicates that you can let go of the pressures of tasks left undone and do something for yourself. Your quiet time may be reading the newspaper or a magazine, playing golf, gardening, sitting doing nothing, listening to music, taking a long bath, or having lunch by yourself. Fifteen or twenty minutes of quiet time twice a day slows your metabolism, lowers your blood pressure, reduces your heart rate, and rests your mind and body. If you think you can't take time to relax, either you're too busy for your own good or you have a mistaken view of efficiency. Taking quiet time can recharge mind and body, increase your energy level, and raise your general level of efficiency and effectiveness.

Alma's Southern mother took a nap every day. About two o'clock, she would undress, put on a nightgown, and get under the covers. Thirty minutes later she would be up, dressed, and ready for the afternoon's activities. At 81, she's still going strong. People who care for themselves during the day have far fewer physical and mental symptoms of stress and are strikingly more resistant to stress than those who do not. Try scheduling a period of quiet time for yourself each day. (If you don't schedule it, it probably won't happen.) Recharging your batteries during the day is an investment in health, happiness, and productivity.

21 | I have an optimistic outlook on life.

Optimism is more than just a frame of mind, it's the basis of the confidence to act. Optimists succeed because they try; they try because they expect to succeed; and they succeed because they try. In short, they cope because they hope. As an old poker partner used to say, "You can't win if you don't get in." Optimists are the "Little Engines That Could" of the world. They handle stress better than pessimists because they do what needs to be done more quickly and confidently and, as a consequence, get out of stress situations quicker.

As we said in chapter 1, stress is in the eye of the beholder. Because they have such positive expectations, optimists view even disastrous events as opportunities for personal growth rather than as sources of stress. Pessimists, on the other hand, see catastrophe lurking around every corner and are the prophets of doom and gloom. These "naysayers" resist taking action because "it won't work." Their prophesies become self-fulfilling. They don't try, nothing changes, and stress grinds on.

Optimists come out of a stressful situation thinking of the positive things they've learned from it, whether it's increased confidence in handling difficult situations in the future, a truer picture of themselves and their abilities, more trust in judging situations or people, or greater ability to obtain help from others. They seem to appraise situations more realistically, understanding the limits that exist in life. They focus on problem solving when situations are under their control and rely on social support or acceptance when they are not.

Studies have shown that optimists have fewer mental and physical symptoms of stress, and are less likely to become anxious or depressed as a result of personal tragedy, natural disaster, or other stressful events. They have more "stress hardy" personalities, having a sense of commitment, challenge, and control. They also have been shown to have a greater tolerance for coronary artery bypass surgical procedures, have fewer complications, and recover faster. They handle the stress of physical injury better and accept physical deformity with more equanimity than do pessimists.[19, 20] Optimists are more likely to drop bad habits and pick up good ones, and don't usually rely on drugs or alcohol to escape stress.

Behavioral evidence suggests that optimism and pessimism are learned and that one's basic orientation can be modified. So, if you're an optimist, you've got something great going for you from the start. If you're not, here are some things you can do to get yourself in a more stress-resistant mindset.

- When faced with a challenge, say to yourself, "I can do it." Say it out loud so you'll be sure to hear yourself.
- Everyone, even the most dedicated pessimists, has had past successes. Think back to earlier successes. Think of what worked then and what might work now.
- Don't overreact in stress situations. Tell yourself to stay calm. Say it out loud.
- Don't overinterpret. Don't chew things over and over. Let them go and relax.
- Optimism is more than just a happy face, but smile every chance you get. Even when you're alone.
- Every situation has an upside and a downside. Look at both as realistically as you can. Try to learn something and gain personal growth out of even the most stressful and difficult situations.

Optimism perpetuates itself. The more optimistic you are, the more likely you will change your life for the better, because you're more convinced your life *can* be changed for the better. With each success, you'll become more optimistic and more willing to try, which will breed more success.

FILLING OUT YOUR *STRESS ACTION PLAN: SUSCEPTIBILITY*

Now that you've gone through the kinds of things that can make you more or less susceptible to stress and have some ideas on what you can do to make yourself less susceptible, finish filling out your *Stress Action Plan: Susceptibility*. We'll cover the problems you can anticipate when carrying out your planned course(s) of action in chapter 20.

N O T E S

1. Belloc, N., and Breslow, L. (1972), "Relationship of Physical Health Status and Health Practices," *Preventive Medicine* 1, 409–21.

2. Veith, I. (1949), *The Yellow Emperor's Classic of Internal Medicine*, Berkeley, CA, University of California Press.

3. Ongoing research at the Biobehavioral Institute of Boston.

4. Brody, J. (1987), *Jane Brody's Nutrition Book*, New York, Bantam.

5. Hauri, P. (1990), *No More Sleepless Nights*, New York, John Wiley and Sons.

6. Faelton, S., and Diamond, D. (1990), *Tension Turnaround*, Emmaus, PA, Rodale Press.

7. Ibid.

8. Skinner, J. E., Lie, J. T., Landisman, C. E., and Fulton, K. W. (1991), The correlation dimension of the heartbeat is reduced by myocardial ischemia in conscious pigs. *Circulation Research* 68, 966–76.

Skinner, J. E., Lie, J. T., and Entman, M. L. (1975), Modification of ventricular fibrillation latency following coronary artery occlusion in the conscious pig: The effects of psychological stress and beta-adrenergic blockade, *Circulation* 51, 656–67.

9. Weisman, A. D., and Worden, J. W. (1977) *Coping and Vulnerability in Cancer Patients,* Monograph, of Massachusetts General Hospital and Harvard Medical School, Boston, MA, Project Omega II.

Weisman, A. D. (1979), *Coping With Cancer,* New York, McGraw Hill.

10. Adams, M. (1976), *Single Blessedness: Observations of the Single Status in Married Society,* New York, Basic Books.

11. Faelton, S., and Diamond, D. (1990), *Tension Turnaround,* Emmaus, PA, Rodale Press.

12. Rippe, J., and Ward, A. (1970), *Dr. James M. Rippe's Complete Book of Fitness Walking,* New York, Prentice-Hall.

13. Health Innovations, Inc., 12355 Sunrise Valley Drive, Suite 200, Reston, VA 22091 (1-800-543-3744).

14. Bailey, C. (1978), *Fit or Fat,* Boston, Houghton-Mifflin.

15. Groger, M. (1985), *E.A.T.: Eating Awareness Training,* New York, Summit Books.

16. Belle, D. (1987), "Gender differences in the social moderators of stress," in *Gender and Stress* (Barnett, Biener, and Baruch, eds.), New York, The Free Press.

17. Williams, R. B., et al (1992), Prognostic importance of social and economic resources among medically treated patients with angiographically documented coronary artery disease, *JAMA* 267, 520–24.

18. Rubin, L. (1986), *Just Friends,* New York, Harper Collins.

19. Kamin-Segal, L., Rodin, J., and Dwyer, J. (1991), "Explanatory Style and Cell-Mediated Immunity," *Health Psychology* 10, 229–35.

20. Seligman, M. E. P. (1990), *Learned Optimism,* New York, Pocket Books.

ANNE'S STRESS ACTION PLAN: SUSCEPTIBILITY

DIRECTIONS: Review your *Stress Audit: Susceptibility* section. Write down an item you rated as never being true of you, describe the problem, set a reasonable goal for change. Stop. Read pertinent section of chapter 3, write down some possible actions that might help. Stop. Read chapter 20, write down your barriers to change. Stop. Read chapter 21, write down your supports for change. *Implement* your plan. *Evaluate* results. *Adjust* your plan.

SUSCEPTIBILITY ITEM: I never get seven to eight hours of sleep at least four nights per week.

DESCRIPTION OF PROBLEM: (Anne's description of her own situation)
I can hardly keep my eyes open after lunch. Sometimes I'm so tired I just put my head down on my desk and take a nap. It's difficult to get up in the morning and I generally oversleep a couple of days a week. I'm late to work so often that it's become a joke, except to my boss. I have to get more sleep, but I have trouble getting to bed at night. I watch television with Mark and get wrapped up in it, or Mom or Mark calls and I talk for hours. If I eat late or drink alcohol or coffee I have trouble getting to sleep and then staying asleep. Because I'm too tired to get things done at work, I often bring work home and stay up late trying to get caught up.

REASONABLE GOAL: Get eight hours of sleep five nights per week. (**Anne sets personal goal.**)

POSSIBLE ACTIONS: (Anne's application of "sleep" portions of chapter 3 to her life)
1) Turn TV off at 10:00 P.M. whether Mark's here or not—no exceptions.
2) Make no phone calls after 9:30 P.M. Let answering machine take calls after 9:30 P.M. Return them when appropriate.
3) No meals later than 8:00 P.M. No caffeine or alcohol after 6:00 P.M.
4) Organize things for next day before 9:00 P.M.
5) Take hot bath by 10:00 P.M. In bed by 10:30 P.M.
6) Do progressive muscle relaxation (PMR) exercise after going to bed.
7) Up at 7:00 A.M. weekdays. Up no later than 9:00 A.M. on weekends. No exceptions.

BARRIERS TO CHANGE: (Anne's application of chapter 20 to her life)

SUPPORTS FOR CHANGE: (Anne's application of chapter 21 to her life)

YOUR STRESS ACTION PLAN: SUSCEPTIBILITY

DIRECTIONS: Review your *Stress Audit: Susceptibility* section. Write down an item you rated as never being true of you, describe the problem, set a reasonable goal for change. Stop. Read pertinent section of chapter 3, write down some possible actions that might help. Stop. Read chapter 20, write down your barriers to change. Stop. Read chapter 21, write down your supports for change. *Implement* your plan. *Evaluate* results. *Adjust* your plan.

SUSCEPTIBILITY ITEM: _____

_____

DESCRIPTION OF PROBLEM: _____

_____

_____

_____

_____

_____

REASONABLE GOAL: _____

_____

_____

_____

_____

_____

POSSIBLE ACTIONS: _____

_____

_____

_____

_____

_____

BARRIERS TO CHANGE: _____

_____

_____

_____

SUPPORTS FOR CHANGE: _____

_____

_____

_____

II

SOURCES: PLAYING HARDBALL WITH STRESS

4 PLANNING A WINNING STRATEGY

Now that you've filled out a *Stress Action Plan* for reducing your susceptibility to stress, you have some idea how the *Stress Action Plan* process works. In this chapter, we'll show you how to get tough with stress and beat it at its source.

GETTING IN TOUCH WITH EXACTLY WHAT IS STRESSFUL FOR YOU

Go over the Sources section of your *Stress Audit* and pick out an item representing a stress point you want to eliminate. Write it down on your *Stress Action Plan: Sources* (p. 119). Next, write a succinct behavioral description of your situation using "I" or "we" statements. Writing it down this way pushes you to view stress behaviorally and emphasizes the choices you have. Moreover, "I" statements help you realize you're the only person over whom you have control. You must work on yourself and not worry about changing other people. As a consequence, the importance of self-regulation in stress management will be more apparent, you'll get a little emotional distance from the situation, and you'll think more clearly and creatively.

Anne's *Stress Action Plan: Sources* is at the end of this chapter. You can take a look at it now to see how she did it. The item Anne worked on, *Trouble with the boss,* comes from the "Job" subsection of the *Stress Audit*. Writing a behavioral description of just how *Trouble with the boss* enabled her to see dimensions to the problem that she hadn't considered before.

Anne's behavioral description of her *Trouble with the boss* item began:

> Charlie, my boss, jerks me around all the time. One minute I'm told to do one thing, the next he wants me doing something else. Then he gets mad and screams at me if everything doesn't get done right on time. He goes ballistic. He interferes with my getting things done when he changes his mind all the time. His disorganization really impacts on my efficiency and could affect my professional career in marketing. Sometimes the tension gets so thick between us you could cut it with a knife.

REVIEW YOUR OPTIONS FOR CHANGE

In writing her problem out in behavioral terms, Anne became aware of a number of ways to manage her job situation. She realized that neither she nor her boss had a clear idea of what her job entailed. Anne now appreciated that Charlie was under a lot of pressure and wasn't handling it well. She recognized some of her own emotional reactions to his behavior, how they influenced her job performance, and began to perceive how to change her situation.

Anne saw that she could communicate better with Charlie if she just stayed calm when she talked with him. She also understood that she needed a clear job description and that she could negotiate one with Charlie. Or, she could take her problem "upstairs" to Charlie's boss or transfer to another job in the company. If none of those options worked, Anne could take a job with a competitor or marry Mark and quit working altogether.

As you write your behavioral description of a situation and how it affects you, you'll also get ideas about how to make your own situation less stressful. After you've written your item and have described its behavioral effects on you, consider your strategic options for making that situation less stressful.

Before you do, however, familiarize yourself with the three basic stress strategies outlined below. Tactics for carrying out these strategies are outlined later in the chapter.

THE "TRIPLE A" SYSTEM FOR REDUCING STRESS SOURCES

The three basic strategies for dealing with the stress in your life at its source(s) are: *altering* situations to make them less stressful, *avoiding* stressful situations, or *accepting* them. Each option has its strengths, each has its weaknesses. Different people use different strategies at different times and switch to others as the situation changes.

You're probably already using some of these strategies without realizing it. Casting your strategies in the "Triple A" framework sharpens your thinking about what it is you're trying to accomplish. Structuring your strategic options in clearer terms also increases your flexibility, sharpens your skills, and makes you a better stress strategist. Let's look at each of your strategic options in detail. You'll get some ideas about when and how your options can be used, singly or in combination, to beat stress at its source.

ALTERING SITUATIONS TO MAKE THEM LESS STRESSFUL

One of the most effective ways of making a situation less of a stress point is to change it. Human beings have for millennia altered the physical environment to make it less stressful, more comfortable, and better suited to their needs. Central heat, air conditioning, elevators, escalators, airplanes, automobiles, and electric lighting are some examples. If our homes or offices are uncomfortable or poorly organized, we move objects around, redecorate, or remodel to make them less so.

We also try to alter our interpersonal situations, usually through problem solving, discussion and negotiation, assertively communicating our requests, or outright bargaining with others to change their behaviors. We even alter our own attitudes, behaviors, and perceptions to make our stress points more tolerable.

Because of their complexity, however, social and personal stress points and circumstances are more difficult to alter than physical ones. We become so tangled up in our emotional involvements and our expectations of ourselves and others that we don't think logically or rationally. We're not always aware of what's going on with ourselves or others and don't know what we or they want, need, or expect of one another. In addition, we all harbor fundamental misconceptions about the basics of human behavior that lead us astray in our interpersonal dealings.

Common Misconceptions About Human Behavior

Many of us have a deep, abiding conviction that others can be made to behave the way we want—from putting down toilet seats, to organizing a checkbook, to being more sensitive and concerned. Guilt, intimidation, force, and manipulation are used to enforce this conviction. Such methods may even produce short-term results. But they're illusory. The desired results continue only as long as the pressure is exerted. Once removed, behavior reverts to what it was before.

You can't *make* anybody do anything. You can't get people to change because you want them to, or because life will be better for you or for them. They will change only if they are motivated to do so.

That's where you're in luck, because all behavior is motivated. You do what you do because you think it will pay off for you in some way. If you're doing something that pays off in some real or imagined way, you keep doing it; if it doesn't pay off, you stop. We all have our own ideas as to what constitutes a payoff. For some people money is the payoff, for others it may be attention, affection, sex, approval, some abstract ideal, and so on.

Sometimes we see something as a payoff because it gets us something we really want. If you're saving to buy a home, money has significance because it leads to an ultimate payoff. You work for money because you have faith that you'll buy a home. At the same time, other motivations compete for our money, time, and attention.

We try to teach this basic concept to all our clients because it is central to understanding human behavior, including their own. We want them to realize that people, including themselves, do only what pays off for them in some way.

In order to motivate others, you first have to know what constitutes a payoff for them. Then you make that payoff contingent upon their behavior. If you have control of payoff contingencies, you can influence what people do and how they do it. If you don't, you can't. But it's only influence. You don't make them do anything, they do it because they want to.

Some of our clients create big problems for themselves because they don't understand that they can only influence, not change, other people. Paul, for instance, was convinced he could make his wife, Sheila, change her mind about getting a divorce if he tried hard enough. He sent her flowers, cards, and letters, and presented rational arguments for getting back together, all to no avail. The harder he tried, the more frustrated he became. He didn't think to ask Sheila what it was she really wanted and couldn't envisage any possible payoff for her in divorcing him.

In our sessions with them, Paul confessed that he had made all the decisions in the marriage and had obsessively controlled everything in the house. For instance, Sheila couldn't write checks because she didn't record the checks the way Paul liked them. He even insisted on the dishwasher being loaded in a certain way. If Sheila arranged something in the house, he would "straighten it up" behind her. Sheila had been miserable living under Paul's obsessive control and had elected to leave. Her payoff in divorcing him was getting out from under Paul's thumb.

When Paul finally understood why Sheila had left and didn't want to live with him any longer, he tried to change. She saw this as just another manipulation. It was too late. Sheila divorced him and now lives alone.

Paul felt hurt and angry but also strangely liberated. If Sheila could make her own choices in life, so could he. In fact, Paul had been just as unhappy as she had been in the marriage, but "Dad made me stick it out." Paul had learned his controlling ways from his controlling father. In his family, people were made to behave in prescribed ways. Paul's father controlled Paul's mother and had raised Paul to follow in his footsteps.

The divorce shattered Paul's basic ideas on human interaction, interpersonal influence, and control. As we talked, Paul discovered the payoffs he had been getting out of his relationship with his parents. He had accepted their behavior because he wanted to "get along with them" and didn't want to anger or "disappoint" them.

Paul decided to change his situation with his parents. But this wasn't easy. His parents couldn't understand why anything should change. They still wanted to tell him what to do and how to do it. When Paul realized that he couldn't alter the situation, he chose to avoid it by moving out of state.

The Problem with Nonassertion

Our own behavior is often the cause of the stress in our interpersonal situations. We're either too passive and submissive and don't get what we want or we're too aggressive and elicit anger and hostility from others. Although we often don't communicate effectively, we expect people to know what we're thinking and feeling, to understand our wants and needs, and to respond accordingly. In our own self-involvement, we don't listen to other people and, consequently, don't have the vaguest idea as to what's going on with them.

Your behavior is the one aspect of life you can control. You can minimize interpersonal stress by behaving assertively and communicating more effectively.

Assertive behavior means expressing to others exactly how you think, feel, and believe in a direct, open, honest, respectful, and nonmanipulative way. If you don't behave assertively, you may find yourself taken advantage of, put down, bullied, or intimidated. People fail to be assertive because they don't think they have a right to be assertive, they fear that such behavior will be seen as aggressive or hostile by others, or because they lack assertiveness skills.

Assertiveness is the balance point of the seesaw between aggression and passivity. When you fail to be assertive, you'll become resentful of the consequences. You won't get what you want, other people will take advantage of you, and nobody will understand you. If you continue being nonassertive, your resentment will grow. You may then swing to the aggressive end of the seesaw.

Your resentment may come out as a furious explosion of aggressive and hostile behavior, as manipulative indirect aggression, or, perhaps, as a sullen, pouting withdrawal from a "hostile insensitive" world. Whatever your outlet, your life will only get worse. Anger and hostility generate anger and hostility in return. Sullen, pouting withdrawal and indirect aggressive behavior infuriates and frustrates others. It doesn't get you what you want and may even prevent you from getting it.

Whether you're assertive, passive, aggressive, or polite often depends on the situation. You may be generally assertive at work or with friends but not with family members or your intimate partner. As we mentioned earlier, Sheila left her husband because of his controlling behavior. Throughout their marriage she never objected to his controlling ways "because it might hurt his feelings." When Sheila finally told Paul how she felt, he was dumbfounded and angrily shouted, "Why didn't you say something? What do you think I am, a mind reader." Sheila replied, "See? I knew you'd be upset, but I don't care now."

Sheila was nonassertive only with Paul. She had no difficulty telling other people exactly what she thought and felt. For his part, Paul had no difficulty being assertive with Sheila, but had real problems with his parents. Your degree of assertiveness is determined by your situation. Notice when you don't speak up and make your wants and needs known.

There are situations, too, that require us to go beyond simple assertive requests if they are to be altered. Sometimes we must defend ourselves against the bullies and the rude clods of the world by taking verbal, physical, political, or legal action. Assertiveness now must include statements of intent if nothing changes. This is in the form of "if this, then that." For example, "If you don't move to the end of the movie line, I'll call the manager"; "If you threaten me physically, I'll move out"; "If you continue to use drugs, you'll have to move out." Then be ready to follow through, with legal action if necessary. Start gradually and use only as much force as necessary to solve the problem.

The Power of Words

The prevalence of the misconception that people can be "made" to do things is evident in the words we use. They not only express what we think about, they determine how we think about it. Often a simple restatement using different words dramatically alters how we think about a situation. Words are much more than just semantics.

One example is the phrase "you make me ———." How different is, "You *make* me angry when you wipe your hands on the tablecloth," than, "I *get* angry when you wipe your hands on the tablecloth." The first instance implies that other people are responsible for your emotions—that their uncouth and boorish behavior "makes" you angry. The alternative phrasing implies that you have control over your emotions, that their behavior is socially unacceptable, and that angry people may behave in angry ways if the behavior is repeated.

You may "get" angry, but other people can't "make" you angry. Similarly, you may "be" happy about something that someone does or doesn't do, but no one can "make" you happy. You, and you alone, are responsible for your thoughts, feelings, and behavior. To believe otherwise places your life in the hands of others and saddles you with the crushing burden of being responsible for the feelings of others.

Confusions, misconceptions, and misperceptions over

personal responsibility for one's thoughts, emotions, and behaviors are at the heart of many marital stress issues. Tina and Sam were involved in an emotional rondeau. Tina was unhappy and Sam was angry. Sam was angry because Tina was unhappy and Tina was unhappy because Sam was angry. Tina's unhappiness started over an argument with a longtime friend. Sam tried to "make" her happy by taking her out more but, predictably, failed. He tried harder. Tina was still unhappy. Sam felt he had failed Tina and was angry that Tina had caused him to be a failure by not responding to his efforts by being happy. Both felt utterly powerless to stop the vicious downward spiral of their relationship.

When they met with us, the confusions over who was responsible for what were cleared away. Tina realized that she either had to patch things up with her friend or just let the relationship go and forget about it. Sam experienced relief when he dropped the impossible responsibility he had taken on, but became aware that there were other things he had been angry about in the situation. Tina's unhappiness had cast a pall over the entire household and he was irritated about that. Also, in her unhappiness over the loss of her friend, Tina was less romantically inclined and their sex life had almost disappeared. Sam realized he had control only over his thoughts, feelings, and behaviors, but that he could make requests of Tina to address her unhappiness because it affected him.

Words and the ways we use them not only reflect our misconceptions, they usually reinforce them. Words are pivotal elements in how we perceive, structure, and think about any situation. It's a circular process that feeds on itself. What we say influences what we think and what we think influences what we say. Those high school English classes on denotation and connotation contained far more than basic language instruction. We didn't know it at the time, but they were also basic courses in thinking and, ultimately, in stress management. Words influence our thinking, our thoughts influence our feelings, and our thoughts and feelings control our behavior.

Changing Your Words Will Alter Your Perceptions

Since stress is largely in the eye of the beholder, one powerful way of altering a stressful situation involves changing the way we think about it. Taking a different perspective is particularly effective in altering our perceptions and reducing the stress of interpersonal situations. More often than not, the difference can be simply in the language we use to describe situations, other people, and ourselves. If we change the words we use, our perception of stress can change radically.

For instance, one of Alma's clients said that losing his job would be a "catastrophe." Alma countered with, "No, losing your job would be unfortunate. A catastrophe is when Mt. Saint Helens explodes in your backyard." Her client got the point—his hyperbole only increased his stress. The subtle shift in language from "catastrophe" to "unfortunate" gave him a more flexible perspective on his job situation. In fact, he didn't lose his job. As so many people do, he was "catastrophizing" or borrowing trouble by agonizing about a future event that never came to pass and by exaggerating and dramatizing current difficulties.

The Tyranny of Shoulds and Oughts

Many people create stressful situations by unconsciously subjugating themselves to a "tyranny of shoulds and oughts." Their language is shot through with "I have to's," "I shoulds," "I ought to's." Just changing their language can restore a sense of control that was mysteriously "lost" without their quite realizing it.

When we find a client laboring under the "tyranny of shoulds and oughts," we have them monitor and write down every time they say "have to," "should," "ought to," or "must." It's a measure of their enslavement. Then we have them substitute "I need," "I choose to," "I want to," and "I'm going to." These are subtle changes, but they bring about big changes in perception, perspective, and behavior.

Separating the Individual from Their Behavior

An inability to separate an individual from his or her behavior is another major cause of many interpersonal problems. A friend, Loyal, made us aware of this when he described how he had maintained a long-term friendship and professional relationship with Mitch, a notoriously difficult colleague. Mitch was warm, charming, and likable as a friend, but was competitive, erratic, disorganized, and capricious as a supervisor. Frustrated and exasperated by Mitch's managerial style, Loyal handled his interpersonal stress by deciding that he liked Mitch as a *friend* but hated the way Mitch acted as his *supervisor*.

Again, the tip-off is in the words used to describe the situation: I hate/love/can't stand him/her; she/he doesn't like me/loves me/thinks I'm wonderful. True, there are people we like or love, dislike or hate, because there is something about them that triggers those feelings in us. It's also true that people behave in ways we like, love, dislike, or hate. It's important for you to keep your reactions to their behavior separate from your reactions to the people. You should also be clear about whether others are reacting to you or to your behavior.

AVOIDING STRESSFUL SITUATIONS

In our culture, avoidance is often seen as a weak, if not cowardly, option for dealing with problems. Words such as *deceit, diversion, dodging, subterfuge, escape, evasion,* and *runaround* are common synonyms that reflect our distaste for avoidance as a strategic option for dealing with problems. The ideal approach is seen as something more forceful and active, where one faces up to one's difficulties and deals with them head-on. For most situations, this is true. But there are occasions where altering a situation isn't worth the time, energy, or effort it takes. When the situation is short-term in nature, you haven't the resources to alter a situation effectively, or you haven't yet decided what to do, often the most intelligent strategy is to avoid the stressful situation.

Avoiding situations where you could be mugged, robbed, or raped is sensible. Avoiding fistfights and fruitless arguments with someone high on drugs or alcohol is reasonable. Other situations we tend to avoid are old, unresolvable arguments with family members, direct power confrontations with superiors at work, or any other situation where the cost or personal risk is high and the perceived benefit is low.

Sometimes avoidance is the optimal short-term strategy. Taking a vacation and forgetting about the office and its politics is a rejuvenating experience. Forgetting your burden of stress and restoring your mental and physical energies makes you more effective in dealing with problems when you return. In classical literature the Greek hero Leonidas, who withdrew, exhausted, from the battle of Thermopylae, says, "I shall lie me down and bleed awhile, then rise and fight again." Refreshed, he returned to defeat the invading Persian hordes.

The Problem with Automatic Avoidance

If you automatically choose "avoid" options in stress situations or once you've adopted an "avoid" strategy that you have difficulty shifting to any other strategy, you could be creating more problems for yourself than you solve. People who always avoid dealing with certain situations may do so out of fear, an inability to assert themselves, or because they lack the skills needed to change.

Paul, whom we discussed earlier, avoided confronting his parents' controlling behavior because he feared their disapproval, and was habitually nonassertive with them. In working with Paul, we helped him realize that he was his parents' adult son, not their child, and that his relationship with them should reflect that difference. And we developed in Paul more assertiveness, by role-playing and designing "scripts" for him to use when talking with his parents.

Soon Paul became aware that he could alter his relationship with his parents. In fact, much of Paul's behavior toward Sheila, his wife, had enabled him to deny that there was anything wrong in his being controlled by his parents. They controlled him and he controlled her and that's the way he thought life should be.

Paul felt that his parents would not or could not change. In the end, he used an avoidance strategy by limiting contact with his parents. He talked less with them on the telephone and limited their visits. He stopped discussing his problems with them. Paul did not want to sever all contact with them, but he decided to avoid their attempts to interfere with his life.

Avoidance and Denial

Denial is a term frequently used in psychology and self-help groups to describe the tendency to minimize undesirable personal characteristics, behaviors, or events. It is frowned upon by mental health professionals and the public alike. Denial is seen as an unrealistic, maladaptive attempt to "wish troubles away" or "sweep them under the rug," which only makes things worse. Most commonly, families are said to be "in denial" when they overlook the substance abuse of a family member or minimize its impact on the rest of the family. In turn, this fosters a passive acceptance of life as it is, allowing such behavior to continue, and leading to harm for both the family and the abuser.

Denial can, in fact, be pathological, but only when it prevents us from recognizing and dealing with situations that require action. It enables us to conduct the affairs of life without worrying about death and the grave. Denying the existence of a life-threatening illness can be deadly, but denying the inevitability of death as its consequence can have a calming effect and allow the body's natural healing and restorative powers to come into play. Our own data on denial indicate that it is, indeed, a powerful strategy for reducing perceived stress.

ACCEPTING STRESSFUL SITUATIONS

There are times when we can neither alter nor avoid a stressful situation and simply have to *accept* things as they are. "If you can't beat 'em, join 'em." "No use beating your head against a brick wall." "That's the way the cookie crumbles." These folk phrases remind us that we must accept life as it comes to us. A simple example involves being stuck in heavy traffic and knowing you'll be late to a meeting. You can't change the amount of traffic. Taking a back way might be just as bad. Ranting and raving, stewing, and imagining the awful consequences of your tardiness only increase your stress. All you can do is relax and "go with the flow" of traffic. Used wisely and appropriately, acceptance pulls you through situations where trying to alter or avoid the situation only makes it worse.

Accepting Reality and Personal Responsibility

John's case involved accepting a situation and getting on with his life. A former bank vice president, John was fired for approving a risky loan that went sour and cost his bank more than a million dollars. At first, John avoided feelings of guilt by denying responsibility for his ill-advised decision. John rationalized, "I had been working too hard and had too much to do. What do they expect when people are spread too thin?"

Furious, he tried to "get even" by telling everyone how "rotten" the bank had been to him. John threatened a wrongful-termination suit. He was going to alter the situation by making the bank not only give him his job back but pay damages for his pain and suffering.

Neither tactic made him feel better, and his lawyer said he had little grounds for a claim. John *had* been less than diligent in reviewing the loan application. Finally, he had to admit to himself that he had been negligent. The demands in maintaining his self-deception were more debilitating than the stress of getting fired. Altering the situation by threatening legal action only compounded his stress. John's blood pressure went up twenty points.

John's physician placed him on medication and referred him to us for stress management. It was apparent to us that John's strategies just hadn't worked for him and there wasn't any way to avoid or alter the fact that he had been fired and was out of a job.

Upside, Downside

We worked on an "upside, downside" analysis of John's situation to see if he could view it in a more acceptable light. The downside, clearly, was that John had been fired for carelessly approving a risky loan and would have difficulty getting another job in banking. The upside was that John had extensive knowledge of banking and finance, had financial resources, and had many influential business contacts. John was now also free to explore other career options if he chose.

After we presented this upside, downside viewpoint, John became calm and considered his options more clearly and logically. He decided to open an office in the financial district, make use of his contacts, and start a new career as a financial analyst and consultant. As John put the humiliation and embarrassment of being fired behind him and concentrated on his new career, his blood pressure returned to normal. In fact, John is a success again, recently bringing several million dollars worth of business to his old bank. He told his client, "It really is a fine bank. They do good work and don't tolerate carelessness."

The "upside, downside" technique is just one way of making an inescapably stressful situation more bearable. Sometimes an upside is difficult to define, but if you look, you can usually find a silver lining. The popular historian Barbara Tuchman even found the upside of the bubonic plague.[1] One-third of Europe's population died, but two-thirds of its population came into an inheritance. The increased wealth of the survivors made the Renaissance possible.

Stress Inoculation

"Stress inoculation" is a preventive technique for reducing the stress of an anticipated situation that can neither be altered nor avoided.[2] There are many variations of the technique, but it typically involves relaxing deeply and then imagining yourself, while in this relaxed state, in the midst of the anticipated stressful situation. One variant of the technique is to imagine the worst possible thing that could happen to you in the situation, but staying deeply relaxed. Another variant is imagining your worst fear and then not having it come to pass.

Our favorite variation on the inoculation theme is relaxed preparation. For example, Walter, a 50-year-old university official, was referred to us for relaxation training and stress management by his psychoanalyst of several years. As he went through his assessment process Walter said to us, "Let me tell you what stress really is. In two weeks, I have to tell the university president that I didn't do something he told me to do six months ago. I thought the assignment was stupid and I haven't done it."

According to Walter, the university president, whom we called "Mr. Bang," was authoritarian, arrogant, egocentric, and given to scathing tongue-lashings. We agreed with Walter that a confrontation with this man would be daunting. However, a stress inoculation would help Walter greatly.

First, we taught Walter how to relax through progressive muscle relaxation, a technique we describe in chapter 13. We helped Walter imagine a somewhat humorous yet realistic picture of "Mr. Bang" having a tantrum. Then we had him imagine presenting his reasons for not completing his assignment to "terrible-tempered Mr. Bang" while staying deeply relaxed.

Role-playing sessions followed, where first Lyle and then Walter played the role of "Mr. Bang." In these sessions, "Mr. Bang" was sometimes outraged at Walter's insubordinate behavior and at other times congratulated him on his good judgment. Walter practiced staying relaxed no matter what was said or threatened. Four sessions one week and one the next made Walter confident he could "handle it."

Walter finally faced "Mr. Bang" and calmly told him he had chosen not to carry out the assignment because he felt it ill advised and told him why. "Mr. Bang" merely frowned and said, "Dammit, why didn't I think of that." He then complimented Walter on his judgment and foresight and invited him to lunch to discuss a new problem.

Anticipatory anxiety and apprehension were frequent problems for Walter. He had to make numerous presentations to trustees, professional groups, alumni, the President's Council, civic groups, etc. Every presentation was preceded by the debilitating trio of sleeplessness, agitation, and anxiety, making it difficult for Walter to prepare adequately. He was plagued by images of catastrophe, fearful that his shaky preparation would expose him as an impostor and that the audience would laugh at him or walk out. This never happened, but Walter continued to be afraid.

For Walter, stress inoculation was a "lifesaving" technique. He began using it to prepare all his presentations, interviews, and significant personal interactions. Preparation became an internal game he loved playing. After a while, he was seldom taken by surprise or was at a loss for words in any encounter. Walter's self-confidence and self-esteem soared. He became as calm and unflappable as he had been anxious and flustered previously. Peers and associates now looked to him for leadership and guidance and he began receiving offers from other universities. After leaving us, he continued to make gains on his own and, in less than a year, he accepted the directorship of a large foundation.

Religion and Faith

Religious faith, philosophical conviction or belief, or dedication to a principle or ideal allows a person to accept stressful situations. Political prisoners, patriots, and religious martyrs, for instance, find a meaning in their suffering that allows them to accept even the most stressful of circumstances. Nathan Hale's famous last words, "My only regret is that I have but one life to give for my country," reflect the kind of fervor that allows patriots to accept mutilation, agony, and death in the name of an abstract ideal. Acceptance and transcendence can be a safety net for you when all other stress strategies fail.

CHOOSING A STRATEGY

Each stress strategy—altering, avoiding, and accepting—has its advantages and disadvantages. What's best at one time and circumstance is not necessarily best for another. You have to choose the right option at the right time to enjoy a strategy's advantages without suffering its disadvantages. Stay flexible enough to switch strategies or try them in combination or sequence. As you master them and become more skillful and flexible in using them, you'll have more control over the stress in your life than you can now imagine.

Keep your strategy practical and simple. Think about your options for altering, avoiding, or accepting the stressful situations in your life as you read through the rest of this chapter and continue working on your *Stress Action Plan: Sources*. As you decide on your best possible options, remember that the primary goal of an effective *Stress Action Plan* is to make your life better. We have to deal with any situation as it is at the moment and we have to deal with it practically as best we can.

CHOOSING A PLAN OF ACTION FOR YOUR SOURCES OF STRESS

In this chapter we've concentrated on examples of demands and pressures that create stress in our lives every day. We've also tried to present a broad range of examples of how to deal with those demands and pressures. At the beginning of this chapter, you selected an item from the Sources section of your *Stress Audit* and described how it affected your life. Now, write out a *Stress Action Plan: Sources* for yourself using an altering, avoiding, or accepting option. Draw on the examples and solutions we've outlined for you and design your own *Stress Action Plan* tailored to your specific situation and needs.

Come up with several different courses of action under each option. Let's go over the characteristics of a good *Stress Action Plan* once more so they'll be fresh in your mind as you work on yours:

- A good *Stress Action Plan* makes your life better.
- A good *Stress Action Plan* can be accomplished in six to twelve weeks.
- A good *Stress Action Plan* has a specific outcome.
- A good *Stress Action Plan* can be stated in behavioral terms.
- A good *Stress Action Plan* is leveraged so you get the "most bang for your buck."

Decide which option and which course of action is best for you right now and try it. If it doesn't work, try another. Once you are comfortable, work on other sources of stress and keep on altering, avoiding, or accepting the demands and pressures of life to make them less stressful. The following chapters offer specific advice on particular items. You may wish to read only those sections which are relevant to your problems.

N O T E S

1. Tuchman, B. (1978), *A Distant Mirror*, New York, Ballantine.

2. Meichenbaum, D. (1986), *Stress Inoculation Training*, New York, Pergamon.

ANNE'S STRESS ACTION PLAN: SOURCES

DIRECTIONS: Review your *Stress Audit: Sources* section. Write down an item you rated 4 or 5 you'd like to work on, describe the situation and problem. Stop. Read the chapter dealing with that problem, write down some specific actions to take. Stop. Read chapter 20, write down your barriers to change. Stop. Read chapter 21 and write down your supports for change. *Implement* your first choice of action. *Evaluate* results. *Adjust* your plan.

ITEM: Trouble with the boss.

DESCRIPTION OF SITUATION AND PROBLEM: (Anne's description of her own situation)

Charlie, my boss, jerks me around all the time. One minute I'm told to do one thing, the next he wants me doing something else. Then he gets mad and screams at me if everything doesn't get done right on time. He goes ballistic. He interferes with my getting things done when he changes his mind all the time. His disorganization really impacts on my efficiency and could affect my professional career in marketing. Sometimes the tension gets so thick between us you could cut it with a knife.

POSSIBLE ACTIONS: (Anne's application of chapter 4's options to her life)

  Alter: (Anne's application of "Alter" portions of chapter 4 to her life)
   1) Sit down with Charlie (during a quiet time when we've been getting along well) and have a real heart-to-heart talk about how we work together.
   2) Negotiate a clear, written job description with Charlie and then make sure we both keep to it. No unilateral renegotiations.
   3) Take my problem with Charlie upstairs to the president of the company and be prepared to fight it out head to head with Charlie.
  Avoid: (Anne's application of "Avoid" portion of chapter 4 to her life)
   1) Request a transfer to another division.
   2) Take the job I've been offered with our top competitor.
   3) Just quit and marry Mark.
  Accept: (Anne's application of "Accept" portion of chapter 4 to her life)
   1) Get so good at relaxing that I can relax anytime, anyplace, and just relax when things get tense.
   2) Understand that Charlie has his problems too and doesn't handle pressure well.
   3) Quit personalizing things so much.

BARRIERS TO CHANGE: (Anne's application of chapter 20 to her life)

SUPPORTS FOR CHANGE: (Anne's application of chapter 21 to her life)

YOUR STRESS ACTION PLAN: SOURCES

DIRECTIONS: Review your *Stress Audit: Sources* section. Write down an item you rated 4 or 5 you'd like to work on, describe the situation and problem. Stop. Read the chapter dealing with that problem, write down some specific actions to take. Stop. Read chapter 20, write down your barriers to change. Stop. Read chapter 21 and write down your supports for change. *Implement* your first choice of action. *Evaluate* results. *Adjust* your plan.

ITEM: _____

_____

DESCRIPTION OF SITUATION AND PROBLEM: _____

_____

_____

_____

_____

POSSIBLE ACTIONS: (Check the ones you'll try first)
 Alter:

_____

_____

_____

 Avoid:

_____

_____

_____

 Accept:

_____

_____

_____

BARRIERS TO CHANGE: (personal, social, financial, practical, etc. Be specific.)

_____

_____

_____

SUPPORTS FOR CHANGE: (personal, family, social, professional, etc. Be specific.)

_____

_____

_____

5 GETTING THE UPPER HAND ON JOB STRESS

Let's start dealing with your job-stress items by returning to Anne and her problems with her boss. Remember what Anne said:

> Charlie, my boss, jerks me around all the time. One minute I'm told to do one thing, the next he wants me doing something else. Then he gets mad and screams at me if everything doesn't get done right on time. He goes ballistic. He interferes with my getting things done when he changes his mind all the time. His disorganization really impacts my efficiency and could affect my professional career in marketing. Sometimes the tension gets so thick between us you could cut it with a knife.

With her description in mind, let's look at Anne's possibilities for altering, avoiding, or accepting a situation in developing a job plan of action. Anne thought she could alter the situation by using her good communication skills to work things out with her boss, Charlie. She could alter the situation by negotiating a clear, written job description with him and making sure he abided by it. Or she could bring the problem to the company president and fight it out with Charlie.

She could also use avoidance options. Anne could limit her contact with Charlie, speaking with him only in brief, impersonal exchanges and communicating as much as possible by memo. She could request a transfer to another division to avoid Charlie entirely, she could leave the company and take a job with a competitor, or marry Mark and quit work.

Anne could also choose a number of acceptance options. She could learn to relax so that she wouldn't get so tense around Charlie. Or, she could understand that Charlie has problems and doesn't handle pressure well. Or, Anne could stop personalizing situations so much, realizing that Charlie yells and screams at everyone.

Trouble with the boss is only one of the many possible sources of stress on the job. We discuss the most frequently occurring problems in the following section. You may have one or several of these job-stress concerns, or some that may not even be covered by the *Stress Audit*. Read through the rest of this section on job stress. Come up with ideas for *Stress Action Plans: Jobs*. With a little thought and creativity, you can create a workable *Stress Action Plan* for almost any job-stress problem.

UNCERTAINTY AND JOB LOSS

In today's economic upheavals, downsizing, layoffs, mergers, and bankruptcies have cost hundreds of thousands of workers their jobs. Millions more have been shifted to unfamiliar tasks within their companies and wonder how much longer they will be employed. Adding to the pressures that workers face are new bosses, computer surveillance of production, fewer health and retirement benefits, and the feeling they have to work longer and harder just to maintain their current economic status. Workers at every level are experiencing increased tension and uncertainty, and are updating their resumés.

The loss of a job can be devastating, putting unemployed workers at risk for physical illness, marital strain, anxiety, depression, and even suicide. Loss of a job affects every part of life, from what time you get up in the morning, to whom you see and what you can afford to do. Until the transition is made to a new position, stress is chronic.

A SENSE OF POWERLESSNESS

A feeling of powerlessness is a universal cause of job stress. When you feel powerless, you're prey to depression's traveling companions, helplessness and hopelessness. You don't alter or avoid the situation, because you feel nothing can be done.

Secretaries, waitresses, middle managers, police officers, editors, and medical interns are among those with the most highly stressed occupations marked by the need to respond to others' demands and timetables, with little control over events. Common to this job situation are complaints of too much responsibility and too little authority, unfair labor practices, and inadequate job descriptions. Employees can counteract these pressures through workers' unions or other organizations, grievance or personnel offices, or, more commonly, by direct negotiations with their immediate supervisors.

Your Job Description

Every employee should have a specific, written job description. Simply negotiating one does more to dispel a sense of powerlessness than anything else we know. It is a contract that you help write. You can object to what you don't want and insist on what you do want. If there is a compromise, it's because you agreed to it. With a clear job description, your expectations are spelled out, as are your boss's.

When Anne negotiated her job description, Charlie jokingly told her that her job was to do whatever he wanted. When Anne objected to his attitude, Charlie was shocked by the callousness of his statement. He began to see himself as a colleague and started soliciting input from his subordinates on what could be done to increase departmental efficiency.

A good job description is time limited. Set a specific date for review and revision based on your mutual experience with this initial job description. If you and your boss can't agree on what your job description should be, look for another job, either within the same company or outside. Even in these tough economic times, it is important that your job be a source of satisfaction and respect.

WHEN YOU'RE A SQUARE PEG AND YOUR JOB IS A ROUND HOLE

Remember the old saying, "Find a job you love and you'll never work another day in your life." Most people spend about 25 percent of their adult lives working. If you enjoy what you do, you're lucky. But if you're the proverbial square peg and your job is a round hole, job stress hurts your productivity and takes a serious toll on your mind and body.

There are many reasons for staying in a job that doesn't fit you or that you don't particularly like. One reason can be "golden handcuffs." A client, David, age 48, told us he couldn't afford to leave his job as vice president of a medical products company because of his high salary, his pension, his benefits, and his "perks," even though job stress had caused him two heart attacks. He felt "marginally qualified" for his job and lived in constant fear that he would be exposed as an "impostor" and summarily dismissed. David "knew" he would never get as good a job elsewhere. David felt his job was too good to quit, but when early retirement became an option after his second heart attack, he retired and opened a specialty craft shop in a local tourist area. In retrospect, he feels his "golden handcuffs" almost killed him and that "the costs of staying there were way too high."

Many of our clients are in jobs they don't like or aren't good at. The quick answer is to get a job they like or one that better matches their skills, abilities, and interests. Easier said than done. Some clients have no idea what kind of job they would like or what kind of job would be better. Worse, they don't have a clue on how to go about finding out this information.

We send these folks to a vocational counselor to learn about their skills, abilities, and talents and the jobs that are more appropriate for them. Next, we help them decide on jobs that interest them. Finally, there's the problem of getting a suitable job. This usually takes time, but understanding about the job-person fit makes it easier to accept their current situation until they find employment.

Suzanne had initially come to us to help her get off the medication she had been on for three years for a panic disorder. We worked on teaching her to cope with her physical sensations of panic while at the same time decreasing her medication. As time passed, it became apparent that her main source of stress and anxiety was career conflict. Suzanne was married with two children, ages 9 and 11. She had been in a fine arts program in college but had not finished her degree. She had been a computer programmer for a couple of years but hadn't liked it. Now that her children were older, Suzanne wanted to return to work. She considered art school or possibly law school. She went to a vocational counselor for testing. The results were a shock to her and to us. The test indicated that she would be well suited as an investigator or a detective. The more she thought about it, the more excited she became. Her father had been a criminal lawyer, and she was familiar with courts and police, but she had ruled out law school. This seemed perfect. When we last saw Suzanne she was working as an investigator for the district attorney's office and was full of stories of stakeouts, tracking missing persons, and investigation of white-collar crime. The self-assurance that came with finding her niche in the work world put to rest her former anxiety.

TRAUMATIC EVENTS ON THE JOB

Some jobs are inherently dangerous and others can suddenly become so. Criminal justice personnel, firefighters, ambulance drivers, military personnel, and disaster teams witness many terrible scenes and are exposed to personal danger routinely. They usually handle such incidents capably. But occasionally a particularly bad episode will stay with them, appearing in memory flashbacks and nightmares. Sleep disturbance, guilt, fearfulness, and physical complaints may follow. Even ordinary jobs can become traumatic: a co-worker, boss, or client physically threatens an employee; a bus crashes on a field trip; an employee is robbed or taken hostage; a shooting occurs. Such events can create post-traumatic stress disorder (PTSD) and result in worker's compensation claims if left untreated by a trauma specialist.

BURNOUT

If in the beginning your job seems perfect, the solution to all your problems, you have high hopes and expectations, and would rather work than do anything else, be wary. You're a candidate for the most insidious and tragic kind of job stress—burnout, a state of physical, emotional, and mental exhaustion caused by unrealistically high aspirations and illusory or impossible goals.

The potential for burnout increases dramatically depending on who you are, where you work, and what your job is. If you're a hard worker who gives 110 percent, an idealistic, self-motivated achiever who thinks anything is possible if you just work hard enough, you're a possible candidate. The same is true if you're a rigid perfectionist with unrealistically high standards and expectations. In a job with little recognition and few rewards for work well done, particularly with frequent people contact or deadlines, you advance from a possible to a probable candidate.

The road to burnout is paved with good intentions. There's certainly nothing wrong with being an idealistic, hardworking perfectionist or a self-motivating achiever, and there's nothing wrong with having high aspirations and expectations. Indeed, these are admirable traits in our culture. Unreality is the villain. Unrealistic job aspirations and expectations are doomed to frustration and failure. The burnout candidate's personality keeps him striving with single-minded intensity until he crashes.

Burnout proceeds by stages that blend and merge into one another so smoothly and imperceptibly that the victim seldom realizes what's happening even after it's over.

These stages include:

The Honeymoon

During the honeymoon phase your job is wonderful. You have boundless energy and enthusiasm and all things seem possible. You love the job and the job loves you. You believe it will satisfy all your needs and desires and solve all your problems. You're delighted with your job, your co-workers, and the organization.

The Awakening

The honeymoon wanes and the *awakening* stage starts with the realization that your initial expectations were unrealistic. The job isn't working out the way you thought it would. It doesn't satisfy all your needs, your co-workers and the organization are less than perfect, and rewards and recognition are scarce.

As disillusionment and disappointment grow, you become confused. Something is wrong, but you can't quite put your finger on it. Typically, you work even harder, to *make* your dreams come true. But working harder doesn't change anything and you become increasingly tired, bored, and frustrated. You question your competence and ability and start losing your self-confidence.

Brownout

As *brownout* begins, your early enthusiasm and energy give way to chronic fatigue and irritability. Your eating and sleeping patterns change and you indulge in escapist behaviors such as sex, drinking, drugs, partying, or shopping binges. You become indecisive, and your productivity drops. Your work deteriorates. Co-workers and superiors may comment on it.

Unless interrupted, brownout slides into its later stages. You become increasingly frustrated and angry and project the blame for your difficulties onto others. You are cynical, detached, and openly critical of the organization, superiors, and co-workers. You are beset with depression, anxiety, and physical illness. Drugs or alcohol are often a problem.

Full-Scale Burnout

Unless you wake up and interrupt the process or someone intervenes, brownout drifts remorselessly into full-scale *burnout*. Despair is the dominant feature of this final stage. This may take several months, but in most cases it involves three to four years. You experience an overwhelming sense of failure and a devastating loss of self-esteem and self-confidence. You become depressed and feel lonely and empty.

Life seems pointless and there is a paralyzing, "what's the use" pessimism about the future. You talk about "just quitting and getting away." You are exhausted physically and mentally. Physical and mental breakdowns are likely. Suicide, stroke, or heart attack are not unusual as you complete this final stage of what all started with such high hopes, energy, optimism, and enthusiasm.

The Phoenix Phenomenon

You can arise Phoenix-like from the ashes of burnout, but it takes time. First of all, you need to rest and relax. Don't take work home. If you're like most of our clients, the work won't get done and you'll only feel guilty for being "lazy."

For example, Harry, a 36-year-old attorney, would regularly load up his briefcase with work, lug it home, and set it down in a corner of the living room, with every intention of doing it after dinner. Too tired to work after dinner, he would try to rest, but the briefcase would "sit there in the corner and glare" at him. The next morning Harry would lug the undone work back to the office.

In therapy, Harry finally realized the futility of what he was doing and stopped taking work home. Now, he could rest and relax in the evening, giving him more energy for work at the office.

Accept your sour attitude, anger, confusion, frustration, disappointment, depression, anxiety, and sense of inadequacy and failure as a normal part of the burnout process and as a necessary step toward your recovery.

Find someone to talk to about your distress—your mate, a good friend, your priest, minister, or rabbi, or perhaps a professional counselor. It is important that both you and whomever you're talking to understand that you are not asking him or her to correct your situation for you, but just to talk with you.

In coming back from burnout, be realistic in your job expectations, aspirations, and goals. Whomever you're talking to about your feelings can help you. But be careful. Your readjusted aspirations and goals must be yours and not somebody else's. Trying to be and do what someone else wants you to be or do is a surefire recipe for continued frustration and burnout.

A final tip—create balance in your life. Invest more of yourself in family and other personal relationships, social activities, and hobbies. Spread yourself out so that your job doesn't have such an overpowering influence on your self-esteem and self-confidence.

WORK SETTING

Sometimes your work setting creates physical stress because of noise, lack of privacy, poor lighting, poor ventilation, poor temperature control, or inadequate sanitary facilities. Settings where there is organizational confusion or an overly authoritarian, laissez-faire, or crisis-centered managerial style are all psychologically stressful.

Act through labor or employee organizations to alter stressful working conditions. If that doesn't work, try the courts, which have become increasingly receptive to complaints of stressful working conditions. Recent rulings created pressure for employers to provide working environments that are as stress-free as possible.

The Occupational Safety and Health Administration (OSHA) is the federal agency charged with monitoring the work environment in the interests of worker safety and health (see p. 135 for further details). If you think your work environment is dangerous to your health and safety from a physical standpoint, give them a call. If nothing helps and the working environment remains stressful, exercise your avoidance option and get a new job. Job hunting can be stressful, particularly in times of high unemployment, but being ground down day after day by work is far worse.

POOR JOB SKILLS

If you don't have the skills to do your job efficiently, you're probably not proud of yourself. Pride in our work is more important than money for most of us. Without pride, work becomes a boring drudge that is inherently stressful.

Specific Job Skills

Take a moment to write down the skills and abilities you think are necessary for you to have pride in your job. Check with your co-workers and get their ideas. After you've come up with a reasonable list, mark the skills and abilities you already possess. Then, go through it again and place an X next to those you don't have but would like to develop. Think about the training you need to develop those job skills and where you might obtain them.

Trade schools, adult education classes, vocational rehabilitation agencies, specialized seminars and workshops, and on-the-job training are just a few of your options. Talk to your employer about getting additional job-related training. Some employers are delighted at the prospect of upgrading their work force and are willing to assist in terms of time off and tuition remission.

Organizational Skills

An organized work space increases your efficiency. Start by making a place for everything and keeping everything in its place. Get rid of clutter—it gets in your way.

Lyle's grandmother had a great way of eliminating clutter in her kitchen that might be useful for your work space. Every spring she would unload everything from her kitchen drawers into cardboard boxes. When she needed something, she would take it from the box, use it, wash it, and put it back in a drawer. Items she used a lot, she put in the top drawers; items she used less frequently she put in the bottom drawers; and items she didn't use at all, she put in a box in the basement. The drawers organized, she'd move on to cupboards and shelves and repeat the process. The last step was to throw away the items left in the basement from the year before. The process would take two months or so, but her kitchen was well organized for the other ten months of the year.

Time Management

You'll need organizational skills for managing your work time as well as your work space. Learn to use lists. Write down what you plan to do during your workday. Sort out which tasks come first. See if certain tasks lead to others. Check them off on your list as you go. You'll find an increasing sense of accomplishment as you march down your list.

For tasks that are not sequential, organize them in terms of the time they take. Set aside uninterrupted blocks of time for activities that require extended periods of concentrated effort. Do the little tasks in the periods in between the big ones. Sometimes do the little activities as a change of pace when larger tasks drag. But make sure you're not using them as distractions to avoid the big jobs.

Goal Setting

Goal setting helps you set priorities on how you spend your time and efforts on the job. Start by deciding your primary vocational goals. If that's too long-term, determine where you want to be five years from now. Keeping these goals in mind, start planning the next year so that it contributes toward those goals. Then break down the upcoming year into months and plan toward meeting the goals of the upcoming year. Think in terms of major goals and minor goals. But make sure they're your goals not somebody else's. You can start by asking yourself: "What do I *really* want to do for a living?"; "How can I get there?"; "What skills do I need?"; "What is the time frame?" Goal-setting skills improve with practice. So keep practicing. A word of caution: Don't get depressed when you do not meet those goals. Check with friends and use the reality-testing skills we discuss later in this chapter to be sure your goals are reasonable.

Social Skills

For many people, their jobs mean much more than merely a paycheck. Work is a place for socializing and making friends. In fact, getting along with co-workers, subordinates, superiors, customers, vendors, and suppliers may be your most important job skill. An unpleasant social situation on the job affects your performance and makes for miserable working conditions. Particularly important is keeping social and business relationships well defined. If you confide in a co-worker as a friend, and he or she fails to keep the confidence, using personal information against you, your sense of betrayal is doubled. Dating co-workers can also become complicated, especially after a breakup. The ability to maintain a businesslike and pleasant demeanor in the face of company politics will defuse many of these situations.

Communication Skills

The most important skill in any social situation is communication. The workplace is no exception. If you score high on both job stress and social stress, pay attention to your ability to communicate with other people.

To improve your communication skills, follow these simple rules:

- Listen to what the other person has to say. *Really* listen. Don't focus on preparing your response. You can practice your listening skills by restating the other person's comments. If you don't understand what he or she is telling you, say, "I don't understand."

- Be assertive in expressing your thoughts and feelings. Use "I" and "we" statements. If you're aggressive or hostile, others focus on self-defense rather than on what you're saying. If you're passive and submissive, they'll ignore you.
- Be honest and direct.
- Be respectful of the other person.
- Be brief.
- Keep it simple.
- Keep it focused on the topic; don't bring in extraneous, distracting comments.

Conflict-Resolution Skills

Conflict-resolution skills are crucial, especially when you are forced to deal with difficult or disagreeable people. It is especially important to listen to the other person's side of the argument to understand his or her basis for disagreement.

Focus on the problem and keep personalities out of it. You may need to let the other person run down before you respond. Avoid personal attack. Don't look for a scapegoat. If the other person does, interrupt with, "Let's focus on the problem," or restate what he says. Turn expressions like, "You stupid jerk, your screw-up cost us that contract," into, "I hear what you're saying. You think I'm a stupid jerk because we lost a contract over something I did wrong. I don't agree with you. I think there were many factors involved. We should be correcting our problems so that we don't lose any more contracts instead of arguing over whose fault it was. I don't like being called names and I get pretty angry when I am. Don't call me that anymore." As with all skills, the more you practice, the better they'll get. See "Communication Skills," for more specific recommendations. *Coping with Difficult People,* by Robert Bramson,[1] is especially useful for work situations.

Reality-Testing Skills

Reality testing is particularly relevant on the job. In this era of rapid and escalating change, it is often difficult to tell what's real and what's illusory. It's an important difference. For instance, you need to know your real value to your company. If you think you're worth more than you really are, you're liable to make unrealistic demands and create problems. If you have no idea what you're worth, you'll get less than what you should.

Use other people as sounding boards to check your view of reality. Ask for feedback from supervisors and co-workers. Don't think you know what separates reality from illusion. Self-deception is seductive and we all do it to some extent. Try to be objective about yourself, your work situation, and how it fits in the grand scheme of things. Be flexible enough to adjust your thoughts and behaviors accordingly.

Thinking and behaving flexibly is invaluable when life isn't working well. Frustration mounts, bringing with it anger and cognitive and behavioral rigidity. A cycle begins of failure, frustration, persistence in failed behaviors, failure, frustration, etc. You're trapped. Step back and say, "This isn't working, I need a different approach, or new insight." Talk to other people for ideas. Try thinking about the problem from a different perspective. Above all, don't keep banging your head against the wall—you'll just get a headache.

AIDS FOR REDUCING STRESS IN THE WORKPLACE

Most companies now have some kind of employee assistance program (EAP). EAPs are great resources for reality testing and their counselors are usually the best people to help with work-related stress problems. EAPs operate in the strictest of confidence, so don't worry that your comments will be passed on to anyone else. If your problems require more time or expertise than EAP professionals can provide, they'll refer you to resources outside the company.

Where there are problems inherent in the organizational structure, or the work setting itself creates stress for you on the job, your best resource for altering the situation may well be a labor union or other employee organization. Talk to them and see what kind of assistance they can provide.

If you think your workplace is stressful beyond the bounds of ordinary employment, consider contacting the Occupational Safety and Health Administration (OSHA) of the federal government. You can reach them at (513) 841-4132. Give them a call stating that you want to make a complaint about stressful working conditions. Your complaint will be taken down on OSHA form 7 and sent to you for your signature. You don't have to sign it, but do return it in any case. OSHA will protect your anonymity to prevent retaliation against you for being a "whistle blower."

If you sign form 7, OSHA will send a team to inspect the work site with no further action on your part. If you do not sign the form, OSHA will send a letter to the company stating that they are aware of stress violations and give the company fifteen days to make corrections. At the end of this time, OSHA will send a team to inspect your work site. Violators will be fined and given thirty days to correct violations. They will be reinspected, and fined again if corrections have not been made. The reinspections continue until corrections have been made.

You might take legal action if all else fails. Should you be incapacitated by the stress in your workplace, you may well be eligible for worker's compensation for stress-related illness, depending on the laws in your state.

The Job Search

Your final recourse in dealing with stress on the job, of course, is to leave and go elsewhere. Don't be impulsive and quit before you have someplace else to go. If your company is downsizing and offering early retirement, it may be your golden opportunity to get out. Many companies provide placement services to employees who choose to leave. Try a headhunting organization or an employment agency for leads. When you are out of work or decide to make a change, approach your job search as if it were a job itself. Stay organized. Schedule specific times to work on this project. Invest time and money if necessary to get good advice. Use informational interviews to explore possibilities you haven't considered before. Most of all, though, tap your personal network for leads and support. Tell everyone you know that you're looking for a job. Don't be shy—friends are a good source for finding out about available jobs. Do not get discouraged. Persistence pays.

There's lots you can do about stress on the job. You're not at anyone's mercy. All you have to do is develop a good *Action Plan* and follow through to get the upper hand on your job stress.

N O T E S

1. Bramson, R. (1988), *Coping with Difficult People*, New York, Dell.

6 MANAGING FAMILY STRESS

Families are a valuable resource in coping with stress, but they are also potent sources of stress for many of us. They can provide a mixture of love, joy, strength, pride, and deep satisfaction, while also causing confusion, irritation, frustration, dissatisfaction, misery, and even violence. Family life is complicated and family stress has many facets. Change brings stress, and the changes that occur within the family constitute stress points that most of us deal with at some time in our lives.

In today's world families have many structures. There are nuclear families of two parents and one or more children, but there are also extended families with grandparents or other relatives, blended families of remarried parents with stepchildren, adoptive families, foster families, gay and lesbian couples with or without children, and co-housing cooperatives of younger and older adults. We use the term *family* in its broadest sense to include those individuals in your life with whom you have a more intimate and loyal connection. As Sister Sledge sings, "We are family." In the end, your family is how *you* define it. If your current family is quite different from your family of origin, you and your partner may experience considerable stress as you develop traditions and patterns that fit your new life.

External demands and pressures affect families as well as individuals. Natural disasters, war, neighborhood feuds or violence, and loss of income are just a few problems families face. These external demands and pressures can draw a family close together and override any internal problems, or they can complete the destruction begun by internal problems. For example, the accidental death or injury of a child can draw a family together, or it can cause acrimonious blaming that ends with the final breakup of a shaky marriage.

NORMAL DEVELOPMENTAL CHANGES

Developmental changes occur naturally within the family, bringing with them ripple effects that touch every member to some degree. Births, deaths, marriages, divorces, separations, maturation of children, aging of parents, etc. alter interpersonal relations, family leadership, and individual responsibilities. Adjusting to these natural changes is very stressful for everyone involved. And everyone *is* involved.

The addition of children to the family, for example, creates many problems of adjustment. Clearly, infants and small children bring a unique set of demands that strains the finances, time, and energy of the entire household.

A less subtle issue of adjustment is what the birth of a child does to the pattern of relationships within the family. When a couple marries there are two relationships (1X2), his relationship with her and her relationship with him. The birth of a child changes the pattern to six relationships (1X2X3). A second child escalates the number of relationships even further to twenty-four (1X2X3X4). The third child increases the number of relationships to one hundred twenty (1X2X3X4X5), making the maintenance of individual relationships within the family cumbersome and difficult.

The birth of a third child places demands and pressures on the family system that go beyond the obvious ones of another mouth to feed, another body to clothe, etc. The pattern of individual relationships often breaks down and the ripples can swamp family stability. Clinically, we have observed that postpartum depressions are more likely to occur following the birth of a third child, disciplinary problems are likely to escalate with older siblings, and parents are more likely to quarrel. Interpersonal relationships strain to the breaking point as family members struggle to maintain a pattern of interaction swamped by the number of individuals involved.

Many families solve the problem by breaking the family into two groups, parents and children. Parents have their relationship between themselves, and the children interact among themselves. The groups interact with each other. In large families where there are more than three children, this becomes a necessary solution.

Interpersonal relationships change when members leave the group. Old patterns don't work anymore. Stress ripples through the family until successful adjustments are made. Increasing adolescent independence and the final (or not so final) move away from home is both emotionally wrenching and a relief. Family conflicts that have smoldered quietly for years erupt when group membership undergoes change. Weddings, funerals, and births are the most likely times of maximum family stress, just when people expect one another to be on their best behavior.

CONFLICT IN THE PRIMARY FAMILY RELATIONSHIP

The biggest area of family stress is conflict between husband and wife. This primary relationship holds the family together. Conflict between spouses spreads through the entire family. Marital difficulties, arguments, fights, violence, and separation mark such conflict.

Marital friction has many causes, but the most common is the waning of the romantic illusions that once enabled partners to ignore faults that they now find intolerable. Sometimes we marry our own creations and are disappointed when dealing with a real person who has a host of shortcomings.

Another major cause of conflict is unrealistic expectations of each other. One spouse, or both, may expect the same treatment they received from their parents when they were children. If they don't get it, they become disappointed, frustrated, and angry, and blame their partner for their unhappiness. These unrealistic expectations have their roots in that primary staple of the psychoanalytic trade, "transference." We choose mates who remind us of our opposite-sex parent, and transfer to our mates the feelings we felt toward that parent when we were children. In time, we may want from our mates what we came to expect from our parents. In some cases, we think our mates should be even better parents than our own and make up for all the disappointments of our childhoods.

Whether we want to or not, most of us end up with marital relationships that mirror our parents' marriages. Observers of family systems find the same issues, themes, and patterns of behavior persisting generation after generation. Or, if we admired our parents' marriage and don't get a similar arrangement, anger and disappointment occur.

We also behave toward our mates in the ways we acted toward our brothers and sisters as children. Eldest children are generally dominant individuals used to being in charge. When two eldest children marry, their lives are often a struggle for dominance, with issues of power and control the flashpoints of their quarrels. Eldest children understand that there can be other views of the world than theirs, but are smugly confident that their view is the only correct one.

Only children can be difficult mates. They can't conceive of there being any way of viewing the world other than their own and are exasperated and frustrated by any suggestion that there is another way.

Middle children are forever competing and comparing themselves to others. Soothing their fragile egos can become their partners' major task in life. Two middle children together can spend their lives endlessly competing with each other as they strive to be on top at last. The middle child understands that there are other ways of seeing the world but is convinced that everyone else is wrong.

The typical youngest child is ambivalent about issues of dependence and independence. They are aware that there are many different views of the world, but are unsure as to whether their own view is right or wrong. They continually seek out authorities. They are used to being looked after and cared for, but they are also used to being bossed and controlled by everyone else in the house. They can't wait to catch up to their older siblings, but never do. And they often spend their lives vainly competing with their older siblings. When youngest children marry, they often spend their time vacillating between wanting to be taken care of and wanting to be the boss. If they and their spouses have cycles of dependence and independence that match, everything can be rosy; if they conflict, both are frustrated, disappointed, and hurt at the other's "insensitivity" and "stubbornness."

When an eldest child marries a middle or youngest child, their expectations and behavior patterns generally match. For example, Lloyd, the big brother of two sisters, got along well with Nedda, the younger sister of three brothers.

The dramas of our lives often seem unconsciously scripted in our childhoods. We recruit others to play roles and parts complementary to the roles we have scripted for ourselves. In casting our life dramas, we select players whose scripts parallel our own closely enough that they meld into an even larger drama with many characters and parts. When our scripts blend smoothly, there are few problems. The fantasies and illusions about ourselves and our mates can continue. When they no longer blend smoothly, or when reality intervenes, we're forced to deal with the people behind the scripts. This can be distressing, but it places us in a position to deal with real life and real-life people.

As illusion fades into reality, communication and understanding are critical in dealing with the many conflicts that inevitably arise. Without good conflict-resolution skills our relationships can deteriorate into quarrels and too often the fighting gets dirty. We call each other names and do our best to hurt, embarrass, or humiliate each other. We personalize the issue and blame each other rather than focus on solving our mutual problems. Dirty fighting can lead to violence as our frustrations with our mates become intolerable.

Instead, partners need to learn how to be good mates. In his book *Love Is Never Enough*,[1] Aaron Beck describes the qualities needed for a happy relationship: commitment, sensitivity, generosity, consideration, loyalty, responsibility, and trustworthiness. Other virtues include the ability to cooperate, to compromise, and to follow through on joint decisions.

FAMILY OBLIGATIONS

Families come with a set of obligations that makes heavy demands on our time, energy, and financial, mental, and physical resources. Obligations that we willingly impose on ourselves and accept from family members would be outrageous when viewed from outside the family. Inside the family, however, they often seem reasonable, ordinary, and expected, because of our notions of what family membership involves.

When we fail to live up to these family obligations, we create stress by feeling anxious or guilty. Unemployment or illness impairs our ability to meet our financial or practical obligations and takes a toll on self-esteem as we see others take on increased responsibilities. Taking on excess responsibilities, and allowing other members to underfunction, can also be damaging. "Martyr moms," for instance, crucify themselves on the cross of family obligation and responsibility. Instead of demanding that family members participate equally in household tasks, they generate guilt and misery in those not sufficiently appreciative of their sacrifices.

Family obligations and the stress they create make themselves felt particularly around family get-togethers such as holidays or vacations. The item most often rated as very stressful is family holidays. While holidays are times of reunion and reconnection, they also carry social and financial obligations. Particularly for young married adults, the inability to meet obligations to both sets of in-laws can generate months of arguments. Whose family do you visit for Thanksgiving? How do you divide up the other holidays? Who gets invited and who gets left out? Some families have difficulty allowing roles to change as the structure of the family alters over time.

One 25-year-old client said, "My mother tells me exactly what food to bring, even what recipe to use. What if I want to make something different this year?"

When ordinary family obligations are compounded by a member's illness or need for chronic care, the strength, resilience, and resources of the family are profoundly tested. At such times, extended family or community support can make the difference between survival and collapse.

PARENTING

The most extensive family obligation is the raising of children. The challenges begin before pregnancy if there are fertility problems and continue through infancy, school years, adolescence, and early adulthood. Each phase has its own demands and rewards.

The problems of parenting create significant stress in many families. Our data show a direct relationship between family stress and the number of children under 5 years of age. The stress is greater for mothers, but fathers are affected also. Parenting is even more challenging when there are disciplinary problems with children, children with special needs, a child leaving home, or unusual child-care responsibilities. Parents, especially mothers, also resonate to the stresses of their children—if their children are having a hard time, parents worry about them.

The three fundamentals for coping with parental stress are teamwork, structure, and discipline. Parents, even if divorced, need to be united as a team and to develop a supportive network. This is particularly true for single parents. An African proverb reminds us, "It takes a village to raise a child." A supportive network includes child-care providers, grandparents, neighbors, the parents of your child's friends, and teachers. Developing such a network for your children enriches their opportunities to learn and to feel secure in the world. Remember, you aren't expected to do it alone.

Structure reduces the feeling that things are out of control. Routines, consistent schedules, and clear expectations help parents and children cope with transitions.

An organized household with set times for meals, homework, daily and weekly chores, and recreation lets everyone know what to expect. You are teaching your children the habits that will help them reduce stress throughout their lifetime. It takes longer to supervise a child's task than to do it yourself, but eventually your children can help you with the hassles of everyday life.

Discipline is the process of teaching children to meet your minimal expectations—good manners, respect for others, and taking responsibility inside and outside the home. This is accomplished primarily through modeling—i.e., living the way you would like your children to live. In creating discipline there are some simple steps to take. Always provide your children with clear instructions. They should be given one at a time and you should spell out what you expect. You should follow this, if necessary, by warning them of the consequences if they don't obey. Finally, if your children do not comply with your request, comes the last phase—correction. Being removed from a situation, losing privileges, or having to make amends to an injured party are all good corrections.

For many parents, correction is the most difficult aspect of discipline. They don't know how to correct effectively or are too frazzled or preoccupied with other demands to follow through. Some parents are paralyzed by the fear that they will make a mistake and do irreparable damage to their children. Stop worrying and making excuses, there are always extenuating circumstances. Be consistent with the process or it won't work.

The confusion between discipline and punishment is often at the base of such parental fears. Punishments such as yelling, criticism, name-calling, or hitting may temporarily interrupt an unwanted behavior but they have negative side effects for both parents and children. Parents feel guilty (sometimes), and children experience loss of self-esteem, anxiety, fear, and shame. Such actions also model for children a negative way to interact with others.

If you correct your children mainly when you're angry and you rely on physical punishment, you teach them not to get you angry, but not a better way to behave. June made this mistake with her three sons when they were small. As adolescents they decided that they were too big and strong to be punished anymore and could now do as they pleased, which to them required increasingly large amounts of money. June's credit cards were "borrowed" by two of her sons and thousands of dollars were charged on them. June and her husband were forced into personal bankruptcy as a consequence.

Some time later, her youngest son, Jimmy, began betting on sporting events by telephone. When the bookies threatened to "break his legs if he didn't pay up," Jimmy went to his mother with the problem and insisted that she take out a second mortgage on her home to pay his gambling debts. Torn between fear for Jimmy and anger at what he had done, June didn't know what to do.

Our counsel was, "He got himself in, let him get himself out. If they break his legs, he will at least learn that he can't do as he pleases with impunity." June was doubtful but followed our advice. Jimmy, terrified, called the bookies and sobbed, "I'm just a little kid. I'm only 15 years old." The bookies relented and let him off with a warning that he was never to place a bet in that city ever again.

Jimmy finally understood that there were limits and that his behavior could have serious personal consequences. Having taken the plunge, June clearly spelled out her expectations of him, the limits she would tolerate, and the consequences for going over those limits. Jimmy tested, but she stuck to it consistently and Jimmy "shaped up." Jimmy is now a practicing attorney. But his older brothers are con artists. All three are putting the lessons of childhood into practice in their adult lives.

SEXUAL DIFFICULTIES

Although they are high up on the list of items couples fight about, sexual difficulties are generally symptomatic of other problems in the family. Couples fight about sex when they're afraid to fight about the real problems. Our stock question is, "What is it you're really angry about?"

When there is hurt, anger, or anxiety about sex, concerns usually involve performance anxiety, approval, rejection, and our partner's fantasized expectations. Once past the emotional issues, the most common problem that makes for sexual difficulties is a skill deficit. Despite the publicity it receives, and our preoccupation with it, most people just don't know much about sex and how to go about attaining a sexually satisfying relationship.

Many sexual difficulties are transient, the result of other stress in your life, including economic demands, fatigue, or lack of time for intimacy. If sexual problems persist, they can permeate other aspects of family life, creating tension around the whole topic of sex. Help is available. There are specific treatments for sexual difficulties. Contact your family physician, urologist, or gynecologist for an evaluation or referral.

FAMILY LOSS

Change is our only constant in life and with change, inevitably, comes loss. Because the family is such a central feature of our lives, loss in the family affects everyone. Whenever family circumstances change—births, deaths, weddings, school graduations—stress is created and can trigger other family-stress problems. These are the moments of failed expectations, loss of illusion, hurt feelings, and the bitter disappointment that generate hard feelings and family feuds. Or, the family may become even closer, providing the warmth, comfort, and support needed to survive.

ALTERING STRESSFUL FAMILY SITUATIONS

Communication

Stressful family situations always involve other people. You have to communicate with those people to alter the situation. Open, direct communication, in fact, makes a family a coping resource; secrets and indirect communication make it a primary source of stress. There are guidelines you can follow in developing more effective family communication. We outlined some of them earlier in our discussion of stress on the job, but they bear repeating and elaboration here because they are so important in our dealings with family members:

• Be brief. Make requests or statements short. Too much discussion can obscure your main idea.

• Be direct and clear. Say what you need or want from the other person. Hints are likely to be missed or misinterpreted. Avoid vague or confusing messages. Be specific.

• Make "I" statements. Speak from your own perspective about how a stressful situation affects you. Steer away from statements about the other person. "You" statements such as, "You should . . ." or, "You should talk," are likely to make the other person defensive or irritated and cut off further meaningful communication.

• Let your family know what effect their actions or words have on you. A good form to follow is, "When you do . . ., I feel . . ." If you say, "When you are late, I get anxious about your safety," you accept responsibility for your reaction and give feedback to your family member about how his or her actions affect you.

• Make sure your verbal and nonverbal messages are the same. Saying "I'm not angry" when you're frowning and speaking in a sharp voice is confusing.

• In addition to practicing good communication skills, be a good listener. Pay attention when someone is speaking to you, keep good eye contact, nod, and encourage further communication by asking for clarification. Give feedback that shows you understood, by paraphrasing what the other person has said or by saying things like, "It sounds like you get upset when you . . ."

Communication skills take practice. One way is to have regular family roundtables where each person gets to speak without interruption for five or ten minutes, using the above guidelines. After all family members have finished, have a discussion where all members get a short period to respond. Remember, one member shouldn't dominate the discussion.

One reason for the lack of good communication is the difficulty of truly understanding someone who is different from yourself. Verbal and nonverbal messages are interpreted in the context of your own experience. Individuals within a family have distinct personalities and individual differences. If the parents are from diverse cultural, religious, or socioeconomic backgrounds, the differences may be even greater. In addition, men and women communicate differently.

It is easy to misunderstand. An example is that of a physician whose son had a learning disorder. The child was bright but couldn't master his schoolwork. The father, to whom learning had come easily, thought his son was lazy. It was only after the learning difficulty was identified through psychological testing that he could stop blaming and start helping his son.

Family secrets—alcoholism, abuse, violence, infidelities, incest—are the biggest obstacles to effective communication. No one talks about them, but everyone knows they're there. Secrets are corrosive and eat away at families. They inhibit open communication and create an atmosphere of secrecy, mistrust, confusion, and frustration that alienates family members from one another. Family tragedies are often rooted in family secrets. Although difficult to talk about, secrets erode family cohesion.

Families don't talk about their secrets because of shame or a fear that the secret, once out, will destroy the family. Families often maintain a conspiracy of silence around their secret and attack any family member who dares break the unspoken vow of silence.

When "family rules" about communication are challenged, problems of control emerge. Family beliefs about assertiveness, aggression, or "keeping the peace" make it difficult to open up communication. Approaching "family secrets" may create tension and anxiety for all parties and require sensitivity and diplomacy. While it is often painful to discuss a family's secrets, relief follows having it "out in the open." The agitation, anger, and anxiety created by letting the secret out can disrupt the family in the short term. There is also the risk of major family disruption. If you're concerned about that, seek professional counseling.

The distinction between privacy and secrecy is important. Some family problems are private matters, best kept within the family. The same is true of private matters between family members. Secrecy means, at best, actively keeping the whole truth from people and, at worst, actually lying or distorting the truth. Privacy connotes a respect for the other person's rights. But don't use privacy as an excuse to continue harboring secrets.

Joe's family situation illustrates how communication failures create stress. Joe, a 53-year-old plumber, came to see us about a year ago for treatment of his impotence after his urologist found no physical cause for his problem. At our first interview, Joe indicated that he and his wife, Betty, 51, had a "very happy" marriage for thirty years. Their three children had done well. The youngest had left home four years earlier. Joe's impotence had become a problem at about the same time and had progressively worsened.

Joe was shy and embarrassed as he sat in our office. He had difficulty talking about anything personal, let alone topics such as sex and impotence. Because male impotence is, in many instances, a symptom of stress and relationship problems, we generally insist that the spouse or partner be included in the treatment. Joe had "no idea" that his problem might involve his wife. Although reluctant to bring Betty into his treatment, we scheduled a second appointment to see them together.

From their interviews and their *Stress Audits*, we quickly determined the causes of their stress and Joe's impotence. Betty scored high on family stress. Joe thought there was no problem. Joe and Betty's marriage had never been happy, they just never fought. Betty glossed over unpleasantness and Joe withdrew into quiet isolation. Betty was angry and resentful because sex had seldom been satisfying for her and because Joe was emotionally distant. She told us she had had only one orgasm in thirty years but was too embarrassed to tell Joe how angry this made her. Besides, she didn't want to "hurt his feelings." So, to "keep peace in the house," she largely ignored him and focused on their children.

Joe was also unhappy about their sex life. He felt Betty was "frigid" and "unloving." He withdrew to protect himself from the frustration and hurt of what he perceived as rejection. Joe had even more difficulty in talking about his feelings than Betty. Even though she never said anything, Joe knew Betty was angry. He had no idea why and was confused and frustrated as to what he could do about it.

Joe had thought that when the children left, he'd get more attention from Betty and their sex life would improve. Instead, she turned her attention to social and church activities. In his anger and disappointment, Joe withdrew even further emotionally and became totally incapable of making love. Betty interpreted Joe's impotence as an indication that she was no longer attractive to him and became even more angry and resentful.

The family situation had become intolerably stressful for both Joe and Betty because of their lack of communication. Neither could express their thoughts, feelings, wants, and needs to the other in an open, direct, honest, and respectful way. They failed to communicate in part because they both automatically chose the avoidance option in handling their difficulties. But more important, they both lacked the assertive skills to speak up and say what they really wanted from each other.

Communication breakdowns like the one Joe and Betty faced are a problem among couples. There are many reasons for this. One is that instead of listening when other people are talking, most of us think about our rebuttal, elaboration, or self-defense and really don't hear the other person. Another reason is that we don't say what's really on our minds, so as not to hurt the other person's feelings or to avoid unpleasantness or conflict. Betty felt that Joe should know how she felt without her telling him. Joe rightly insisted that he was not a mind reader and that Betty would have to tell him if she wanted him to know what was going on with her.

We sent Joe and Betty to separate assertiveness-training workshops and gave them Manuel Smith's excellent book *When I Say No, I Feel Guilty*[2] to read. We also had them practice an exercise where each spoke uninterrupted for twenty minutes and the other just listened.

Joe and Betty's secret was that their marriage wasn't perfect. They couldn't and didn't talk about it. As a consequence, their sex life was never defined as a problem and went unaddressed. It was painful and anxiety provoking to deal with their sexual secrets, but it ultimately brought them closer together. Joe, for the first time, understood Betty's frustration and disappointment; and Betty saw Joe's hurt and isolation. They still have their problems, but they can talk about them and they understand each other better now. Joe's potency has returned, and they recently went on a "second honeymoon."

Conflict Resolution and Problem Solving

If communication and understanding are improved, there still remains the question, "What do we do about it?" Some families talk a lot but fail to offer solutions and to agree on a plan. Just as you have to make and implement a *Stress Action Plan*, families have to make decisions and follow through. Otherwise, the problem just sits there, continuing to create conflict.

For most of us, conflict is stressful in and of itself. Whenever people come in contact, disagreements emerge around values and opinions. This is particularly true in families. How comfortably families resolve their differences depends on the level of their conflict-resolution skills. Some families avoid overt conflict at all cost. They may have difficulty solving chronic problems because the problems are rarely identified, and solutions are not openly discussed. Other families are conflict ridden because even minor problems are blown into major arguments, including insults and put-downs. Poor communication is distressing to all concerned and seldom addresses the problem itself.

There are several guidelines for effective conflict resolution.

• Identify the problem. Let each person state how he

or she sees the issue. Avoid blaming others. Maintain respect for each person involved in the discussion.

• Stick to that one issue. Stay focused on the issue at hand, the one that is here and now. Don't bring up old complaints from the past. We call that "gunnysacking." Imagine that old hurts and conflicts are not dealt with but tossed into an imaginary "gunnysack" over your shoulder. Then when an argument starts, you argue not only about today's issue but dump the whole sack of grievances onto the table. Then you really have a mess!

• Keep your comments simple and clear. Too much talk can confuse or blur the real problem. Take turns in defending the different positions. Focus on how each family member is interacting with everyone else in sharing responsibility for the disagreement as well as its possible solution.

• Generate options for a solution. Ask each other, "What can we do to make it better?" "What do you suggest we try?" Be careful not to automatically evaluate or criticize any family member's ideas.

• Agree on an action plan. Think how the plan would affect each family member and what might happen if the family tried other possibilities. Respect the suggestions of all members of the family, pointing out the consequences of a suggested plan of action rather than ridiculing an idea or dismissing it without serious consideration.

• Try your action plan for a short period. See how it works. Don't say "I told you so" if it doesn't. Change plans that don't work. Keep the good parts and make adjustments to make them better.

Anger, defensiveness, or anxiety derails any discussion. Family members must recognize when they are so angry that communication is impossible. When you're so mad you can't think straight, you won't solve anything.

Certain signals warn of destructive interactions. Loud voices, swearing, accusations, and labeling ("You're a jerk") don't help. Aggressive body posture and facial expressions either shut down the other person's ability to communicate or create similar aggressive posturing. Mean what you say, say what you mean, but don't be mean when you say it.

If your family agrees ahead of time to minimize destructive anger, each member is expected to cope with his or her own anger. Take a break from the discussion if it gets too heated. Or take a deep breath, count to ten, or make coping statements to yourself such as, "Keep calm"; "Think how you can get your point across better"; or, "Stick to finding an answer instead of trying to prove her or him wrong."

If you have to leave the room, a statement such as, "I have to cool off for a few minutes so I can think straight," is better than just walking out. Reassurance that the discussion will continue at a later time until some resolution is found allows other family members to support your "time out" choice.

Negotiating Deals with Family Members

Another way of altering stressful situations in the family is through contracting and making agreements. There are always things we want other family members to do or not to do. Sometimes they comply with our stated wants and needs, but many times they don't. As we mentioned, you can't *make* anyone do anything, you can only influence them by making it worth their while. If you want a family member to do or not to do something, make a deal. Write the agreement out as though it were a legal contract. Be careful not to promise too much. You'll have to stick by your end of the agreement if it is to work. It's important to renegotiate periodically and allow room for escape clauses in your agreement.

Sarah and her 10-year-old son, Pete, were continually squabbling over Pete's reluctance to practice his violin. Pete liked taking lessons and performing but hated practice. Every day after school, Sarah would insist that Pete practice and Pete would resist. He'd dawdle and stall, sometimes spending long periods of time in the bathroom as part of his avoidance strategy for handling the stress of Sarah and practice. Sarah would nag, Pete would pout, and both would end up angry and in tears.

We helped Sarah work out an agreement with Pete whereby Pete had to practice the violin to earn TV viewing time. In addition, if he learned a piece of music it was worth money. They started at ten dollars per piece, but had to renegotiate when Pete began finishing a piece every other day. Then there was a significant prize to be won with the completion of each book of music Pete was assigned.

Sarah was now less involved in Pete's musical life. He practiced as long as he wanted, when he wanted. It was up to him. The "deal" eliminated a major source of stress between mother and son. Both are happier about violin lessons now. Pete, Sr., is even happier that he no longer has to "referee" their daily shouting and sulking matches. When Pete started resisting school homework, Pete and his mother promptly whipped up another "deal" before they got to the tears.

AVOIDING STRESS IN THE FAMILY

Picking the Right Time and the Right Place

There are times when the best way to manage family stress is to avoid it. Certain predictable situations, people, or topics are bound to be difficult if brought up at the wrong time or in the wrong place. Family arguments frequently occur in the kitchen prior to dinner. Family members are hungry and tired and in the middle of preparing a meal. Avoid difficult discussions by saying, "I'd better not talk about this now, I'm not in a good mood. Can we talk after dinner is over?" A constructive discussion may occur when things are calmer.

There are times, however, when we are unsuccessful in postponing such discussions and arguments ensue. You can end them by excusing yourself and walking out. Or, you can refuse to become embroiled in the argument until the other party gives up on the argument.

Moving Out and Moving On

Sometimes the only intelligent approach to reducing your stress is to move out and move on. This is a difficult step to take and often is as stressful, at least at first, as staying. It's hard to do. Carole, whose story we presented in chapter 3, had known for a long time that her relationship with Ray would never get any better before she finally found the strength to move out and move on.

It's time to move out and move on when the situation you're in is psychologically or physically damaging to you if you stay. If you can, avoid any relationship that you feel is abusive. But even the most wary sometimes find themselves enmeshed in physically or psychologically damaging relationships. If this is happening to you, and there is no promise of it getting better, move out and move on at your first opportunity. If it takes legal action to get out, take it. File a complaint with the police, get a restraining order, sue for divorce—do whatever you must in order to take care of yourself by stopping the abuse and getting away from the abuser. Be aware that leaving sometimes escalates the abuse, so seek help from social and human services before planning your exit. For facilities and organizations in your area that can help, look in the Yellow Pages under social services or check with local churches and hospitals.

Moving out and moving on also can be a decision based on personal growth. When children come of age can be a difficult time for families. Grown children want independence and freedom, but they also want the comfort of the parental home. The parents want their homes to themselves after years of raising children, but they also want to keep their children with them as long as possible. The ambivalence on both sides creates stress for all concerned until it is resolved, generally by the child moving out and moving on.

Moving out was part of the natural growth process for Carole. For the first time in her life she realized her inner strength, that she could maintain herself in the world without a man to protect, defend, and provide for her. The boost in self-esteem she felt as she established her independence and realized she was a competent, effective person carried her through graduate school. It helped her become a professional counselor for women trapped in abusive relationships.

If you decide it's time for you to move out and move

on, look before you leap. Have a place to move to. Make sure you're financially able to go it alone. Let your friends help and support you in changing your life.

When Denial Helps and When It Hurts

Some families insist on working out every problem in detail. Obsessive concern about resolving every little issue is stressful. Many small problems resolve themselves if left alone. When Lyle became chairman of an academic department he was advised by a friend who had chaired a number of departments, "Never do today what you can put off until tomorrow."

Denying the existence of a problem reduces its importance and makes it less stressful. Raising children is an example. Children go through phases where they are rebellious, the "terrible twos," for instance. You can turn every confrontation into a wearing and stressful power struggle, or you can occasionally ignore the defiant behavior and let your child and yourself pass through the phase more peacefully.

Anyone can be grouchy and difficult to deal with at times, your family included. It's not necessary to deal with these occasional bouts of ill temper to "work things out." Let them slide, ignore them, deny their importance. Most of the time, they'll go away on their own.

When denial becomes a way of keeping a family secret, however, it hurts much more than it helps. Problems that paralyze a family and create stress for everyone in it do not get addressed because everyone spends their efforts and energies denying that problems such as alcoholism, drug addiction, and violence exist. Carole, for instance, kept the abusive relationship with Ray secret, even from herself, by denying that it was a problem.

When we first started seeing Brendan, a 41-year-old civil engineer, for his stress-related hypertension, it was apparent that his problem was related to his being an overly responsible, adult child of an alcoholic (ACOA). He admitted that his mother, now in her seventies, had a "drink now and then," but denied that it had ever been a problem.

Brendan had problems at work and at home. At work he assumed excessive responsibilities and a heavy workload. He was always the first in and the last to leave work. This made him unpopular with co-workers because he pushed subordinates as hard as he pushed himself. He had been the target of several union grievances, some of which had been upheld. As a result, he had been reprimanded and told to change his managerial style.

Home was not a haven for Brendan. He pressured his two children, 8 and 10, about their schoolwork and railed at them for being "lazy and irresponsible." They countered with sullen resentment and withdrawal. His wife, Mildred, who joined Brendan in therapy with us, complained that Brendan created an atmosphere of angry tension in the house. Mildred also criticized Brendan for being cold, unemotional, and unfeeling. She blamed it on his "hypocritical WASP family" that had trained him to be "just like them."

Mildred insisted that her mother-in-law was "a drunk" and that the family "protects the old harridan by acting as though she's perfectly normal." When asked to estimate his mother's alcohol intake, Brendan blandly guessed "maybe a fifth of scotch every other day or so." With this evidence, we agreed with Mildred that his mother was an alcoholic. We also explained how his family maintained their denial through the family rules: *don't* feel; *don't* talk; *don't* change. Anyone who violated the rules faced ostracism and exile. Brendan was angry and canceled their next three appointments.

When they came back in, Brendan's denial was no longer working for him. He had "kissed the concrete of reality." His mother, in a drunken stupor, had made a scene at a family gathering. Brendan now realized she was an alcoholic.

In our sessions, Brendan told of childhood episodes of coming home from school to find his mother unconscious on the living room couch or slumped over the kitchen table. One incident in particular spoke eloquently to the level of the family's denial. His father had come home from work in the early afternoon to find Brendan's mother and Brendan's Uncle Ivan tipsy after "having a few cocktails." Angry, the father silently went to the refrigerator to get ice to prepare himself a drink. When he opened the refrigerator door he found the ice tray empty. Brendan's father exploded in rage, scattering the contents of the refrigerator onto the kitchen floor because "nobody ever fills up the goddamned ice trays after they empty them." No mention was made of his wife's intoxicated state, or of his brother's unexplained presence on a weekday afternoon. The incident was never mentioned again.

As an adult, Brendan's father could escape the intolerable home situation by retreating to the office and working long hours. Being a child, Brendan couldn't. As an adult, though, he followed his father's example and spent as much time at work as possible. The family rules of don't feel, don't speak, and don't change produced the manager, husband, and father characterized as cold, unfeeling, undemonstrative, rigid, harsh, and demanding. Brendan's blood pressure was a silent reflection of the stressful job and home he created for himself through his behavior.

ACCEPTANCE

Self-improvement has long been an American preoccupation. Sometimes even perfect isn't good enough for the gurus of motivational pop psychology. Many of our clients have put themselves and their loved ones through torture by demanding more of themselves and their loved ones than they can possibly give.

Lower Your Standards

Our counter to the cult of perfectionism is, "Lower your standards and relax. You don't have to be perfect." Accepting someone we love "as is" is one of the greatest gifts we can give them and ourselves. If you're unhappy with loved ones, lower your expectations and accept them for who and what they are. Let go of your ideas of perfection, particularly as they apply to other people. Accepting your loved ones, however, doesn't mean you have to accept what they *do*.

Had Brendan been able to accept his mother's lack of perfection, he wouldn't have denied her alcoholism. The problem would have been addressed and, perhaps, resolved many years before it was.

Supporting Other Family Members

Support is the sincerest form of acceptance. Support means understanding what members of your family are going through and letting them know that it's all right for them to feel the way they do. It's not insisting that they be different. It's saying you know who they are and where they are and that you love them. Too often we confuse support with cheering someone up when they're down and trying to make them feel good. That's not support. It's an attempt to make ourselves feel better. We say things such as, "Don't be mad," and "Don't cry," because we feel uncomfortable when people are upset. A friend told us that when his mother died, his aunt came up to him at the funeral and told him, "Your father is crying. Do something about it." He said, "What do you want me to do about it? Doesn't he have a right to cry?" Remember, people have the right to feel upset or bad, so accept their feelings.

Taking Responsibility for Your Own Feelings

Everyone is responsible for his own feelings and no one else's. When we assume responsibility for someone else's happiness, we communicate a lack of respect for their competence as human beings. By the same token, you can't expect anyone else to be responsible for your happiness. It is a crushing and frustrating burden for that person and it disempowers you. If a loved one is not happy, don't assume it's your fault, nor is it his or her fault if you are not happy.

SKILLS FOR COPING WITH FAMILY STRESS

There are a few vital skills necessary for dealing with family stress. These include:

- *Communication.* Practice using the guidelines we

outlined earlier in this chapter to develop your communication skills. You might also be interested in reading Deborah Tannen's book[3] on communication styles and how they affect relationships.

• *Self-assertion.* Skill in asserting yourself, graciously, appropriately, but firmly, is vital in maintaining productive and rewarding interpersonal relationships. You don't want to be a hostile, aggressive ogre, but you don't want to be a wimp either. Assertive skills keep you somewhere in the middle. They are invaluable in any situation in which you have to deal with other people. They're worth their weight in gold in the family situation. You might read Manuel Smith's *When I Say No, I Feel Guilty* and Jacubowski and Lange's *The Assertive Option* for more on how to develop your assertive skills.[4, 5]

• *Conflict resolution.* There's nothing like a family fight and they happen all the time. If a family never disagrees, quarrels, or fights, something's wrong. The problem is not the conflict itself but learning how to resolve conflicts. We gave you some of the guidelines we suggest to our clients earlier in this chapter. Go back and take another look at them. Conflict is inherent in any situation involving people. You can improve the quality of all of your interpersonal relationships by sharpening your conflict-resolution skills, but they're particularly important in the family setting.

• *Parenting.* You're not born knowing how to be a parent, you need to learn. There are many wonderful books on child rearing. Most communities have parenting workshops you can attend. Also check with your child's school and pediatrician for recommendations.

• *Forbearance.* Sometimes we just have to put up with people, and we all have family members who fall into that category. Accept the fact that they're not going to change and you'll have to live with them as they are. Forbearance is a skill that improves dramatically with practice. It's liberating not to have to worry about how other people behave.

• *Get organized.* Getting a family organized is like running a small business. If the daily tasks are organized and routine, everything is easier. Have a schedule for meal preparation and cleanup, transportation needs, and chores. Hang a big calendar in the kitchen for posting events and upcoming commitments. Have a place for leaving notes and messages. A blackboard over the phone is marvelous. Organize household storage or work space (with labels if necessary) so that things are where you can find them. When your space overflows, don't get more storage. When in doubt, throw it out, or recycle it to others who may need it. Make a plan for the exchange of money so that each transaction does not create an argument. Find time for brief "staff meetings" to update everyone on the inevitable changes in the system.

• *Financial budgeting.* Family finances can be problematic when they get out of hand. It doesn't take a lot of skill to sit the family down around the table and list the money that comes in and the money that goes out. Yet, many families don't do this. Be mindful that differences in basic values surface during discussions about money. Your conflicts with money interact with other family members' competing needs. As a result, many families never face the budget openly. Instead, they fight over each purchase. Getting those figures together can be a chore, but do it. They are central to the budgeting process. You can't get started without them. Negotiate who contributes how much, and how money is to be allocated. Set aside what you need for fixed-cost essentials, such as mortgage or automobile payments. Next, set aside what you estimate will be needed for variable-cost essentials such as food, fuel, clothing, repairs, cleaning, etc. If there's anything left, negotiate allocations for nonessentials, luxury items, savings, and investments. Teenagers and adult children living in the home who have an income should be included in this planning.

• *Sharing.* Fairly allocating common resources is a key part of family life, drawing people closer in mutual interdependence. All members benefit from sharing tangible resources such as space, food, and money, as well as the work involved in keeping a household functioning. An old proverb says, "Many hands make light work." Discussing ideas, feelings, and experiences, whether difficult or pleasurable, creates a bond of understanding among family members. On the other hand, too much sharing may mean little privacy, conflict over personal ownership and competition for scarce resources. What is the balance in your family? Correctly weighing communal life and privacy doesn't come naturally. You may have to work on it.

RESOURCES FOR COPING WITH FAMILY STRESS

• *Your extended family.* This is often the first resource people tap. It can be either easy or hard, depending on your relationship with your relatives. This resource depends on trust and reciprocity to function. Don't borrow money you can't pay back or incur obligations you don't want to reciprocate. Don't allow resentments over an imbalance of exchange to ruin these most important relationships. And don't pull your extended-family relatives into an internal family feud.

• *Family therapy.* Sometimes family stress and family problems get so far out of hand that you need help. Family therapy can be of great assistance in getting your life back on track and running smoothly. Family therapists are trained specifically in family therapy. They come from diverse professional backgrounds—psychology, social work, psychiatry, and pastoral counseling, to name a few. In selecting a family therapist, interview several before you make up your mind. Check their credentials and experience, particularly with the kinds of problems your family is having. You might even ask for references. A family therapist shouldn't take sides in family conflicts or problems; rather, the focus should be on the problems and their resolution. Everyone should be comfortable in the situation and not feel under attack if the therapist is doing his or her job.

• *Assertiveness training.* Assertiveness training is usually conducted in group settings and is offered by a variety of mental health facilities, clinics, hospitals, and community organizations. They generally involve didactic lectures and role-playing, sometimes videotaped for playback, in which you apply the concepts from the lectures to your personal situation. Call your local mental health facility or state psychological association for a referral to a group in your area.

• *Bibliotherapy.* Self-help books are available on many facets of family stress. Check your local bookstore or library for books on your particular family stress points. We have listed a number of them in appendix II.

• *Legal system.* When all else fails, there are always the police and the courts. Where violence, drug abuse, criminal activity, or physical abuse is creating stress in the family and all other efforts have failed, call 911. If the time has come to dissolve your marriage, get a divorce lawyer. When child support is insufficient, delinquent, or lacking entirely, seek out the appropriate agency in your area and institute proceedings.

• *The welfare system and private charitable organizations.* The federal government and all states have systems for supporting families in need. In addition are many charitable organizations that aid families. If you need help, ask for it. It can lift you over a rough spot and give you the time to regroup and get back on your feet.

NOTES

1. Beck, A. (1988), *Love Is Never Enough*, New York, Harper & Row.

2. Smith, M. (1975), *When I Say No, I Feel Guilty*, New York, Bantam.

3. Tannen, D. (1990), *You Just Don't Understand*, New York, Ballantine.

———. (1990), *That's Not What I Meant! How Conversational Style Makes or Breaks Your Relations with Others*, New York, Ballantine.

4. Smith, M. (1975), *When I Say No, I Feel Guilty*, New York, Bantam.

5. Jakubowski, P., and Lange, A. (1978), *The Assertive Option*, Champaign, IL, Research Press.

7 OVERCOMING PERSONAL STRESS

Personal stress develops from situations that affect your relationship with yourself. A strong and positive sense of self is a powerful asset in coping with the stresses of life. Events or experiences that shake your self-image have a negative impact on your ability to overcome external challenges in your life. Being uncomfortable with how you see yourself is also a major stress point.

Personal stress comes from success and achievement or personal setbacks and failures. Trauma such as an injury or illness, being assaulted or robbed, or minor violations of the law, such as a speeding ticket, test your endurance and well-being, thereby creating personal doubts, self-examination, anxiety, depression, and illness. Worries about attractiveness, weight, aging, or physical changes in your body as a result of injury, illness, or time destroys peace of mind and affects your relationships with yourself and other people.

Personal stress is difficult to address with self-help measures. You're so close to the concerns causing your stress, they're hard to see. Often, you're unaware that stress influences how you see yourself and how you feel about what you see. And even when you become aware of personal stress, you're often so enmeshed with its causes that you feel powerless to do anything.

FAILURE TO MEET OBLIGATIONS TO YOURSELF

The most pervasive aspect of personal stress in our clients is trying to meet their obligations to themselves. Some of our clients feel guilty about being "selfish" while being resentful about getting "short-changed" by life. This conflict is created by your being overly involved with career, family, fame, fortune, the needs of others, or maintaining your lifestyle; you are never alone, or get personal things done, or pursue your personal goals and aspirations. It comes from your feelings of failing to live up to what you really are, for giving up your dreams, for "selling out," or "settling." Shakespeare expresses this universal truth in Hamlet, "And this above all: To thine own self be true."

Loss of self-esteem and self-respect or regaining it is a persistent theme in art. Edward Hopper's painting *Boulevard of Broken Dreams* and Arthur Miller's play *Death of a Salesman* illustrate how loss of self-esteem and self-respect makes life empty and meaningless. The movie *Rocky*, on the other hand, portrays the joy, elation, and deep satisfaction that come from following your dreams and living up to your potential.

LOSS OF PERSONAL AUTONOMY

Limitations on personal freedom—going where they want, when they want, and how they want—and autonomy are the second most common type of personal stress affecting our clients. Personal freedom is central to most of us. Biological limits on personal autonomy are particularly troublesome for women. An unwanted pregnancy, for some women, is like nine months in jail. Sexual difficulties or starting menopause can be equally stressful.

Jail or prison terms, by definition, threaten or limit our personal autonomy and freedom. Changes in recreational or religious activities often reflect a loss of freedom of choice. Limitations on our personal autonomy are so stressful for us that we will fight against them to the death rather than tolerate them. The New Hampshire state motto, for instance, is "Live Free or Die."

LIFE CHANGES

Change always creates stress and life always involves change. Change is an inevitable part of normal development and growth. As we grow and mature from childhood to adolescence to adulthood to maturity and senescence, we go through changes in residence, in our living conditions, and in our personal habits, interpersonal relationships, and recreational activities. These changes involve leaving something familiar and moving on to something new and unsettling in its uncertainty.

Often, the demands and pressures of life changes create further personal stress by diverting our energies and resources. Sometimes we have difficulty meeting our obligations to ourselves. Drug and alcohol problems develop as we seek relief from the stress.

PERSONAL APPEARANCE

In our culture, we overemphasize looks and appearances. If you compare yourself to the airbrushed, slick magazine versions of masculine or feminine "perfection," you're bound to be disappointed. Nobody looks like that. Many of our clients try, and end up feeling miserable when they fail.

The narcissism of failed perfectionism is a particularly difficult area of personal stress, because it leads us to feel ugly, undesirable, fat, or old and worn out. One client, Michelle, was devastated when we pointed out that her distress over her "faults" was a bigger issue than the "faults" themselves. She saw her perfectionism as a "character flaw" that would prevent her from being as perfect as she really "should" be.

Allegra's reaction to breast-reduction surgery illustrates how these problems generate stress in all areas of life. Referred to us by her family physician, Allegra was depressed and suicidal because she was convinced that her husband, Dante—a "very handsome man" several years younger than she—was going to leave her because she was "old and ugly."

Even in her depressed and saddened condition, Allegra was still attractive, dressed well, and looked considerably younger than her 48 years. We wondered what her mirror was telling her that we weren't seeing.

When we spoke to Dante he seemed genuinely surprised to hear Allegra's fears. He denied wanting to leave, insisting, "She's not just a beautiful woman, she's a lovely person and I love her." He admitted to recent tension in the relationship and indicated that they had quarreled "more over nothing" in the last year or so than in their previous five years put together.

As we talked, Dante realized that everything had been "fine" between them until Allegra's breast-reduction surgery. Allegra had been big busted since she was a teenager. Proud of her breasts, Allegra had received a lot of male attention because of them. In her late thirties and early forties, however, she had gained weight, and had developed chronic upper-back pain due to the increased weight of her breasts. She tried losing weight, wearing special bras, doing exercises to strengthen her upper back, and taking medication for her pain. Nothing worked. Finally, on the advice of her doctor, she turned to breast-reduction surgery.

Afterward, she was horrified by the results. She hated the shape of her new breasts. They seemed odd-looking: one was "perky," the other "sagged." Her scars were bigger and more noticeable than she had expected. She felt "disfigured and ugly." She was furious at her surgeon. Although Allegra never talked about it to her husband, she thought Dante felt the same way.

Allegra tried to conceal her "disfigurement" with loose-fitting clothing. She refused to let Dante see her undressed. She even hated the way she looked with clothes on. She became obsessed with her "ugliness" and increasingly fearful that her husband would leave her.

The first *Action Plan* we worked out with Allegra was for her to get a padded bra and to start wearing nice clothes. Next, we set up a thought-stopping program, restricting Allegra's thoughts about her body between 11:00 A.M. and 4:00 P.M. and between 8:00 P.M. and 10:00 P.M. Along with this, we had her schedule an hour of "mourning"—from 5:00 P.M. to 6:00 P.M.—where she was to think of nothing else but her body and her feelings about her surgery. In a couple of weeks she started feeling better about herself.

Allegra and Dante scheduled daily talks about her body and his feelings about her. We had her look in her mirror, write down ten things other than her breasts that she liked about her body, and discuss them with Dante. Allegra found that she liked her hair, her teeth, her eyes, and the shape of her nose. Surprisingly, she found that Dante liked her eyes and her smile and had never really thought much about her breasts. We extended her thought-stopping program to include thoughts of Dante leaving her.

We then had Allegra write a letter to her surgeon expressing her anger and disappointment over her surgery. The letter didn't change anything, but she felt much better. Allegra scheduled an appointment with another doctor to explore the possibility of a surgical repair, but didn't keep it after deciding, "it's not bad enough to go through that again."

Allegra and Dante's marriage is back on track. Her depression has lifted. Allegra's focus has changed from staying the way she was to enjoying the way she is. She's a lot happier now and has dropped her painful focus on being perfect.

PERSONAL SUCCESS

Most of us are taught that success is our reward for hard work. Success, however, often brings demands from yourself and/or others that you continue achieving at that same high level. That's not always possible. Success often brings changes in lifestyle and self-image that are difficult to maintain unless you continue performing at that same high level.

When you're successful, there are the problems of what to do for an encore and how to cope with the personal stress that comes with your success. Drugs and alcohol are frequent solutions. Many sucessful people would agree with comedian Richard Pryor when he said, "Cocaine is God's way of telling you you've got too much money."

PERSONAL TRAGEDY

The stress that occurs from physical changes due to aging—hair loss, weight gain or loss, diminished athletic or sexual prowess, injuries or scars—can be particularly severe when they result from personal tragedies such as accidents or illness.

When you're maimed, disabled, or disfigured by trauma or illness, there's more stress involved than from the damage to self alone. Many times, tragedy makes it difficult or impossible to do what you used to do that you identified as part of yourself. A disabled athlete like Bo Jackson has to deal with the personal stress of living with an infirmity and no longer being a professional athlete. If his primary personal identity was as an athlete, the stress could be intolerable.

PHILOSOPHICAL CONCERNS

Most people have their own ideas and convictions about how the world works and their place in it. Some of us are rigid and unyielding about our particular views and myth systems while others are flexible and frequently change their views.

Philosophical or religious preoccupations, questions about our basic beliefs and concepts, and concerns about right and wrong and personal morality, make up an element of personal stress. Our views relating to these basic issues are part and parcel of who and what we are. When they are challenged by circumstances, ourselves, or others, the threat is to something basic and vital about ourselves.

ALTERING PERSONAL STRESS

The key to handling personal stress is to build your self-esteem. Write a list of ten things you like about yourself. Pay yourself compliments: "I really did a good job on that"; "I may not be the best, but I'm awfully close." If you have difficulty accepting compliments, keep practicing until you can. Look at yourself in the mirror and say the things to yourself that would make you feel good if someone else said them to you. Another way of limiting your personal stress is to try looking at your situation from a less immediate perspective. Take a long-term view of life, particularly your own. Nothing in your life is wasted; every experience prepares you to cope with situations later on.

Look at your parents' lives or their friends' lives. Draw on older people's experiences for examples of how changing your perspective can reduce the stress of your current situations. Two books we often recommend in this regard are *Passages*, by Gail Sheehy, and *Seasons of a Man's Life*, by Daniel Levinson.[1,2]

Be assertive about your personal privacy, freedom, and autonomy. Examine your goals and directions, and make sure you're doing what you want to do, going where you want to go. Are your goals your own or someone else's?

Decide what you want to be doing and where you want to be in five years, then figure out what will get you there. This can be tough on relationships. You may have to decide which is more important, the relationship or your freedom.

If you're feeling bad about not meeting obligations to yourself or berating yourself for being a failure and not having lived up to your potential, take time out for a reality check. With whom are you competing? To whom are you comparing yourself? Young people often compare themselves to people ten or twenty years older. Whose aspirations are you reaching for—yours or someone else's? Your parents'? Your spouse's? Your teachers'? How much of your feelings of failure have to do with disappointing others? Quit competing, quit comparing yourself to others, and follow your dreams. Make a list of your achievements, successes, and accomplishments. Chances are you'll be pleasantly surprised at how much you've done.

How much of your personal stress has to do with impossibly high standards others have set for you or you've set for yourself? How much comes from overestimating your talents, abilities, and capacities? Do you tend to overestimate, underestimate, or accurately estimate what you can and cannot do? Get in touch with reality. Ask someone you trust and respect for an honest appraisal of your abilities. Consult a career counselor or headhunter. If you've got it, go for it. If you don't, back off on your standards and give yourself a break.

If too much success is the problem, just slow down. You don't have to aspire to an image of success. You don't have to exhaust yourself to live up to your past achievements. Take it easy and don't assume more than you can handle. You don't have to live up to someone else's ideas on how much is enough or what you should do with success when you get it. You might want to take a look at whether your advancement is worth the hassles it brings.

Sometimes success loses friends, arouses jealousies, or makes enemies. Greg, for example, was deeply hurt that his best friend for years, Jeremy, was jealous of his good fortune. Jeremy sarcastically referred to Greg as his "rich and famous friend." Another client of ours made numerous enemies in his company when he was promoted over them. Sometimes success can be more than you can bear.

Altering personal stress can be a daunting task and everyone needs a little help with it from time to time. Tap your friends or family. If you need more support, get in touch with a good counselor or therapist.

AVOIDING PERSONAL STRESS

The first step here is to stay away from people and situations that place unreasonable and unwelcome demands on your time and limit your personal freedom. Avoid people and situations that leave you feeling bad about yourself. Don't buy into someone else's ideas about who you are and what you should or should not be doing with your life.

You don't want to avoid success, just the stress it creates. So, limits the changes success creates in your life. And don't make too many changes at once.

Prepare for the developmental changes that will occur over the course of your lifetime. Foresight is an invaluable means of avoiding stress. If you know what to expect, you can plan for change, making it less stressful when it happens. You will get older, you will be less beautiful, you won't be as quick or as strong. The transitions, however, will be gradual and you'll have plenty of time to adjust. The better prepared you are for them, the less stressful they'll be for you.

Don't have unrealistically high expectations for yourself. Be the best you can be. But you'll make yourself miserable if you anticipate too much. You'll agonize about not being other than what you are and create unnecessary pain for yourself. Try to see the humor in your personal situation, and don't take yourself too seriously.

ACCEPTING PERSONAL STRESS

Life isn't fair and bad things happen to good people. Personal loss and tragedy are a part of life and are always stressful. We can't alter or avoid them. Our only option is to accept them when they happen and move on.

In her book *On Death and Dying*, Elisabeth Kubler-Ross defined the phases of grief we experience with personal losses and tragedies.[3] The first phase we go through is disbelief. We deny the loss or tragedy; we can't believe it could happen to us. We clutch at straws that prove it didn't really happen.

Next we go through a bargaining phase. We try to make deals with people we want to believe have the power to change events so that they didn't really happen. We call on our gods, our doctors, our politicians, or our powerful friends to intercede. We have fantasies of turning back the clock and taking steps to prevent the occurrence of our particular personal loss or tragedy.

Then comes anger. "It's not fair" is the watchword here. We need to blame and punish someone else. We search for scapegoats and rail at our fate. We elevate our blood pressure as we angrily search for ways to "get even." Much of the anger we experience during this phase is directed at ourselves for having been so "stupid," for not having been sufficiently superhuman to have foreseen and avoided the loss or tragedy.

Grief and depression come with the realization that the loss or tragedy did occur, that bargaining won't change anything, and that your anger and rage are useless. That is the most devastating phase in adjustment to tragedy or loss. It's the time when suicide most frequently occurs, when stress-related illnesses erupt, when we're barely able to cope with the ongoing stresses of everyday living. It's an extremely painful but necessary phase. There's no way to avoid it. In fact, denial of the grief and depression only compounds the problem. Denial or avoidance makes the final, healing phase more difficult to complete. Don't go for the antidepressant medication. Look at your misery as a positive experience; it leads to acceptance of your personal loss and tragedy and a return to inner peace.

The final phase of adjustment is acceptance. You'll get to it sooner and easier if you have philosophical or religious beliefs that help you integrate tragic events into a perspective of life as an unfolding process. Accept yourself for who and what you are, imperfections and all. Lower your standards to a realistic level. Good enough is good enough. Look yourself in the eye and tell yourself that you don't have to be perfect. Accept the fact that those romantic, idealized visions are just that and have little to do with who and what you are.

SKILLS FOR COPING WITH PERSONAL STRESS

Self-Discovery Skills

Discovering who and what you really are is a lifelong process. The key to self-discovery is honesty—with yourself. Take a few hours when you will be undisturbed and take an honest look at yourself. Tell yourself that whatever you find will be okay. Be truthful with yourself about your wishes and desires, fears and angers. Get your feelings out on the table and be comfortable with them.

If you're feeling blue, don't get depressed and agitated because you "shouldn't" be. Accept it and do something about it. One of our friends say that when she gets the blues, she gets into a warm bath, thinks about her miseries, and she has a good cry. She says it makes her feel a lot better. She understands that occasionally feeling blue means she has a well-rounded emotional life.

Don't overdo it. Remember your discoveries, but don't obsess about them. Otherwise, it becomes a little too easy to paralyze yourself with self-doubt and narcissism.

Self-Assertion Skills

Assertiveness is an important skill for dealing with personal stress. If you're not assertive, you'll be taken advantage of by your nearest and dearest. You'll spend a lot of time regretting your inaction. One patient described himself as a "gutless wimp" because he could never speak up when other people put him down.

One of our clients, Donna, felt bad about "being only a housewife" after having worked as a marketing director at a bank. She and her husband, Ari, a newly appointed professor at a Boston university, were subjected to a seemingly endless series of welcoming social events and cocktail parties. Everyone knew of her husband and his accomplishments. When asked about herself and what she did, Donna would apologetically reply, "Oh, I'm just a housewife." A common reaction was, "That's too bad. It must be awfully boring for you." Donna would feel crushed. And for days afterward she'd berate herself for not having defended her choice to stay home.

After working with us on her assertiveness skills, Donna hit on just the right tack at the next dinner party. When she was asked what she did, Donna made her usual reply. When the "Oh, that's too bad" comment came back, she said, "It's given me more time for myself than what I was doing before." That easily led into discussion of her former as well as current interests. Donna felt great that people now knew about her accomplishments but felt even better for standing up for herself and being graciously assertive.

If you're having problems being appropriately assertive, look at a couple of the books on assertiveness we've mentioned in other sections. We recommend *Your Perfect Right*, by Alberti and Emmons, and *When I Say No, I Feel Guilty*, by M. Smith.[4, 5] They'll give you some great tips on how to overcome uncertainty and anxiety when faced with disagreements.

Goal-Setting Skills

Before you can deal with personal stress you have to know what it is that you want to accomplish. If you're not sure, sit down and think about it for a while. Once you've come up with your overall goal, set up subgoals that will lead you to achieve it. Don't start until you know what it is you want to accomplish for yourself and how you want to go about it.

Reality-Testing Skills

Keep your goals within the bounds of reason. Don't try to do the impossible or irrational. Check with friends to see if they think your goals make sense. Make use of experts. Reality testing is a skill that can be developed. Sharpen yours and use it before you jump into anything that may backfire on you and create more stress than it eliminates. A good *Stress Action Plan* is one that really helps the situation. Your reality-testing skills help determine if your plan is a good one.

Cognitive-Flexibility Skills

Stay flexible as you try to work out a course of action that will reduce your personal stress. If your first plan doesn't work, think of something else. Be on guard about getting into a thinking rut, particularly about yourself. Brainstorm with yourself about yourself. Put limits on your internal censor and explore some of those "wild" thoughts that may come into your consciousness if you let them. Some of them might turn out to be just the ideas you need.

Behavioral-Flexibility Skills

Flexibility should be extended to your actions as well. If you always do what you've always done, you'll always get what you've always got. David Burns's *Intimate Connections* has a number of techniques for overcoming the fears and confusions that often underlie the behavioral rigidities that keep us acting the same ways in the same situations, causing the same stresses and strains that make life more miserable than it need be.[6]

Self-Acceptance Skills

It may seem strange to think of self-acceptance as a skill, but it is. Like all skills, it takes practice and application to keep it sharp and working. One way to develop and maintain self-acceptance skills is to look in the mirror and say out loud, "You're just fine just the way you are," or to echo the cartoon character Popeye: "I ams what I ams and that's all what I am. I'm (———), the (———) woman/man."

Self-Esteem Enhancement Skills

If you don't feel good about yourself, you need to develop some self-esteem enhancement skills. One way is to say some positive things about yourself. Look in your mirror and tell yourself how good you are. It may seem silly at first, but affirmations have a way of catching on. You'll have to keep at it for a couple of weeks or so, but you'll be surprised how much better you feel.

Another way is to write a list of five good aspects about yourself every night before you go to sleep for a week. No repeats. At the end of the week, pick out the ones you like best, make a new list, and stick it on your mirror or someplace where you'll see it frequently.

For more on self-esteem enhancement we suggest you read David Burns's *Feeling Good*.[7] It will help you get away from thinking about yourself in negative terms and put you through a string of exercises that will enhance your self-esteem.

Organizational Skills

Organizational skills are important in keeping ourselves together, in making sure we save enough time for ourselves, and in ensuring that we have sufficient resources to be good to ourselves. Our friend who finds crying in a hot bath important in accepting her blue periods has organized her life well enough that she has the time to do that.

You can't set priorities or achieve goals if you don't get organized. We recommend making a list to get yourself organized. Make sure you schedule times for self-examination, crying in a hot bath, sleeping late on the weekends, or just "vegging out" in front of the TV. "If you don't have time for yourself, you're going to experience personal stress; you have to be organized to find time."

AIDS FOR COPING WITH PERSONAL STRESS

Personal stress is difficult no matter how many skills you have for dealing with it. Most of us need outside help to enhance our personal skills and address specific stress concerns. Outside help includes the following:

Psychotherapy

Psychotherapy increases your awareness of deep-seated psychological problems, minimizes the emotional "baggage" you carry, and helps you develop a more realistic view of yourself and your relationship to the rest of the world.

Ask your family physician for a referral to a psychotherapist, or contact your state psychological association, state psychiatric association, or state social work association. Get at least three referrals and interview these therapists before you begin any therapy with one of them. The best indicator of whether a therapist is the right one for you is your degree of trust of him or her. If you're not comfortable or find a therapist difficult to talk to, move on. You owe it to yourself to get that right therapist.

Cognitive-Behavioral Therapy

Cognitive-behavioral therapy focuses on the irrational thoughts and ideas that lead to a loss of self-esteem and create self-defeating attitudes. Changing the way you think makes it possible for you to change the way you feel and behave. Check with your local mental health professional organizations for an appropriate referral.

Counseling

Sometimes you don't really need therapy, you need to talk about your problems and get professional advice on what you should do and how you might do it. Again, check with your local mental health professional organizations for a referral to a counselor.

Group Therapy

Group therapy can be helpful in establishing a realistic view of yourself. Other group members' reactions and comments may provide you with ideas and viewpoints about yourself that you never would have thought about in other settings. One of the powerful elements in group therapy is that you can get good ideas about your impact on other people without jeopardizing existing relationships or creating psychological vulnerabilities for you in your everyday life.

Bibliotherapy

We have been impressed by the proliferation of excellent self-help books in the past few years and make bibliotherapy a regular element in our treatment programs. There is a list of the ones we think are particularly good, organized by category, in appendix II. Since you're reading this self-help book, you must have some faith in bibliotherapy. Take a look at our suggestions—you might find something that's perfect for you and your personal stress points.

N O T E S

1. Sheehy, G. (1976), *Passages: Predictable Crises of Adult Life*, New York, Dutton.

2. Levinson, D. (1978), *Seasons of a Man's Life*, New York, Knopf.

3. Kubler-Ross, E. (1969), *On Death and Dying*, New York, Macmillan.

4. Alberti, R., and Emmons, M. (1982), *Your Perfect Right: A Guide to Assertive Living*, San Luis Obispo, CA, Impact Publishers.

5. Smith, M. (1975), *When I Say No, I Feel Guilty*, New York, Bantam.

6. Burns, D. (1985), *Intimate Connections*, New York, Signet.

7. Burns, D. (1980), *Feeling Good: The New Mood Therapy*, New York, New American Library.

8 DEALING WITH SOCIAL STRESS

Social stress comes in many different shapes and sizes. Social estrangement and isolation, what the great sociologist Emile Durkheim termed *anomie*, is perhaps the most prevalent. Social and geographic mobility have brought a sense of freedom, autonomy, and liberty to Americans but not without cost.

It is not unusual for people to move hundreds or even thousands of miles for college or career. Each move brings a fresh sense of social estrangement and isolation. Old relationships end, new relationships begin. People feel disconnected, unwanted, and alone. As relationships are stretched by social and geographic distance, special care is needed to maintain them. Often this effort cannot be maintained.

Loneliness is the clearest sign of social isolation. It strikes when we lose our sense of connectedness with people who understand us, when we lose a good friend or partner, or when life changes disrupt our social networks. You can combat loneliness by rebuilding your sense of connectedness. That's never easy, but if you're shy, socially anxious, or have limited social skills, building networks can be overwhelming.

Jerri had been lonely ever since she moved to Boston from Indiana. Her family had lived in the same community for years and she knew everyone in town. Jerri and her two sisters were popular and led active social lives.

The transition from high school to college had been easy. She attended a local college with several longtime friends and lived at home the first two years. Her first job after college was as a local journalist. Jerri always felt she belonged. When she went into town or to the mall, she usually ran into people she knew. She was accustomed to the phone ringing and a steady calendar of social activities.

Jerri came to graduate school in Boston to further her journalistic career. At first she relished the anonymity of the big city but that soon changed. She made few friends in school and worked hard in her courses. Homesick, she spent a lot of time on the phone with friends and family.

After a while, Jerri started to build a social network. She attended a number of church and school functions. She made a few more friends, but something was missing. It all seemed so superficial and transient.

After getting her master's degree in journalism, Jerri took a job with a public relations firm. Soon thereafter, she began experiencing physical and mental stress symptoms. She became increasingly depressed and lonely and started gaining weight. Tension headaches and upper-back pain forced her to seek medical help. Her physician referred her to us.

Jerri's *Stress Audit* results and her personal history made it clear that social estrangement and isolation were her major problems. Accustomed to a rich and varied social network at home, Jerri felt close only to her boyfriend and to her roommate in Boston. Unhappy in her job, she made no attempt to befriend her co-workers.

Jerri had great social skills. She could talk to anyone. Her problem was developing a deep sense of connectedness with other people. Because a meaningful social network was so important to her, Jerri presented a polished, "perfect" social appearance. She couldn't relax and just be herself with people. The harder she tried, the more tense she got.

It was difficult for Jerri to admit to herself that she had no "real" friends. Her feelings of depression made it even harder to make friends because telling the truth meant expressing negative feelings, which meant she was less than perfect.

Another problem was finding people she could relate to, who shared similar values. As we talked, she realized that she clung to the small-town values of her childhood, disdaining the materialism and fast pace of the big city. For Jerri, a move back home seemed the best long-term solution, and that's what she finally resolved to do. She decided she wasn't a "big-city girl after all."

Issues of social alienation and isolation are particularly difficult for ethnic and racial minorities. One of our colleagues, Eddie, was elected to the Phi Beta Kappa Society at a predominantly white liberal-arts college. As the only black person at the induction ceremony and banquet, he told us he had felt like "a blackbird sitting in a snowbank" and was miserable during what was for everyone else a moment of pride and achievement. Now a highly respected professional, Eddie doesn't feel as isolated as he did back then. He belongs to a number of professional organizations and is active in community affairs and local politics.

There are certain times when we are at greater risk for social isolation—after a move, after a change of status, or during times of other stress. A change of residence isolates you from even the simple social connection of being recognized at the corner grocery store. Leaving home for school or a job strips you of an identity built up over many years.

A change of status also leads to social isolation. In a divorce, who gets the friends is often as traumatic as who gets the house. Going from having a partner to being single may mean having to build a new social network. Moving from student to worker or from a child-free couple to parents with small children can dramatically affect your social life. Changes in financial status may affect recreational activities—dropping softball for golf as you move up the corporate ladder—further removing you from old friends. New job interests may mean that friends grow apart.

Special times of stress may bring friends closer or may mean neglect of friendships. An illness or tragedy may increase contact with a few good friends. More often, though, we retreat during difficult periods, concentrating on survival and coping. We don't have the time or energy to cultivate old or new acquaintances. When both partners in a family are working, neither may have the time to spend socializing on the telephone or planning special events.

People who feel shame about some aspect of their lives are especially vulnerable to social isolation. Their shame may be about someone in their family, for instance an alcoholic mother or a grandfather with mental illness, or it may be personal, such as a history of rape or sexual abuse. People feel ashamed about many things, often what others shrug off as unfortunate. One person may feel acute shame about financial loss while another thinks it's merely inconvenient. One woman can accept having an abortion or giving up a child for adoption, while another feels a terrible shame about it.

For people with shameful secrets, letting anyone in to know the details of their lives is threatening. Fear of being found out and fear of rejection hampers relaxed social interaction. As long as the guard is up to protect the secret, intimate social conversations are tense and fraught with danger.

THE STRESS OF SOCIAL OBLIGATIONS

The support and feeling of connectedness that comes from a solid social network is powerful, but you can have too much of a good thing. Belonging to a group brings obligations that take up considerable time, energy, and resources. For some, however, the costs far outweigh the benefits.

Being identified as the leader or spokesperson for a group can be particularly stressful. Being responsible for or to a social group can become an unwanted burden. Leading a group can be a frustrating experience. Often you feel a need to follow along with a group consensus even though it's against your better judgment. Sometimes being the leader of one group can exclude you from other groups. As a leader, you often end up with too much work and don't enjoy the freedoms and privileges of other group members.

One of our clients, Claudia, had particular problems with the stress of social obligations. Claudia enjoyed her social life and belonged to a number of religious, civic, and social groups. She went to synagogue regularly and was active in Hadassah. She was a leading fund-raiser for her local museum and a member of its board of trustees.

She entertained regularly and often gave small dinner parties. Even though she worked part time in her husband Arthur's business, she talked on the phone daily to her friends. When Arthur joined the country club for business and social reasons, Claudia became chairperson of the social and entertainment committee.

Then Claudia got pregnant and had twins. She had looked forward to having children and now her life was just perfect. Or was it? Her social obligations wouldn't go away. After a few weeks of rest, Hadassah, the museum, the country club, and her friends expected her to pick up where she had left off. Claudia just wanted to stay home with the twins but felt she couldn't say no to these groups and friends.

In a short time, Claudia was exhausted and "stressed out of my gourd." Referred by a friend, she came to us for help. Claudia knew her problem—something had to go. But she didn't know what, or how to do it.

We had her list the pluses and minuses for each group, the upside, downside exercise. Afterward, Claudia understood clearly that the museum and the country club took up too much time. But how to tell them? We enrolled her in an assertiveness training group and had her read Manuel Smith's *When I Say No, I Feel Guilty*.[1] We role-played how Claudia could graciously decline offices and memberships without closing the door on future involvements or hurting anyone's feelings.

Once she straightened out her priorities and repaired some basic social skills, Claudia handled her social demands and obligations well. The twins are now in school, and Claudia has increased her level of social activity again. But this time she knows how to keep it from getting out of hand.

Odessa's social demands were somewhat different from Claudia's but just as burdensome. Odessa had raised seven children, two grandchildren, and helped out with neighborhood children whose mothers worked outside the home. She belonged to a close-knit black community centered around her church and neighborhood. This network of kinship and friendship was an important source of emotional and practical support for her family. However, it often seemed to demand more than she could handle.

Whenever someone was sick, Odessa felt obligated to send food or drop by to visit. When someone died, she shared the family's grief. When one of the neighborhood teenagers got in trouble, she sympathized with the parents. When there were baptisms, weddings, or graduations, she attended the parties and always brought a gift. While it felt good to be at the hub of a strong social network, Odessa paid a price in time, emotional energy, and financial drain. What sometimes made it worse was the nagging feeling that if she needed help, she wouldn't get it back in kind.

Odessa went through the same assertiveness training, bibliotherapy, and role-playing routine as Claudia. Odessa is still a cornerstone of her community but she doesn't pay the price she used to because she knows how to set limits on social demands and expectations.

The circumstances were different for each of them, but the issues were the same: Social demands and obligations got out of hand and were draining them physically and mentally.

SOCIAL CONFLICT AND ALIENATION

Interpersonal relationships are particularly stressful because of emotional and social ramifications. Conflict is seldom pleasant, but it's much more painful to quarrel with friends than with strangers. Fighting with friends is different from fighting with relatives. Relatives usually stick through upsetting disagreements, whereas friends or acquaintances walk away. Conflict or stress in friendships may also affect your relationships at work, with other friends, your recreational patterns, and other family relationships.

Social conflict can also lead to social alienation, with its problems of social discrimination, prejudice, exclusion from social groups, and feeling unwanted and alone. Feelings of alienation can be heightened when a close friend moves away, when there are significant changes in your social activities, or when you don't have the freedoms and privileges your friends and acquaintances enjoy.

In addition, social conflict can result in social alienation on the job and interfere with your productivity and effectiveness. One young woman, Kit, began dating a co-worker, Stephen, after he persistently showed interest in her. He invited her to go with him to the company Christmas party. Their appearance together announced to everyone on the job that they were an "item."

Two months later, they broke up after an angry spat, but they still had to see each other every day at work. Stephen was angry and sought support from co-workers. Hurt by the breakup, Kit pretended she didn't care, but her work was affected. She had difficulty concentrating and started making mistakes. Kit began to worry about losing her job. She was unsure with whom she could be friends at work, not wanting to put co-workers in the middle of her conflict with Stephen.

Stephen's work also suffered. He finally left and took another job. For Kit some of the friendships were never the same, and some of Stephen's friends blamed her for his departure from the company.

Conflict can threaten an entire social network. For example, Margie and Troy were part of a network of couples who had socialized together for years. After her divorce, Margie found out that Troy had had an affair with one of the other women in her social group. Margie was so furious she decided to never see that woman again. Then their friends faced a dilemma whom to invite to parties, because if one was invited, the other would stay away.

Not wanting to put her friends in this awkward position, Margie decided not to go to big parties, confining her visits to small luncheons with close friends. Although this reduced tension, Margie lost an irreplaceable support network.

ALTERING SOCIAL STRESS

There are a number of ways to alter stressful social situations depending on the nature of the stress involved, but they all boil down to these basic principles:

• Be assertive but gracious. You have to stand up for your basic rights as a human being but do it in a way that doesn't alienate other people unnecessarily. This is particularly true in situations where social demands get out of hand.

• Seek out people who share your interests; people you understand and who understand you.

• Remember to smile. Be open with people and be yourself. Allow other people to be themselves. Get to know them and accept them for who they are.

• Work on your social skills and use them. Talk to people and be friendly. To make a friend, many times you must be a friend. Don't be bashful and shy about taking the first step.

Reducing your social isolation and loneliness calls for a plan of action and requires a number of skills. Your first step is to identify some of the causes of your isolation. Is it because you have moved or changed your life recently? Have others moved, died, or taken a different path from yours? If so, include steps to reach out to rebuild your social network in your *Action Plan.*

Is the problem a more longstanding one of shyness or social anxiety?

Dealing with shyness and sensitivity to rejection helps overcome social isolation. To make connections, you must approach others, initiate conversation, establish that you have something in common with them, create a connection, and follow through to deepening the friendship. For more information on overcoming shyness and social anxiety read *Conquering Shyness*, by Jonathan Cheek, Bronwen Cheek, and Larry Rothstein,[2] and *Intimate Connections*, by David Burns.[3]

Do you have difficulty trusting others or sharing the details of your life? Mistakes and tragedies of the past can be dealt with and accepted, thus freeing you to be more open to making friends. Approaching others requires trust and a sense of safety and reassurance. Working through fears of rejection, nonacceptance, or vulnerability that may have developed during early life in the family or during school years can greatly reduce a chronic source of social isolation.

AVOIDING SOCIAL STRESS

One way of avoiding social stress is by staying in touch with people you already know. Keep the friends you've got. Use your telephone and don't be afraid to call to say hello. The person you're calling will be glad to hear from you. If your friends are geographically distant, run up your long-distance bill. It's good therapy. If you have friends close by, try getting together regularly for lunch or dinner or just an evening of television.

If there are rifts or misunderstandings with friends, do what you can to repair them or straighten them out. Don't wait until you run out of friends before you start doing something to keep those you already have.

Continue smiling and stay upbeat and positive. No one likes to hang around a grouch or a whiner. This doesn't mean you can't be yourself, just don't expect your friends to be unfailingly understanding and therapeutic. Don't strain friendships by expecting friends to be therapists. It's not fair.

On the other hand, listen to their views and to their problems, but don't try to be a therapist. Don't feel obligated to do something about a friend's troubles. If your friend's problems strain the relationship, suggest that he or she see a professional.

Be careful about how much you promise to friends and associates. Don't agree to do more than you can or are willing to deliver. You'll be labeled unreliable and lose friends. Promises can be unspoken, so be careful what you say by your actions as well as your words.

Be diplomatically assertive with friends and associates. Don't wait until you're angry before you put limits on your friends' and associates' demands on your time, resources, and energy. When conflicts erupt, resolve them as amicably and as quickly as possible. The longer conflicts go on, the more bitter and disruptive they become.

ACCEPTING SOCIAL STRESS

There are times when there's nothing you can do to avoid or alter social stress. Accept that sometimes people won't like you no matter what you do or don't do. When it happens, don't take it personally. Develop a thick skin. Take pride in your ability to tolerate isolation, alienation, and social conflict.

Remind yourself that self-respect and integrity come first. To be alone is not necessarily to be lonely. Schedule time to be by yourself. Don't wait until you're having someone over to make your living space warm, pleasant, and inviting. Keep it that way for the most important person in your life—you. Do it for yourself. You deserve it.

SKILLS FOR COPING WITH SOCIAL STRESS

Social Manners

Manners are a primary social skill. They are not just stilted etiquette, which fork to use or how much to tip or when to write a thank-you note. It's knowing what to say or do and when and how to say or do it. The best book we've come across for boning up on this important social skill is *Miss Manners' Guide for the Turn-of-the-Millennium*.[4] This is a witty and engaging book of advice for correctly and graciously dealing with most social uncertainties.

Assertiveness Skills

Personal assertiveness is essential in every situation involving other people. It is an essential skill for dealing with family, social, work, financial, and environmental stress. If you're not assertive, you'll be taken advantage of, even by those who are nearest and dearest to you.

If you're having problems being appropriately assertive, take a look at a couple of the books on assertiveness we mentioned earlier in other contexts.[5] They'll tell you how to overcome uncertainty and anxiety when faced with disagreements. The combination of assertiveness and good manners should take you through almost any social minefield.

Self-Esteem Enhancement Skills

You can tolerate a good bit of social stress if you feel good about yourself. If you don't, you must develop self-esteem enhancement skills. As we said in chapter 7, practice affirmations in the mirror. One client, Joel, who was a salesman, would tell himself how great he and his product were and how sorry he felt for those who didn't realize this. As Joel repeated his affirmations in front of his mirror, he found more and more items to compliment himself and his product. His self-esteem and sales soared. Sounds hokey, but it works.

For more on self-esteem enhancement we suggest you read David Burns's *Feeling Good.*[6] It will help you get away from thinking about yourself in negative terms and recommend a string of exercises to enhance your self-esteem. We also suggest you read Burns's *Intimate Connections*[7] for more concrete tips on how to improve your social effectiveness through feeling better about yourself.

Cognitive-Flexibility Skills

As with any kind of stress, you'll have to stay flexible as you try to work out a course of action that will make things better. If the first one doesn't work you'll need to think of something else, and to do that you'll have to stay flexible in your thinking. We recommend Edward De Bono's *Six Thinking Hats*[8] for suggestions on handling problems in different ways.

Behavioral-Flexibility Skills

You not only have to think flexibly, you have to act flexibly. If you always do what you've always done, you'll always get what you've always got. Again, *Intimate Connections* has a number of techniques for overcoming the fears and confusions that often underlie the behavioral rigidities that make life more miserable than it needs to be.

AIDS FOR COPING WITH SOCIAL STRESS

Professional Help

Consider getting professional help if you have difficulty developing an appropriate set of skills for alleviating the social stress in your life. Check with your state psychological association for referrals for social skills training, cognitive-behavioral therapy, behavioral desensitization, group therapy, and assertiveness training.

Bibliotherapy

There are many excellent self-help books on the market. We use bibliotherapy regularly in our treatment programs. See appendix II for our suggestions and select one or more books that would be appropriate for helping you with your stress item.

NOTES

1. Smith, M. (1975), *When I Say No, I Feel Guilty*, New York, Bantam.

2. Cheek, J., with Cheek, B., and Rothstein, L. (1990), *Conquering Shyness*, New York, Dell.

3. Burns, D. (1985), *Intimate Connections*, New York, Signet.

4. Martin, J. (1990), *Miss Manners' Guide for the Turn-of-the-Millennium*, New York, Pharos Books.

5. Alberti, R., and Emmons, M. (1974), *Your Perfect Right*, San Luis Obispo, CA, Impact.

Smith, M. (1975), *When I Say No, I Feel Guilty*, New York, Bantam.

6. Burns, D. (1980), *Feeling Good: The New Mood Therapy*, New York, New American Library.

7. Burns, D. (1985), *Intimate Connections*, New York, Signet.

8. De Bono, E. (1985), *Six Thinking Hats*, New York, Penguin Books.

9 BEATING ENVIRONMENTAL STRESS

Our environment is both a concern and a potent source of stress for many of us. Destruction of animal habitats, vanishing wildlife, shrinking rain forests, pollution, acid rain, oil spills, etc., and their implications for future life on this planet distress us all. Less obvious environmental destruction includes violent crime in your neighborhood or threats to you or your loved ones.

American society has undergone sweeping changes over the course of the twentieth century and stress is an unavoidable byproduct. Geographic, social, and financial mobility have disrupted the semisettled society of 1950, leaving us with the challenging and highly stressful task of forging a new society for the twenty-first century. Conflicting political agendas, competitions among societal factions, breakdown in the social order, constant flux in our cities and neighborhoods, discordant community values, and shifting social mores all contribute to creating social discord.

NEIGHBORHOOD HASSLES

You experience the stress generated by societal discord in everyday neighborhood hassles. As population densities increase, our neighborhoods become increasingly crowded and stressful. Construction work disrupts our daily routines and brings the stress of noise, dust, and dirt to our doorsteps. Declining quality in local schools, inadequate public services, and dilapidated recreational facilities further disrupt the ordered routines of daily life.

Neighbors who fail to maintain their property or are noisy or unfriendly make a neighborhood unpleasant. Add violent crime, vandalism, and other minor crimes and neighborhood stress becomes intolerable. When this happens, good people move, bringing even greater disruption and more stress for those left behind.

But even those who move do not escape. Moving takes time, energy, and money. New neighborhoods can be more stressful than old ones. You have to adjust to new neighbors, new traffic patterns, new stores, and new schools. No neighborhood is hassle-free. You deal with unfamiliar problems with depleted resources. You may look back wistfully to the old neighborhood you couldn't wait to escape.

HOUSING HASSLES

Controlling environmental stress begins at home. For most of us home is a haven, a safe harbor, where we can lick our wounds, rest and restore our energy before returning to the fray. Hassles in the house rob us of this haven. When the kitchen sink is piled with dishes, the table is covered with magazines and mail, the floor strewn with toys, and the cat box hasn't been emptied all week, home is no haven.

Home renovation, construction, or remodeling brings noise, dust, dirt, and disruption into our living rooms, kitchens, and bedrooms. There's no escape. Even ordinary home maintenance can be a challenge. Painting, papering, repairing, planting, watering, mowing, clipping, and trash removal all take time and energy. Repairing damage from vandalism or other minor crime in the neighborhood adds to the struggle. Struggles with city hall over zoning laws, permits, and municipal services or utilities disturb the tranquility of your little haven. The congestion of rush hour traffic exacerbated by road crews puts you over the edge.

It takes effort to control or avoid these daily hassles; postponing or neglecting them rarely helps in the long run. Instead, you can create soothing and beautiful surroundings to reduce your stress and provide you a place for renewal.

BEN'S HYPERTENSION AND WHY HIS DOG BIT HIM

Whenever we think about environmental stress, we remember our client Ben and his dog, Bing. Ben, the president of a major company, had moved to an exclusive suburb to escape the crowding, crime, noise, dust, dirt, and other agitations of the city. After some initial adjustments, life in the 'burbs' became quite comfortable. Ben's children were doing well in school, his neighbors were friendly, and he had a big yard where he could play fetch with Bing, his black Lab.

We first heard about Ben from his physician. Ben was having problems with high blood pressure and his physician thought stress might be a cause. Ben wouldn't come to see us because he didn't believe stress was causing his blood pressure problems. He changed his mind after Bing bit him.

Here's what happened. One evening when Ben returned from work, Bing, ball in mouth, greeted him in the driveway looking for a game of fetch. Preoccupied and irritable, Ben kicked Bing out of the way with the side of his foot. Bing nipped Ben's ankle and ripped his pants. When Ben's wife, Vashti, jokingly praised Bing for protecting the family from "Godzilla," Ben exploded and demanded an immediate family meeting. His children confirmed Vashti and Bing's reaction—Ben had become an ill-tempered tyrant. After that meeting, he called us for an appointment.

As we went through Ben's *Stress Audit*, it became apparent that traffic was his biggest stress point. Every morning he would leave his quiet suburban home at eight o'clock to be in his office by nine. About a mile from home, traffic would start getting heavier and slower. Typically, there would be a few "narrow misses" by the time he made it to the highway.

Once on the highway, traffic was faster but still crowded and made dangerous by frantic commuters desperate, like Ben, to get to work on time. Ben's adrenaline level would climb higher and higher whenever he was cut off by a recklessly speeding "lane hopper." His anger would escalate to the point where he was cursing and gesticulating wildly at his fellow travelers.

After his highway workout, Ben would fight his way through downtown traffic. Finally arriving at his parking garage, he would often find his space occupied and the attendant absent. Having parked in someone else's slot, he would hurry the two blocks to his office and arrive, out of breath, five minutes late for a standing nine o'clock meeting with his department heads. Still boiling, he would be abrasive and contentious, a tone that seeped down through all levels of the company, disrupting morale, efficiency, and productivity. As the morning wore on, his adrenaline level would subside and by lunchtime he would be as congenial as ever. But the damage was done.

At five o'clock, Ben would leave the office to face the reverse of his morning traffic ordeal. Transformed into his enraged and furious alter ego, he would arrive home at six (on a good day) and snarl at his wife and children until he calmed down sometime after dinner.

After hearing his story, we suggested to Ben that he implement an avoidance strategy by escaping rush hour traffic. Ben objected that he couldn't do that because of company responsibilities. We pointed out to him that, as president, he could arrange his schedule to suit himself. Ben decided to come in an hour earlier and leave an hour earlier, when his commute would be a less intense experience.

This worked. Not only was traffic less harrowing, but he saved twenty minutes in travel time. Getting to work an hour earlier gave Ben time to prepare for his nine o'clock meeting with his department heads and enabled him to set a tone of friendliness that filtered throughout the departments of the company. Getting home earlier in the afternoon gave him time to play fetch with Bing again. When he had to work late, Ben simply stayed at work until rush hour traffic had cleared.

It took time, but company morale and productivity came back to where it had been and Ben became "Dad" at home again. A treatment program of caffeine withdrawal, progressive muscle relaxation (PMR, see appendix I), biofeedback, and hand-warming exercises helped lower the dosage of Ben's antihypertensive medication and eventually helped him discontinue it.

SKILLS FOR COPING WITH ENVIRONMENTAL STRESS

Political Skills

Political skills can be invaluable in dealing with environmental stress. You don't have to be a born politician to create change. All you have to do is convince other people that something should be done in a particular way. It's like creating a *Stress Action Plan*. Identify the problem, describe how it affects you in behavioral terms, examine your strategic options, decide on a plan of action, overcome resistances, and follow through.

If you're trying to get other people to do something you want done or to go along with you on something, remember that you have to make it worth their while. Other people have to see that it's in their best interests to back your plan. Ask yourself, "Why would anyone want to support this?" If you can't give yourself good reasons, others might not listen.

Be congenial. Don't get angry if people don't agree with you or see things the way you do. Look for areas of agreement and build alliances. Work up petitions to present to those who can do something about the environmental issues that concern you. Be assertive in following through.

Property Maintenance Skills

Keeping your home environment orderly is perhaps the most effective way of avoiding the stress associated with housing hassles. If you have skills, it's easier. If you know how to clean, mend, and straighten up, you've got the basics. If you can paint, take care of minor plumbing repairs, hang a picture, drive a nail, replace glass, tend your yard, you're in even better shape. If these are skills you don't have and you can't afford to hire someone to do home maintenance, look in the home-improvement section of your local bookstore or library. Also, adult education classes in many cities and towns teach various home-maintenance skills.

Organizational Skills

If you intend to do something about neighborhood hassles or general societal discord, you'll have to get organized. You'll need to manage your time effectively and learn how to delegate authority and responsibility. Don't do the whole job at once or by yourself. Divide it into small tasks and decide what needs to be done first and who can do it best. Get other people to take a piece of it and report back when they're through. Set up committees. Give them goals and make sure they follow through.

Social Skills

We talked about social skills earlier, in chapters 6 and 8. The same rules apply here. If you're going to do anything about societal discord or neighborhood hassles, you'll have to work with other people.

Goal-Setting Skills

You have to know what it is that you want to accomplish. If you're not sure, sit down and think about it for a while. Once you've come up with your overall goal, set up subgoals that will lead you to achieve it. Don't start until you know what it is you want to accomplish and how.

Reality-Testing Skills

Keep your goals within the bounds of reason. Don't try to do the impossible or irrational. Check with friends to see if they think your goals make sense. Talk with others as well. Make use of experts. Read up on whatever it is you're thinking about. See how it was done and what is useful for your situation. What are the realistic pitfalls of your goal and how can you avoid them? Reality testing is a skill that can be developed. Sharpen yours and use it before you jump into anything that may backfire on you and create more stress than it eliminates. A good *Action Plan* is one that helps the situation. Your reality-testing skills can determine if your plan is a good one.

Cognitive-Flexibility Skills

Stay flexible in your thinking. Don't get stuck in a rut. Remember, there's more than one way to skin a cat. If your first plan didn't work or wasn't feasible, try another. Look at the problem from a different angle. Brainstorm. Don't rule out anything at this stage. Ideas that sound ridiculous at first sometimes pan out in the end. Often when we get frustrated, we get fixed in our thinking. The more frustrated we get, the more rigid we become. We find ourselves insisting there is only one way to solve the problem—the way that has failed repeatedly.

Behavioral-Flexibility Skills

Just as we need to stay flexible in our thinking, we have to stay flexible in our behavior. Frustration leads not only to rigid thinking but to rigid behavior. We keep blindly doing the same things over and over even in the face of repeated failure and frustration. If you always do what you've always done, you'll always get what you've always got. Don't go on automatic pilot and react in a reflexive way. Step back and take a look at what you're doing and how you're doing it. There's usually some other way of behaving that is more effective.

AIDS FOR COPING WITH ENVIRONMENTAL STRESS

Use your skills effectively but also take advantage of the aids you might have available to assist you in seeing your *Action Plans* through to fruition. Look for civic or environmental organizations that could help you achieve your goals. The Lions, Kiwanis, Chamber of Commerce, Rotary, Sierra Club, Appalachian Mountain Club, Wilderness Society, National Park Service, etc., are just a few places you could start. See if there are neighborhood associations that could help. If there aren't any, you might want to start one.

There are also political organizations. If you have a political party affiliation, solicit your party for assistance. Check out city, county, state, and federal agencies for one that might be responsive to your needs. Be assertive. Remember, they work for you. Make them do their job.

10 CONQUERING FINANCIAL STRESS

Most of us have strong feelings about money. Just thinking about it generates anxiety, depression, and anger, the three stress emotions. When nearly 20,000 people were asked what emotions they associated with money, *Psychology Today* found that 71 percent chose anxiety, 52 percent listed depression, and 51 percent picked anger (multiple choices were permitted). Money is more than economics. Rightly or wrongly, it is also the currency of self-worth for many of us. Uncertainty about our financial future translates into uncertainties about ourselves and our self-worth.[1]

More family fights are over money than any other issue. Worry about money is a primary source of stress. And it doesn't have anything to do with how much money you have. It's a problem on all socioeconomic levels. Not having enough money to meet basic expenses is particularly worrisome. Financial ups and downs are emotionally devastating. When we can't pay our bills, we're embarrassed, ashamed, and humiliated.

Money won't buy you love or happiness but it eliminates worries about food, shelter, clothing, educational opportunities, and so on.

Money influences where and how we live, who our friends and associates are, and even those we marry. In many instances it becomes the final arbiter of value and worth of property, goods, services, other people, even of ourselves.

Few events are as stressful as a financial setback or loss. When it's tied in with loss of a job or a demotion, it is doubly stressful. Financial reversals are stressful due to the changes they engender in our lives and lifestyles. These changes, however, are exacerbated by blows to our dignity, pride, and self-respect.

In general, the higher your income, the lower your stress. However, a major financial gain such as an inheritance, or large winnings from gambling, the stock market, or the lottery, could be just as disruptive and stressful as a major financial loss. The secret of happiness is the stability of your income. The more stable it is, the fewer changes you're likely to make in your lifestyle.

THE WILSONS WIN THE LOTTERY

The Wilson family provides a particularly tragic example of the havoc and stress a major financial gain can bring into your life. The Wilsons lived a quiet, peaceful existence among lifelong friends—until everything changed when Grace Wilson won the state lottery.

Prior to her windfall, Grace and her husband, Sean, had raised five children and lived in a modest home in the urban neighborhood where they had both grown up. Grace's mother was "just down the street" and her sister lived next door. A hair stylist at the local beauty parlor, Grace socialized with her friends and neighbors as she did their hair. Sean had been a bus driver for twenty-five years; his route for the last ten years had included his own neighborhood. He enjoyed chatting with his regular passengers as he drove. The Wilsons knew everybody and everybody knew them.

Life hadn't been perfect for the Wilsons. They fought about money. They liked nice things, but there was never enough money to buy them. Over Grace's objections, Sean had financially assisted several of her relatives at one time or another and Grace resented it.

Grace had a dream of moving to a beautiful home in the suburbs, one with landscaped grounds and a wide curving driveway. Every Saturday she would invest ten dollars in the state lottery and imagine herself greeting friends and neighbors at the door of her home newly purchased with her winnings. But years passed, and except for occasional forty-dollar winners, Grace's dream went unfulfilled. But one day she bought a ticket at her local drugstore. A week later, she won $2.3 million in the lottery!

Fun-loving folks, the Wilsons held several celebratory parties. It was too much for Grace's mother. She died of a heart attack after a gala late-night dinner. Grace and her mother had been close, and Grace went into a deep depression that required a short hospital stay and anti-depressant medication. She couldn't wait to leave the neighborhood where she was reminded of her mother at every turn. Sean took early retirement, Grace quit the beauty parlor, and they moved to a large, beautiful home in an elegant Boston suburb. The mortgage was large, but so was their annual income from their winnings.

Their children loved the house. So much so that one daughter, Victoria, separated from her husband and moved in with her three small children "for a few months." A son, Richard, who was "between jobs," showed up with his belongings asking to "come back home till I get back on my feet." Their friends from the old neighborhood, however, didn't seem to care for the new house and never came to visit. Their new neighbors weren't friendly. In fact, they saw the Wilsons as interlopers.

Grace's relatives began asking for loans. Some of Sean's estranged relatives also tried to cash in on his new wealth. Their children began quarreling. One faction insisted that the settled-in son and daughter move out; Victoria and Richard felt otherwise. Richard and his brother Michael got into a fistfight on the beautifully curving driveway.

Grace became increasingly bitter and had to be hospitalized once again for depression. Sean began to drink and started having problems with hypertension.

As the fabric of their family and social lives disintegrated, Sean and Grace faced financial problems. They couldn't handle the expense of Grace's hospitalization and four extra people in the house. Sean's loans to relatives were not repaid. They had to borrow against their next annual lottery payment to meet the mortgage.

The stress and turmoil were too much for Grace. One morning Sean found her dead from an overdose of her sleep medication.

Sean sold "Grace's big house" and bought a condominium in Boston. He drank heavily. His friends, children, and relatives continued to ask, sometimes beg, for money. He tried to escape by traveling to Florida, the Caribbean, and Europe, but he was lonely.

Now in his early sixties, he married Jean, a woman twenty years his junior. His children were furious and refused to accept her. Sean's hypertension became uncontrollable and he had a minor stroke.

Jean, a former client of Alma's, brought Sean to us to "get some help with this mess." We ended up seeing the entire family, sometimes individually, sometimes in groups, and sometimes all together. The sessions were raucous but productive, as lifelong rivalries among the children were addressed for the first time and Jean's place in the family was defined and acknowledged.

A distribution of Sean's estate was negotiated and agreed upon with his children. Sean wrote a will containing clear provisions for each of them. Jean won the family's heart by offering to forgo any part of Sean's estate. She had told the family earlier that she had married Sean because he was a "good, kind, gentle man" and because she loved him, but they hadn't believed her. Now they did, and there were many hugs and tears as they apologized for the "awful things" they had said about her.

With peace and stability restored, Sean's blood pressure began responding to medication and the residual signs of his stroke almost disappeared. Problems among the children came up from time to time, but Sean and Jean stayed "above the fray" and were not distressed by them.

This all happened a few years back. Recently we heard from Jean that Sean had died of a heart attack at age 67. She said, "Winning the lottery was the worst thing that ever happened to Sean and Grace. It was too much money and they didn't know what to do with it. It killed them both." We're inclined to agree.

ALTERING FINANCIAL STRESS

Here are some practical things you can do to get things back under control if you are having financial problems: (1) make a budget; (2) construct a realistic five-year financial plan; (3) hold family business meetings; (4) get financial advice from someone trained and equipped to deal with finances, such as a banker, an accountant, or the Consumer Credit Counseling Service in your area.

Protect yourself from the further aggravation and stress of fending off bill collectors. You have rights, even if you are short on cash. You are protected from harassment by bill collectors by the Fair Debt Collection Practices Act, which prohibits them from bothering you at unreasonable hours, annoying you at work, or otherwise hounding you about unpaid bills. You can get a copy of the Act from the Division of Credit Practice, Federal Trade Commission, Pennsylvania Avenue at Sixth Street, Washington, DC 20580.

AVOIDING FINANCIAL STRESS

Perhaps the best way of dealing with financial stress is by avoiding it. There are a number of ways you can do that. Number one is to build the habit of living within your means. Don't overextend yourself or your budget.

Number two is to put aside money from each paycheck for emergency budget busters such as auto repairs, unexpected trips, medical bills, and so on. If you have a little "cushion," you're much less likely to fall apart when something out of the ordinary happens. You'll save money much more easily and painlessly if you do it automatically and regularly. Join a payroll savings plan and put a percentage of your paycheck into savings. If you can manage it, 10 percent is a good figure to shoot for; if you can't, try 5 percent.

You should also have savings that are separate from your emergency fund. Long-range savings for a home, retirement, education, and the like provide a means to improve your quality of life; emergency funds are a means to continue it.

If your financial situation makes it impossible for you to save, look for a job that pays better. If that's not an option, take a hard look at your expenses to see what you can cut out or economize on. Change your shopping habits by trying different stores and looking harder for bargains. Cut back to bare necessities if you have to, but balance income and expenses so you can put something aside.

Think about a sideline or a part-time job to make a little extra. Check the help-wanted sections of your local paper. Brainstorm with friends and family to come up with ideas to make extra money. It could even be fun to do something different with your spare time.

ACCEPTING FINANCIAL STRESS

The most important element in accepting financial stress is finding a more accurate and reliable way of measuring your self-worth. Friendships, community work, religious or spiritual involvements, teaching, etc., are more reliable and constant elements in the calculus of self-esteem than money. Quit measuring your worth in dollars.

SKILLS FOR COPING WITH FINANCIAL STRESS

Organizational Skills

As with most things, the first step to getting your finances in order is to get organized. Start with taking a look at where the money comes from and where it goes. Write it down. You might try carrying a pocket notebook and record every expenditure. Once you've done this for a month or so, you'll have a better idea about what needs to be done. Keeping records is a necessity. Read some of the excellent financial-planning books in your local bookstore or library for tips on record keeping.

Goal-Setting Skills

You'll need to set goals to get your finances in order. Most of us plan and save better and easier if we know what we're planning and saving for. Decide on your overall goals and then set up short-term subgoals that will lead to them. Think in terms of five-year plans. Break the five-year plans down into one-year plans. Cut the one-year plans down into six-month plans. Give yourself lots of subgoals so you'll have plenty of markers to indicate whether you're on track and moving in the right direction.

Reality-Testing Skills

As you're setting financial goals for yourself, be realistic. Don't spend more than you can afford. Watch credit cards and charge accounts. They have a way of taking over your life. Pay your bills and your taxes on time. Ignoring them won't make them go away. When you make up your budgets and set up savings plans, don't cut things to the bone. Be sure you keep out enough for recreation, entertainment, and vacations. You are your own most important financial asset. You have to take care of yourself first. The secret is in knowing what's fat and what's muscle. Don't save so much that you create other stresses for yourself.

Once you have saved up what you consider a significant amount, you'll probably start thinking about investments. Don't get carried away with "get rich quick" schemes or investments that you know little about. You're probably not going to become financially secure overnight. It takes time. If something looks too good to be true, it probably is. Check it out with your local Better Business Bureau or talk to someone at your bank about it before you invest any money.

Economic Knowledge

When it comes to financial stress, the more you know about economics and finances, the better off you'll be.

Become knowledgeable about money and how it works. Take an adult education course on financial planning and personal economics. Join an investment club. Check your local library or bookstore for books on money, finances, and economics.

Budgeting Skills

Setting up a budget is essential if you're going to reduce your financial stress. It takes time and some organizational skill, but it's worth it in the long run. Remember to leave room for slippage in the system. Set down your fixed costs first, then what you'd like to save, then your variable costs. Don't forget to include entertainment, recreation, and vacations. If you are unable to set up your budget, ask your financial adviser to give you a hand or do it for you.

For those who are in severe financial difficulty, there are consumer credit agencies who help consolidate loans and make arrangements for payment plans to creditors. One example is Credit Improvement and Debt Counseling of America. You can also call the Support Centers of America at (202) 296-3900. They have offices throughout the U.S. that offer free and reduced rate financial advice. Finally, you might call your local society for CPAs.

Communication Skills

In many instances, your financial woes will involve other people—your spouse, children, friends, and family. When this is the case, it's not enough to get your financial affairs in order, you have to involve others in the program. You have to make them understand what it is you're trying to do and why, and what your goals are and how you intend to reach them. To do that, you have to communicate. You have to talk to the people who are involved and make sure everyone is pulling in the same direction.

It's particularly important to communicate with your creditors when you get behind in your payments. Most of them will be willing to work out some kind of schedule with you if you'll just talk to them. Let them know that you're not a deadbeat. Regular payments, no matter how small, go a long way in communicating good faith.

Vocational Skills

You have to have marketable skills if you expect to generate income. Vocational skills can translate into financial security for you and your loved ones, if the skills you have are in demand. If your vocational skills do not command the kind of income you need, try retraining in something that will pay better. Before you do that, however, take a look around and see if you might market your current skills more effectively.

Cognitive-Flexibility Skills

As you work through various *Action Plans* to reduce your financial stress, remember to stay flexible in your thinking. If one plan doesn't work, try something else. Brainstorm and keep your options open. If you always do what you've always done, you'll always get what you've always got.

AIDS FOR COPING WITH FINANCIAL STRESS

Financial Counseling

The most obvious aid for dealing with financial stress is financial counseling. Talk to an accountant, a banker, a financial planner, or some other professional trained to deal with personal finances and equipped to advise you. You might look up in the phone book your local Consumer Credit Counseling Service, a community-sponsored, nonprofit group providing low-cost, confidential services.

Educational System

Investigate your local adult education program for classes on management of your finances. This is a major resource that frequently gets overlooked. Check with your local public school systems, colleges, and universities for any community courses they might offer.

Vocational Training or Rehabilitation

If you need to upgrade your vocational skills to increase your earning power, see what's available through local and state vocational training and vocational rehabilitation programs. If they don't have anything suitable, they may be able to direct you to something that is.

Cognitive-Behavioral Therapy

If you get stuck in your thinking and can't find your way out of your problem, you might want to seek out a cognitive-behavioral therapist. Sometimes just the slightest little twist on something you've been thinking about can open up whole new vistas.

Bibliotherapy

Don't forget your local libraries and bookstores as aids in your struggles with financial stress. Bibliotherapy may be just the ticket for dealing with financial stress. The proliferation of excellent self-help books in the last few years has made high-level, practical expertise available to everyone at a relatively low cost.

NOTES

1. Rubenstein, C. (1981), "Money Discontents," *Psychology Today*, 15, 36–38.

III

SYMPTOMS: SOOTHING THE BODY, CALMING THE MIND

11 THE BODY'S DELICATELY BALANCED ECONOMY

In chapter 1, "Stress Points," we talked about what stress is, what it isn't, and how it works. In this chapter we'll continue that discussion by focusing on how stress creates symptoms. We have some definite ideas on this topic that are a little different from those you may see elsewhere.

The first is that the different kinds of stress generate different kinds of symptoms. The second is that you may experience different kinds of stress simultaneously. Your stress points can be complex or simple, as can the stress symptoms you experience.

As we described in chapter 1 with the Biobehavioral Model of Stress, when you mobilize your resources to deal with demands and pressures, you become physiologically aroused. If your level of arousal gets too high, it enters a danger zone. The particular pattern of stress symptoms you develop depends on how frequently you enter that danger zone and how long you stay there.

Fortunately, your body has built-in mechanisms for repairing the damages wrought by overarousal. These natural recuperative and healing processes restore your body and chase away your symptoms of stress if you just give them a chance. There are times when you'll have to slow down, lower your level of arousal, and let them take over. There are a number of techniques for doing this, which we'll explain as we go through the different symptoms systems in this section.

Just as you designed *Action Plans* in sections I and II, you'll tailor an *Action Plan* in this section for calming your mind and healing your body.

STRESS AND THE MIND-BODY CONNECTION

It all starts with the mind-body connection, which is central to the most current thinking on stress. A mythology has grown around this connection similar to the mythology around stress itself. Sometimes the two mythologies become intertwined in a very confusing way. So, just as we debunked some of the mythology surrounding stress, we'll dismantle some misconceptions about the mind-body connection.

Myth 1: There is a mind separate from the body.

False. The mind and body are one and the same. The organ of the mind is the brain and the brain controls the rest of the body as it sees fit. The brain receives information about the external world and from inside through the senses, interprets it, makes decisions about what to do, and directs the rest of the body to respond accordingly. Anything that affects the body is perceived and interpreted by the brain. The brain is a curious organ in that it can perceive and respond to its own activity. Thoughts are the product of brain activity and are also perceived by the brain. They can have a powerful effect on the body.

Myth 2: If a physical complaint is rooted in mental processes it isn't real—it's imaginary.

Mental processes can disrupt the body's functioning to the point where there is actual structural damage to tissue and organs. The physical problems rooted in disruptive mental processes are no less real than is a broken leg. The stomach ulcer caused by the influence of thoughts and feelings on gastric secretions is a physical reality.

Myth 3: Since the brain controls the body, all physical complaints are really under mental control.

Not so. That same stomach ulcer we mentioned above may have been caused by the stomach's reactions to thoughts and feelings, but it will require medication for relief in the short run. Successful long-term treatment would include modifying the thoughts and feelings that produced it, as well as medication to provide symptomatic relief during the healing process.

Myth 4: Mental as well as physical complaints are due primarily to chemical imbalances and are best treated by prescriptions.

All bodily processes are chemical in nature and they get out of balance from time to time. Hunger, for instance, is caused by an adaptive shift in chemistry that makes us want to eat. Our bodies have built-in mechanisms for bringing things into balance. But we don't give them a chance to work because it takes time. Medication is a quick and easy answer, but it doesn't restore chemical balance—it creates a chemical imbalance of its own. Medication may make symptoms disappear or make them more tolerable, but the introduction of any foreign substance may create side effects worse than the symptoms. Short-term medication sometimes helps calm us enough to reestablish effective self-regulation, but in the long term, reliance on external chemical control can be more damaging than helpful.

Myth 5: We potentially have total control over our minds and our bodies and are therefore responsible for anything that befalls us. If we get sick, it's our own fault because we didn't take care of ourselves or think the right thoughts.

This particular myth can lead to guilt and self-flagellation. Life is an interplay of self and circumstance. We can control many things, but the list of things we can't is a long one. Most of us do the best we can most of the time. Control over our bodies and our minds comes through developing our knowledge, skills, and abilities. No matter how well we learn to self-regulate, many circumstances remain beyond our control.

Myth 6: The power of mind, faith, or spirit can cure anything.
Mind, faith, and spirit are indeed powerful and can heal many mental and/or physical problems. But they can't cure everything. When you suffer from virulent infections, genetic diseases, traumatic injuries, and poisonings, your mind and body need external treatment. Knowing when to use a certain medication or treatment is what is important.

YOUR BODY IS A BUSY PLACE

Now that we have discussed the myths surrounding the mind-body connection, what does go on? Over the years, we have been struck with how little people really know of themselves and their bodies. Given an understanding of how stress affects their bodies to produce symptoms, though, they readily engage in our stress management and self-regulation treatment programs.

Your body is a busy place. Raw materials for the manufacture of body parts such as blood, bone, muscle, skin, and hair, and for their maintenance, repair, and replacement, are taken in, converted to usable form, and distributed to the appropriate construction sites. Food is turned into energy to fuel this biological economy and waste products are carried away. All this activity runs automatically and requires only minimal attention from us. If we provide food, water, oxygen, and a safe, external environment, and we avoid trauma and are reasonably good at self-regulation, our bodies will manage very well on their own.

Beneath your skin, many intricate, interacting biological systems carry out their life-sustaining functions from birth to death. Depending on what goes on around us, some systems speed up, some slow down, and some become inactive. Since the world around us is constantly changing, these systems must adjust continually to the perceived circumstances of the external world and to one another. But this is not a state of uncontrolled chaos. The brain and the nervous system form a command and communications network that choreographs the body's intricate balance of change and adaptation to change.

When life is tranquil and calm, we seldom notice what is going on inside our bodies. Everything purrs along smoothly, quietly, and evenly. However, when our bodies, our resources, or our self-esteem are threatened or challenged, alarms go off and our bodies mobilize their defenses according to the magnitude and kind of the perceived danger.

Then we become more aware of what's happening inside our bodies: our hearts pound rapidly, our hands get sweaty and cold, our mouths become dry, our blood pressure soars, our muscles tense, our thoughts race, we may feel an urge to void our bladders or bowels, and so on. These physical reactions to a perceived threat or challenge have been termed the "fight or flight" response. It mobilizes our resources and energies for either fight or flight, depending on the circumstance. Psychologically, we experience these internal events as the emotions of anger, fear, or anxiety.

The brain orders these reactions according to the magnitude of the perceived threat or challenge. Fueled by adrenaline, they are as automatic as the less obtrusive bodily activity associated with peace and tranquility. Like a song that lends itself to many interpretations and variations, the "fight or flight" response is different for each of us.

HOW STRESS AND THE MIND CAN DISRUPT BODILY PROCESSES

Anne, whom we discussed earlier, illustrates how stress creates trouble by disrupting the body's delicately balanced economy. Basically uncertain of who she was and what she wanted out of life, Anne's major problems involved a conflict between marrying Mark, and thereby pleasing her mother, and succeeding in her career. Both were extremely important to her. Anne experienced any threat to either as a direct threat to herself.

When her mother or Mark talked of marriage and family, Anne felt her career being jeopardized; when her career became demanding, Anne felt her chances for marriage and a family were lessened. Anne's pattern of physical reaction to threat was an involuntary tensing of her abdominal muscles as though anticipating an attack or a body blow. A rapid, shallow breather, tensing her abdominal muscles forced Anne to breathe even more shallowly. If the threat persisted, her breathing would become shallower and faster still until she hyperventilated. Anne's "heart attacks" and emotional distress were generated by her hyperventilation.

Hyperventilation sets in motion a chain of events that disrupts the oxygen supply so necessary to life at the level of the individual cell. We inhale to bring oxygen into our lungs, where it is picked up by the hemoglobin in our red blood cells and carried away to the rest of our body's cells. On the return trip, blood moves carbon dioxide (produced as a waste product of cellular metabolism) back to the lungs, and we breathe it out into the environment when we exhale. The concentration of this waste product in our bloodstream controls how easily blood unloads oxygen to our body cells and also influences our blood pressure. When we hyperventilate, we decrease the concentration of carbon dioxide and reduce the efficiency of oxygen released to cells. Frequently, we also experience a drop in blood pressure as blood vessels dilate to increase the flow of blood through tissue. The fall in blood pressure, however, just reduces circulation.

When this happens, we're hit with the double whammy of reduced circulation and lowered oxygen release. The cells of the body don't get enough oxygen to carry out their functions, resulting in dizziness, numbness, and tingling sensations. They let us know about it, particularly the nerve cells that make up the brain. Our heart beats faster and harder as it tries to get our blood pressure high enough to restore circulation to the brain.

We breathe faster and faster to get more oxygen into the system, but only make things worse as we exhale even more carbon dioxide. Our hearts are pounding rapidly and as our chest muscles tire from the rapid breathing they start to ache. The combination of Anne's rapidly pounding heart and her aching chest muscles convinced her that she was having a heart attack and threw her into a panic that only increased her stress and hyperventilation.

PATTERNS OF STRESS, PHYSIOLOGICAL AROUSAL,* AND SYMPTOMS

For most of us, different patterns of intensity and duration in our levels of physiological arousal result in different sets of stress symptoms. Some sets of symptoms tend to develop early, whereas others tend to appear later on. In the figures below, you can see the different sets of symptoms that, in general, go with specific patterns of intensity and duration. The vertical axes of the four patterns shown represent your level of physiological arousal; the horizontal axes represent time.

Everyday Stress

Figure 1 (page 220) illustrates a principle of physiological arousal—a baseline level of physiological activity goes on at all times in our bodies. Increases in physiological arousal start from this baseline level. The illustration shows four small increases and one large increase in arousal, none of which reach the danger zone, and then return to the baseline level of arousal. This is everyday stress. There's an increase in your level of physiological arousal that you're probably aware of, but it's not intense enough, nor does it last long enough, to create stress symptoms.

This kind of stress occurs, for example, when you get locked out of your car and can't make your school car pool pickups on time. Some of the children's parents denounce you because they have to leave to get their children. It's an upsetting and unpleasant incident, but your life returns to normal in a few hours and so does your level of physiological arousal. You don't need professional help because you don't have any major stress symptoms.

---

*We are aware that "arousal" is an obsolete physiological concept that greatly oversimplifies the actual physiological events involved in the appraisal of situations and resultant physiological stress reactions. We use it here solely for descriptive and heuristic purposes.

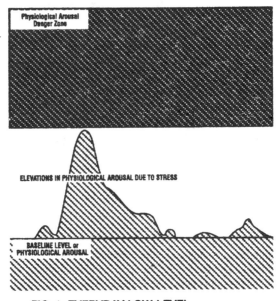

**FIG. 1. EVERYDAY LOW-LEVEL
STRESS, NO SYMPTOMS**

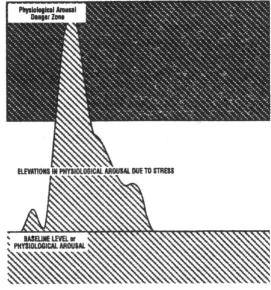

**FIG. 2. ACUTE STRESS EPISODE, MS
AND PNS SYMPTOMS**

Acute Stress

Figure 2 illustrates another familiar type of stress reaction—the "fight or flight response"—where an acute episode of physiological arousal is intense enough to get into the danger zone for symptoms. Symptoms involving the muscular system (MS) or the parasympathetic nervous system (PNS/stomach, gut, and bowel) are generally associated with such single-episode, acute stress reactions. Most people treat these symptoms by using limited amounts of nonprescription medications such as aspirin, antacids, or laxatives. Such acute stress reactions accompany major moves, career decisions, or conflicts in your primary love relationships or on the job.

Recurrent, Episodic Acute Stress

Shown in figure 3 (page 222) is the pattern of physiological arousal involved in recurrent, acute stress episodes. Notice a major difference—these two stress episodes start from a different baseline of physiological arousal. Episode 1 begins from a baseline level of ordinary, everyday physiological arousal; but episode 2 starts from a baseline of episode number one's declining level of physiological arousal. Thus, a relatively minor stress episode keeps you in the danger zone longer because it picks up where the first episode left off. Like the straw that breaks the camel's back, the additive, cumulative nature of stress shifts the pattern of symptoms from muscles and gut to heart and blood vessels.

Recurrent, episodic acute stress is serious. It produces symptoms involving the sympathetic nervous system (SNS) (heart, blood vessels, sweat glands), the cognitive (COG) system (thinking, memory, judgment, decision making), and the emotional (EM) system (moods, feelings, and emotions), which can be incapacitating and life threatening. These symptoms send people to emergency rooms or to cardiologists, psychologists, or psychiatrists. They can be severe enough to require palliative medication or even hospitalization.

The symptoms of recurrent, episodic acute stress are usually not recognized as stress related because we are

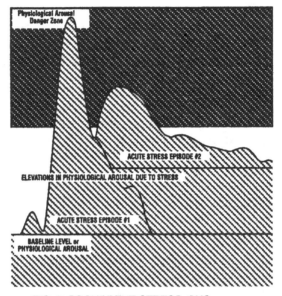

FIG. 3. RECURRENT STRESS, SNS, COG, AND EM SYMPTOMS

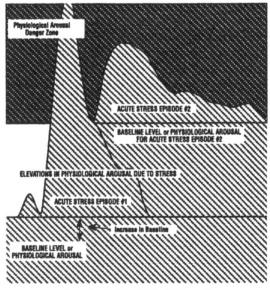

FIG. 4. CHRONIC STRESS, END AND IMM SYMPTOMS

so used to stress in our lives. In addition, the cognitive and emotional symptoms of recurrent, episodic acute stress cloud our ability to think our way out of the stress situations. Consequently we stay at a dangerous level of physiological arousal far too long because we fail to identify and deal effectively with the sources of our stress.

Who is most prone to recurrent, episodic acute stress? "Type A," cardiac-prone personalities, for one. Their hostile, competitive nature subjects them to recurring episodes of acute stress. Nonassertive people also experience recurrent episodes of acute stress because they can't put limits on other people or get themselves out of stressful circumstances. Disorganized people make up another group because they never get themselves organized well enough to cope effectively with stress.

Chronic Stress

In the last example, figure 4, the baseline is higher than in the three earlier examples. Your baseline level of physiological arousal can change daily depending on your use of chemical stimulants, degree of sleep deprivation, nutritional status, and general level of excitement. The result is that it takes less of a physiological reaction to demands and pressures to push you into the danger zone for symptom development.

In the example shown, physiological arousal never gets out of the danger zone. This is the malignant pattern that accompanies chronic stress. This is the stress we are least likely to recognize as causing our symptoms. Often we don't even know this stress is there until it lets up. Then we miss the feeling of constant pressure and experience the let-up as a foreign, uncomfortable feeling.

Chronic stress is deadly. It creates systemic illness by affecting basic body systems through its impact on our endocrine (END) and immune (IM) systems. Chronic stress reactions are found in the unrelenting stress of poverty, miserable marriages, neurotic preoccupation with problems from our past, and being trapped in painfully unrewarding work situations. Chronic stress brings a sense of helplessness, hopelessness, and defeat.

DESIGNING YOUR *STRESS ACTION PLAN: SYMPTOMS*

In treating our clients, we have learned that some symptoms respond better to one kind of behavioral treatment while other symptoms respond better to other treatments. No universal treatment works equally well for all symptoms or for all people.

Meditation, for instance, works well on cardiovascular and immune symptoms for people comfortable with passive relaxation procedures. For those who prefer a more active technique, progressive muscle relaxation or guided imagery may work. However, for a symptom involving the muscular system such as muscle contraction headache or temporomandibular joint (TMJ) pain (described in the next chapter), progressive muscle relaxation and electromyographic (EMG) biofeedback (described in chapter 19) are the treatments of choice and work well for almost everyone.

In this section, we'll show you how to pair your symptoms with the treatment plan that gives you the most effective and lasting relief in the least amount of time. We'll also help you create a plan to deal with your stress symptoms.

Let's start by referring to Anne's *Stress Action Plan: Symptoms* form at the end of this chapter. The particular symptom bothering her was *shortness of breath*, an SNS item. Look at your own *Stress Audit: Symptoms* section and find an item that you rated as particularly troublesome (4 or 5). Note its body system. This is important because the treatment of your symptom will be specific to the body system (muscular system, sympathetic nervous system, etc.) in which it occurs.

Next, write down exactly how your symptom affects you in behavioral terms. Describe how and when it starts, what makes it better, what makes it worse. Study Anne's description below as an example of what we mean.

> Whenever I get real upset and nervous like when I have a fight with Mark or my boss, I start having trouble breathing. Then I start to hyperventilate, trying to get my breath. I feel strange and dizzy. It just gets worse

and worse and I get so scared I think I'm going crazy. My heart starts racing like crazy and I start getting numb. Sometimes I get pains in my chest and I think it's my heart going bad and that I'm going to die any minute. What's worse is that I worry so much about it happening that sometimes I think I make it happen.

Once you've finished your description, read the chapter that discusses the body system that includes your particular symptom and the self-regulatory techniques to treat it. Write them down as possibilities on your *Action Plan*. Read more about the self-regulation techniques you've chosen in chapter 19, "Calling on the Healer Within."

We'll discuss Anne's *Stress Action Plan: Symptoms* in detail in chapters 14 and 15. The following chapters discuss symptoms and their systems in the order in which they appear in the *Stress Audit*. You can go straight to the symptom chapter that concerns you most and read the others later, if you like.

ANNE'S STRESS ACTION PLAN: SYMPTOMS

DIRECTIONS: Review your *Stress Audit: Symptoms* section. Write down a symptom rated 4 or 5 you'd like to work on, describe it in terms of when, where, how it's a problem, what makes it better, what makes it worse. Stop. Read chapter 11 and the following pertinent chapters, write down some actions that might help. Stop. Read chapter 20, write down your barriers to change. Stop. Read chapter 21 and write down your supports for change. *Implement* your plan by trying out the easiest and least expensive treatment action you've written down. *Evaluate* the success of that action and try the next choice if necessary.

SYMPTOM: Shortness of breath

SYSTEM: Sympathetic Nervous System

DESCRIPTION: (Anne's description of her symptom and how it affects her)
Whenever I get real upset and nervous like when I have a fight with Mark or my boss, I start having trouble breathing. Then I start to hyperventilate, trying to get my breath. I feel strange and dizzy. It just gets worse and worse and I get so scared I think I'm going crazy. My heart starts racing like crazy and I start getting numb. Sometimes I get pains in my chest and I think it's my heart going bad and that I'm going to die any minute. What's worse is that I worry so much about it happening that sometimes I think I make it happen.

POSSIBLE ACTIONS: (Anne's application of chapters 14 and 15 to her symptoms)
1) Remember to breathe through my nose slowly and evenly. I'll need to practice that. (chapter 14 and appendix I)
2) Stop the catastrophizing thoughts, the "what if . . ." thoughts. (chapter 15 and appendix I)
3) Remember to stay in the moment, don't worry about what might happen. (chapter 15 and appendix I)
4) Make myself a relaxation tape with a special emphasis on diaphragmatic breathing. (chapter 14 and appendix I)

BARRIERS TO CHANGE: (Anne's application of chapter 20 to her life)

SUPPORTS FOR CHANGE: (Anne's application of chapter 21 to her life)

STRESS ACTION PLAN: SYMPTOMS

DIRECTIONS: Review your *Stress Audit: Symptoms* section. Write down a symptom rated 4 or 5 you'd like to work on, describe it in terms of when, where, how it's a problem, what makes it better, what makes it worse. Stop. Read chapter 11 and the following pertinent chapters, write down some actions that might help. Stop. Read chapter 20, write down your barriers to change. Stop. Read chapter 21 and write down your supports for change. *Implement* your plan by trying out the easiest and least expensive treatment action you've written down. *Evaluate* the success of that action and try the next choice if necessary.

SYMPTOM: _____

DESCRIPTION OF SYMPTOM (when, where, and how it's a problem, what makes it better or worse):_____

_____

_____

_____

POSSIBLE ACTIONS: _____

_____

_____

_____

BARRIERS TO CHANGE (personal, social, financial, practical, etc.):_____

_____

_____

SUPPORTS FOR CHANGE: _____

_____

_____

12 YOUR ACHING BACK, HEAD, JAW, ETC.

Almost everyone has experienced muscular aches and pains. A slip on the ice pulls a muscle in your back. You exercise too strenuously after a sedentary week and are bothered by stiffness the next two days. The repetitive motions from long periods of typing or from painting the ceiling leave you with a sore shoulder. Any of these can cause muscle pain.

So can stress. Increased muscle tension is an important part of the "fight or flight" stress reaction to demand and pressure. Noradrenaline from the sympathetic nervous system alerts the muscles to tense up in preparation for action. Tense muscles get set to act quickly in response to threat or danger. You move faster and have greater strength during an emergency because of this boost.

If no action occurs, muscle tension may remain. You adopt an "on guard" posture that lasts as long as you feel threatened: shoulders up, arms slightly forward. Waiting for the "pain in the neck" supervisor's evaluation may bring on a knot in your upper back. The frown from worry about your taxes may create a tension headache.

Stress also contributes to inattention to your body's signals, increasing the likelihood that you will sit, stand, or move in ways that strain your muscles. Most people under stress are less likely to continue their exercise program, leaving their muscles vulnerable to strain when called upon for strenuous effort.

The skeletal muscular system is comprised of more than six hundred and ninety-six separate muscles. It accounts for more than 40 percent of body weight.[1] Any one of these muscles can become overly fatigued, injured, or can develop spasms. Muscle fibers are designed to tense and then relax. A muscle can go through this tense/relax cycle indefinitely. As you walk, one set of muscles tenses while the opposing muscles relax. However, a muscle under sustained tension without an alternating relaxation phase eventually develops spasms and pain. Sustained tension from emotional stress, poor posture, or certain repetitive movements does not allow this relaxed phase to occur.

Unrelieved muscle tension leads to tension headaches, back pain, and TMJ, temporomandibular joint (jaw), pain. Chronic muscle tension pulls on the muscle's tendon and can lead to pain where the tendon is attached to the bone and can pull the body out of balance, creating new pains. This may also cause an inflammation of the tendons, resulting in the painful condition called tendonitis. Chronic muscle tension can result in a deterioration in muscle health, strength, and conditioning. When weakened muscles are pushed beyond their physical limits, they spasm, which we experience as cramps in large muscles.

Conditioning, stretching and relaxation can reduce muscular symptoms of stress. Strong, healthy, well-conditioned muscles tolerate much more tension than weak, poorly conditioned ones. Muscles need nourishment, exercise, and rest if they are to work without complaint.

If you suffer muscular symptoms only occasionally, an anti-inflammatory painkiller such as aspirin may be your best solution. If they occur regularly, however, reduce your level of muscle tension through some of the techniques described at the end of this chapter.

TMJ PAIN

A common stress-related muscle symptom is jaw joint or TMJ pain. People who habitually clench or grind their teeth often experience pain in their jaw. TMJ pain is a leading dental problem in this country.

One TMJ client, Karen, would resolutely "set" her jaw when faced with adversity. She struggled through, clenching her teeth every step of the way. Even when her problems had passed, the habit of clenching her teeth persisted. In addition to reducing her stress situations, we taught Karen to relax her jaw with EMG biofeedback and progressive muscle relaxation exercises described in chapter 19 and appendix I. Her TMJ pain subsided somewhat, but came back after she had been out of treatment for a few weeks. We found out that Karen's jaw felt so good after her first series of treatments that she had started chewing gum again. Her pain disappeared when she stopped chewing gum for good.

Another TMJ client, Marla, was a "nocturnal bruxer" (she ground her teeth in her sleep) and woke every morning with a sore jaw and a throbbing headache at her temples. Relaxation and EMG biofeedback worked quickly with this patient and we wondered why. A no-nonsense pragmatist, Marla told us she had simply quit bruxing in her sleep. When asked how, Marla said that once she understood what the problem was she simply told herself to quit bruxing and if she did she would wake herself and say "stop it." It took Marla two weeks to do away with a problem she'd had for many years.

Not all TMJ problems are resolved this quickly. Some TMJ symptoms are related to dental misalignment. However, before you have surgery or permanent, expensive dental work, try several weeks of biofeedback and relaxation therapy.

YOUR BODY'S BALANCE

Remember that stress is additive. There may be other factors that contribute to chronic muscle tension. Incorrect posture and repetitive motions alone or in combination with emotional tension may push you over the pain threshold.

Biomechanics is the study of how the body moves in relation to gravity and other pressures. Body build, posture, and overuse of particular muscles affect your biomechanics. Biomechanical stress that places a chronic strain on muscles can produce symptoms by itself, or make it easier for low levels of physiological tension to trigger symptoms.

Your body build, for instance, can place particular twists and strains on your muscles. An example is the difference in leg length found in about 71 percent of the population.[2] Let's say your left leg is shorter than your right leg. When standing, your hips will tilt sideways, with the left side lower than the right. This places a twisting, torsional strain on the muscles of your lower back. Your left shoulder will be lower than your right. If you're like most people, you'll raise your left shoulder so that your shoulder line is straight. This places a torsional strain on the muscles of your upper back and tilts your head to the right. Again, if you're like most people, you'll compensate by tilting your neck to the left to keep your eyes at the same level. This places a torsional strain on the muscles of your neck.

With your spine bent in an S curve and the muscles in your lower back, upper back, and neck already tense from the torsional mechanical forces imposed on them, it doesn't take much stress-related physiological arousal to generate back pain, stiff necks, and muscle contraction headaches (described below).

One way to tell if you have one leg longer than the other is to look at the hemline on your skirts, or the length of your trouser legs, or your belt line. If one side is higher than the other and you're having back problems or muscle contraction headaches, consult your physician or podiatrist for a possible corrective insole or lift in your shoe.

Another common biomechanical source of muscle strain is head posture. If you carry your head too far forward or too much to one side, you place an unnatural strain on the muscles of your neck and upper back. You probably don't realize it, but your head weighs approximately ½ of your body weight. For a 120-pound woman that comes to over 17 pounds; for a 180-pound man it's almost 26 pounds.

Your head, in fact, is much heavier than a bowling ball. Consider that your head is balanced on your spinal column like a bowling ball on a broomstick. The only structures that keep your head from flopping over when it gets out of balance are the muscles of your neck and upper back. When you keep your head in a balanced, gravitationally neutral position there is little strain on your muscles. Once it gets out of gravitational neutral, however, those muscles in your neck and upper back strain, causing stiffness and pain.

You're also likely to get muscle contraction headache pain in the back of your head, your forehead, and above and behind your eyes.

One way to maintain your head in gravitational neutral is to keep your ears lined up with your shoulders and your nose lined up with your breastbone. Calculate the weight of your head and remember it. It'll be a helpful reminder to keep it in gravitational neutral.

One of our clients, Luke, age 49, had muscle contraction or "tension" headaches not just once in a while but almost every waking hour of every day for years. Owner of a chain of furniture stores, Luke was a wealthy man and had spent a fortune seeking help from physicians and from famous medical centers. Luke was sent to us by his psychiatrist, who had told him that his tension headaches were a muscular expression of an "unresolved Oedipal rage" directed toward his wife and mother-in-law.

At our first interview, Luke told us he had suffered "unremitting tension headaches for the last seven years." As he related his story, Luke thrust his head forward, out of gravitational neutral, frowning gravely as he talked about his headaches. From the deeply etched lines in his forehead, we knew that Luke frowned a lot.

When we asked Luke why he frowned so much, he looked surprised and asked, "What do you mean?" We pointed to a mirror on the wall in front of him so he could see what we were talking about. Frowning and poor head posture had become so habitual that Luke was totally unaware of it. Moreover, he didn't realize that his habit of thrusting his head forward and continual frowning created a constant, debilitating tension on the muscles of his upper back, neck, and head, pushing them into the danger zone frequently and keeping them there for long periods of time. His headaches were caused by chronic muscle contraction and muscle spasm, not by an "unresolved Oedipal rage."

We taught Luke how to sit and stand in a straight, easy, natural way. We helped him to relax the muscles of his upper back, head, and neck by practicing progressive muscle relaxation exercises daily. We made an audio tape of PMR exercises for Luke so he could do them when he traveled. Using electromyographic (EMG) biofeedback we showed him the effects of relaxation and frowning on the muscles of his forehead. We broke his frowning habit by having him put mirrors in strategic locations in his office and home where he could see himself easily and correct his expression when he caught himself frowning. Finally, we had Luke get his wife, children, and employees to remind him to relax whenever they saw him frowning.

Luke still gets occasional muscle contraction headaches but they're far milder than they used to be. He still takes his relaxation tape with him when he goes out of town. His years of daily headache pain were ended by changing something as prosaic as his posture and a habitual facial expression.

REPETITIVE MUSCLE INJURIES

Violinists, typists, industrial workers, or anyone who performs repetitive motions for long periods may develop muscle spasms and pain. They may be able to tolerate such demand on their muscles during times when they are healthy and otherwise relaxed. However, if demands increase, rest or stretching periods are fewer, or other tensions occur, muscles may be unable to relax sufficiently, ultimately going into spasm or tendonitis.

In addition to medical treatment, progressive muscle relaxation exercises can help the individual learn to notice increased muscle tension before it gets painful, and to relax the muscles completely on breaks from activity.

SELF-REGULATION TECHNIQUES FOR MANAGING MUSCULAR SYMPTOMS OF STRESS

Many techniques are effective in reducing muscular symptoms of stress. None are foolproof. What works for one person may not work for another. We've listed the simplest and easiest to use first and the most involved last.

You can use some of these techniques by yourself; others may require help. Several of them are described further in chapter 19. Those techniques that induce deep relaxation tend to lower your metabolic rate and general level of physiological arousal. They may affect your need for prescription medications. If you are taking a medication for a seizure, cardiovascular, diabetic, or endocrine disorder, ask your physician to monitor your medications more carefully as you integrate these techniques into your lifestyle.

Because pain is a warning sign of possible injury or disease, your physician should diagnose any structural or organic problems before you proceed with a behavioral program.

Postural Adjustment

Make sure your sitting and standing posture is straight, easy, and natural. Keep your head in gravitational neutral when sitting or standing—keep that bowling ball balanced. Your spine should be straight, front to back and side to side. Use a mirror—full-length is best—to check your posture.

A postural exercise you might find helpful is to imagine that your body is suspended on a string connected to the center of your head. Let your body relax and become a weight hanging from that string. You'll find yourself straightening up and putting yourself in gravitational neutral almost automatically.

Progressive Muscle Relaxation (PMR)

PMR is the most powerful technique for reducing muscle tension and for increasing body awareness. It involves tensing and relaxing muscles in a progressive series and is often taught as an introduction to biofeedback (discussed below). After a muscle has been tensed, it tends to relax even more when the tension is released. Learning muscle relaxation also teaches you to notice small levels of tension before they reach a painful state. Scanning the body for tension on a regular basis and letting go of tightness will prevent an escalation of muscle symptoms. For a full description of PMR, see appendix I, which details a script that can be repeated on a tape for playback, or purchase the tape from the Biobehavioral Institute. (See the order form at the back of the book.)

Moist Heat

There is nothing like soaking in a hot bathtub after a long day of exercise. Moist heat also works on tension-related aches and pains. The moist heat of a hot shower, bath, face cloth, or heating pad dilates the small blood vessels in your muscles, improving circulation. The warmth also relaxes the muscle fibers.

Massage

Facial or body massage also improves circulation and loosens muscles. One client with headaches reported several hours of relief after having a facial at her beauty salon. Massage manually stimulates circulation of blood through the muscles, bringing fresh oxygen and carrying away waste products that cause soreness. This restores the chemical balance of the muscles and the surrounding tissue. Massage also realigns muscle fibers, decreasing the tendency for muscle spasms. Deep pressure on the muscle tends to stretch it, after which the muscle relaxes.

A massage can relieve tension, but it cannot keep you from tensing up again. If you are in the habit of holding tension in a particular muscle, your tightness will return. Relaxation training will help you recognize tension as it builds, and to let it out often throughout the day, developing the habit of relaxation in that muscle.

Massage is best done by massage specialists, but you can get it at home if there is a pair of willing, able, and competent hands available. You can massage those parts of your body within reach yourself, especially your forehead and upper shoulders, which are common areas of tension.

Exercise

Stretching exercises increase the flexibility of muscles and tendons, developing elasticity and increasing mobilization of the joints. Muscles usually relax even more after being stretched. Stretching prior to exercise is critical to prevention of injury. Do not hurry your workout by skipping the warm-up stretches. It's better to have a few minutes less of the aerobic exercise and a little more preparation of your muscles.

Yoga and other physical disciplines such as Tai Chi complement traditional stretching exercises. Yoga relaxes muscles by slow, continual stretching and relaxing of different parts of the body in sequence. Yoga training usually includes proper posture and breathing. Most communities have yoga classes available.

Strengthening exercises serve several functions. Strong, flexible muscles are less prone to tearing or injury. Gradually increasing exercise also increases circulation in the muscles, bringing nourishment to them and clearing out pockets of irritating metabolic wastes such as lactic acid.

Relax completely after exercise. Lie down if possible and let your body become like a rag doll. Let the energized muscles unwind completely before resuming your normal activities.

You may need to consult an exercise specialist or physical therapist to create an effective exercise program. For example, there are specific exercises for back spasms and specific ones to avoid. In addition, some injuries are caused by overworking one set of muscles but neglecting another set, which counterbalances the first. You may tend to favor, and thereby weaken, a part of your body to protect it from pain.

MAINTAINING PROGRESS

Once your muscular aches and pains disappear, continue to use these techniques to make sure your discomfort doesn't come back. We have found that clients tend to discontinue their successful techniques when they no longer have problems. When their symptoms return, they conclude that the treatment didn't really work, rather than realize the need for regular maintenance of a successful program.

Theodora was in an automobile accident three years ago that left her with chronic back pain. She had great success in a pain management program at a rehabilitation hospital and had been pain-free for one year. She was referred to our services when her pain returned. It turns out her home life was becoming increasingly stressful. Her son and daughter-in-law were unable to handle their two small children, and Theodora took over their care. She no longer took the time to do her relaxation and back-strengthening exercises. She was also lifting the children, ignoring her physician's advice. Interestingly, when out of town to visit a relative, her pain disappeared. When she arrived home at the airport, her pain returned. The emotional stress of her new responsibilities increased the tension on her damaged back just enough to start the pain cycle again. Our role was to reinforce her previous program and remind her to do what she already knew to do.

PROFESSIONAL HELP

Electromyographic (EMG) Biofeedback

EMG biofeedback works through a sensor that listens to the electrical activity of the muscles below the skin where the sensor is placed. This minute electrical activity, measured in microvolts, is amplified and displayed so that you can see the tension in particular muscles. The EMG signals can be transformed to sounds (auditory feedback) or onto a computer screen (visual feedback). You can then easily hear or see how a muscle tightens with a certain movement, posture, and state of emotion.

Next you practice the stretching, pressure, massage, or relaxation techniques that bring down muscle tension. Given this kind of feedback, most people learn to reduce muscle tension to very low levels. Progress is followed up by daily home practice. Biofeedback is best done professionally, but once you've learned the basics, you can do it yourself with a home biofeedback training instrument. To find a biofeedback specialist in your area, contact the Association for Applied Psychophysiology and Biofeedback, 10200 W. 44th Avenue, Suite 304, Wheat Ridge, CO 80033, (303) 420-2902.

Physical Therapy

Physical therapists know muscles. They tend to use things such as moist heat, controlled exercise, stretching, posture, and gait training to help condition and strengthen debilitated muscles that are prey to stress. Professional physical therapists are licensed or certified in each state. Ask your physician for a referral or look in the Yellow Pages for one. Your local hospital probably has a physical therapy department you can call.

Myotherapy

Myotherapy is a method of releasing muscular cramps or contractions through the use of brief sustained pressure on a "trigger point," cooling and stretching the muscle, and mechanical adjustment of the body, followed by corrective exercises. The techniques of myotherapy were developed and made famous by White House physician Janet Travell, M.D., who treated President John F. Kennedy's back pain.

A trigger point is a hypersensitive focus in the muscles or the membrane (fascia) that covers them. As you press along a sore muscle, you may find an especially sensitive knot, about the size of a pencil eraser. Manually compressing this trigger point with a knuckle or thumb for five to seven seconds often releases the tightness. A muscle may have several such trigger points.

Myotherapy requires a professional myotherapist, a person highly trained in muscular anatomy and physiology. These therapists are sensitive to biomechanical problems and will teach you how to release your own trigger points.

Locating a myotherapist may not be easy, but they can be found in most major metropolitan areas. They work only on referral, so ask your physician for some names. You may also write to the National Trigger Point Myotherapy Association, c/o Box 68, Yarmouthport, MA 02675, the National Chronic Pain Outreach Association, 7979 Old Georgetown Road, Suite 100, Bethesda, MD 20814-2429, or the American Academy of Pain Management, 3600 Sisk Rd., Suite 2D, Modesto, CA 95356, (209) 545-0754.

Neurology, Physiatry, and Rehabilitation Medicine

Physiatrists are doctors trained in rehabilitation medicine who specialize in the treatment of muscular aches and pains. Many are either trained in behavioral medicine or have behavioral medicine specialists on their staffs. Physiatrists, as physicians, can determine if further diagnostic information is necessary and can make appropriate referrals when your muscular symptoms are due to a more medical problem. They can be found through your local hospital. Many neurologists also specialize in the diagnosis and treatment of muscle pain.

N O T E S

1. Bardeen, C. R. (1921), "The Musculature," Section 5, in Morris's *Human Anatomy* (C. M. Jackson, ed.), Philadelphia, Blakenston's Son & Co.

2. Beal, M. C. (1950), "A Review of the Short Leg Problem," *Journal of the American Orthopedic Association* 50:109–121.

13 WHEN IT GETS YOU IN THE GUT

The parasympathetic nervous system (PNS) is part of what's called the autonomic nervous system. The PNS generally decreases physiological arousal. The other piece of the autonomic nervous system, the sympathetic nervous system (SNS), which we'll discuss in the next chapter, increases physiological arousal. Between them, they handle the general housekeeping of the body and do so fairly automatically. Hence, the term *autonomic*.

The PNS takes care of the "vegetative" or domestic chores of the body. It handles details like heart rate, digestion, excretion of urine and feces, and sexual functions. PNS symptoms such as indigestion, heartburn, "acid stomach," gas, flatulence, diarrhea, constipation, irritable bowel syndrome, colitis, difficulties with urination, and sexual dysfunctions develop as a consequence of the physiological arousal associated with acute stress.

PNS symptoms of stress involve irritations of stomach, gut, and bowel tissue, and disruption of smooth-muscle functions. Symptoms can persist long after the stress that caused them has vanished. Even when the irritation or dysfunction is minimal, the tissue or muscle is often sensitized to recurrences. It thus takes less and less stress to generate symptoms. If these symptoms run in your family you may have a genetic predisposition to this type of disorder. A prior illness or irritation may also have weakened the tissue. Acute stress then exacerbates that weak link. With each recurrence, the possibility of permanent tissue damage increases and severe conditions such as ulcerative colitis, Crohn's disease, urinary retention, or cystitis may occur.

Your PNS symptoms of stress, therefore, may become increasingly severe or may change over time depending on the amount of damage created by earlier acute stress episodes. For instance, what started as "acid stomach" may lead to heartburn, which may lead to ulcers. It depends on how frequently you experience stress and how great the cumulative damage to tissue and smooth muscle created by each acute episode.

FRANK'S ULCER

Frank's PNS symptoms, for instance, escalated in just that way. Frank, 53, came to us on referral from his gastroenterologist, who thought stress had a lot to do with Frank's ulcer. She was right.

Frank was a chubby, jolly man. He was proud that he "didn't have an enemy in the world." Friendly to everyone and everyone's friend, Frank had moved up the ladder in a midsize multinational corporation by diligence and hard work. Now corporate comptroller for American operations, he was in line for a promotion to vice president of finance. Two of his long-term colleagues were also under consideration, but Frank was the front-runner.

Frank tried to downplay the competition but admitted to us that it was "pretty fierce." Although he was the front-runner, he was ambivalent about the position. Every promotion he had received over the last twenty years had been traumatic. He wasn't sure he was willing or able to go through it one more time.

Frank had started out with the company as a bookkeeper. By going to night school, he became a certified public accountant and was elevated to manager of his department with a big raise in pay. His co-workers were jealous, and there was some initial tension, but it subsided in a few weeks.

The raise meant a new house in a new neighborhood. Frank was nervous about maintaining the mortgage, but his wife, Dorothea, insisted that it was best for them and their three children. She also insisted on remodeling and refurnishing the house. Turmoil reined for a while but dissipated after a few months.

Frank recalled this as his first experience with "indigestion." He remembered having heartburn in the middle of the night and burping a lot. He started keeping a bottle of "pink stuff" in his desk drawer at work and frequently took antacid tablets to relieve his stomach trouble. At the time, he had related his symptoms to the disruption in his schedule and his diet.

Three promotions later, Frank began seeing the company physician for prescription medications for his stomach trouble. He was advised to watch his alcohol and coffee consumption and to quit smoking. He did so and his symptoms went away.

With his next promotion, Frank and Dorothea built a new house in a posh suburb and joined a country club. His stomach problems started up again, but came back under control after a few months on medication.

Every promotion had been a traumatic transition for Frank because he couldn't tolerate change. He wanted to be friends with people and "get along," but colleagues were resentful when he moved ahead of them. Frank was constantly placating people or apologizing about something.

Promotions brought even bigger transitions at home. Dorothea expected Frank to enjoy his new positions and raises by moving up in the world. To her this meant a bigger house, a more expensive car, a nicer neighborhood, better schools, and more powerful friends. On the other hand, Frank liked life to go along smoothly. Moves and adjustment were very stressful for him.

Now Frank was being pressured to take on a fast-track job coveted by two people he had worked with for years. Dorothea wanted him to take the job because he "deserved it," and besides, "it's a lot more money." Frank had been agonizing over his situation for about a week when his stomach trouble came back in full force. His gastroenterologist found an ulcer, began treating it with medication, and sent Frank to us for stress management.

The first step we took was to help Frank establish a connection between his symptoms and the acute stress episodes he had experienced with each promotion. We explored in some detail his need to get along with everyone and sent him to an assertiveness-training workshop.

In addition, we had joint sessions with Frank and Dorothea. She was amazed that their moves had been so traumatic for him. She had enjoyed them and had thought they were "fun." In one session, Frank surprised everyone by explosively expressing his anger and resentment at Dorothea for pressuring him to take the promotion without listening to his reasons for not taking it. She had no idea he felt that way because he had "never said anything before."

Frank learned some deep relaxation and imagery techniques that helped lower his level of physiological arousal. He worked on these procedures at home and at the office. Frank saw images of cool, soothing milk flowing over the lining of his stomach and gut. His symptoms subsided, but, on his physician's advice, he stayed on his medication for a few months to make sure they didn't come back.

In the end, Frank decided to take the promotion. But this time he didn't move into a new house. He talked with his two friends before he accepted the position, telling them that he'd rather they be angry at him because he took the promotion than be angry at himself because he hadn't. The deciding factor for him, though, was that he thought the job would be fun and he could handle the pressure.

BLADDER AND BOWEL

Voiding difficulties, problems with urination, constipation, or diarrhea, are sometimes made worse because people tend to ignore their body's signals when they are under stress. One client, Alicia, whose bladder was so badly stretched that she no longer could hold urine, was referred to us by her urologist. Alicia told us she was too busy at work to go to the bathroom. If she had an urge to urinate, she would suppress it, and shortly the urge would pass. Then Alicia would forget to go later. Unfortunately, two things happened: her bladder stretched so much that she lost muscle tone and began to experience urinary leakage; and second, Alicia lost the feeling that told her when her bladder was full.

Alicia's treatment had three stages. First, she had to understand and appreciate the wisdom of her body that informed her when to void. Her physical needs had to take priority over work. We pointed out that Alicia wouldn't be much use at work if she was sick at home. Second, she practiced PMR and autogenic imagery (refer to appendix I) twice a day, especially tuning in to physical sensations in her lower body. Third, Alicia worked on issues of perfectionism and fears of inadequacy that drove her to put work performance over her health.

TECHNIQUES FOR MANAGING PNS SYMPTOMS OF STRESS

The techniques we describe in this section lessen the discomfort, distress, and pain of PNS symptoms but are in no way a substitute for competent medical care. If you're having PNS symptoms, see your physician or gastroenterologist first and discuss using these techniques to reduce your distress and pain. Used as a synergistic element in an overall medical treatment plan, they are powerful tools.

You can use some of these techniques by yourself but you may need help with others. Since many of these techniques involve relaxation, they lower your metabolic rate and general level of physiological arousal. This may reduce the amount of prescription medications needed to treat your condition. If you are taking a medication for a seizure, cardiovascular, diabetic, or endocrine disorder, be sure to have your physician monitor your medications regularly as you institute these new techniques. For more information on these techniques and how to use them, see chapter 19.

Self-Monitoring

Keep a daily record of your symptoms, your stress levels, and the related things that may irritate your system such as certain foods or activities. If particular foods seem to trigger your symptoms, eliminate them for a few weeks and see what happens. Coffee, alcohol, and nicotine are common offenders, as are highly. acidic, spicy, and fried foods. Eat regular meals on a schedule, avoid frequent snacking, and consume adequate amounts of fruit, fiber, and vegetables to keep your bowels functioning well. Make connections between your diet and all your PNS symptoms, not just those that affect your digestive system. Once you have a sound diet that gives relief from your symptoms, stick to it.

Quiet Time

You can't be quiet and aroused at the same time, so set aside some quiet time for yourself every day, especially before and after meals. Don't rush your meals. Blood is directed away from the stomach during physiological arousal. The body digests food best when physical arousal is slow and blood is directed to the stomach. If possible, pick a place where you can be by yourself, undisturbed, a place where there are no phones, no business conversations, just peace and quiet. One of our clients spends his lunch hour in his car in the company parking lot.

Deep Breathing

Deep breathing slows the body and quiets the mind. Under duress, gastrointestinal needs for oxygen are partially postponed. Oxygen is directed away from the digestive tract to the large muscles, in preparation for "fight or flight." Digestion slows down or stops. As you quiet the body and mind through deep breathing, the efficiency of your cardiovascular system in delivering vital oxygen to your gastrointestinal tract returns.

Progressive Muscle Relaxation (PMR)

PMR is a powerful technique for releasing physical tension and for becoming aware of your PNS symptoms (see appendix I and order form). As your muscles relax, your overall physical arousal slows, allowing activity in the stomach and bowel to normalize. Some tensions that interfere with sexual arousal can also be reduced through PMR. This technique sets the stage for using meditation, biofeedback, autogenic imagery, hypnosis, and affirmations in the healing process.

Meditation

Sitting meditation has similar effects of slowing the body's processes, allowing the organs to resume normal functioning. Spiritual beliefs in your ability to be healed may further energize your body's natural restorative abilities.

Electromyographic (EMG) Biofeedback

EMG biofeedback (explained in chapter 12) can be used to deepen muscle relaxation in the treatment of PNS symptoms. You can listen to bowel sounds with a regular stethoscope. However, more refined biofeedback of gastrointestinal activity is difficult and has generally been limited to research clinics. Autogenic and hypnotic imagery in connection with PMR are preferred.

Autogenic Imagery

The body responds to the suggestions of your mind. As you relax with PMR, conjure up images of cooling relaxation surrounding the distressed tissues of your body. Frank, for example, used images of cool, soothing milk running over the angry, red, irritated lining of his stomach. Another client with irritable bowel problems used images of his intestines as a knotted rope in a tug of war between two groups of large, powerful men. As they pulled, the knot would get tighter and his cramping pain would increase. Then he would envision the men falling, losing their grip on the rope, and the knot loosening and untying itself, and his cramping pain would lessen. Try different images until you find one that appeals to you and works. (See appendix 1 and order form.)

A common reaction to chemotherapy for certain types of cancer is nausea and vomiting. Some patients develop nausea even on the way to treatment in anticipation of the chemotherapy side effects. Training in relaxation and autogenic imagery has been shown to dramatically decrease this reaction.

One client's imagery for nausea was, "Let me feel fresh, cool mountain air filling my lungs. Bit by bit, let my stomach become quiet and relaxed. As all my muscles relax, my inner organs will also relax."

Hypnotic Imagery

The effects of imagery can be enhanced through the deepening of concentration that occurs in a hypnotic trance. A trained hypnotist can teach you self-hypnosis and help you refine your healing imagery. Some hypnotherapists make audio tapes of your sessions so that you can practice at home.

Affirmations

Before ending your relaxation or hypnotic exercise, allow a few moments to say to yourself certain statements affirming your intention to be healthy. The suggestions you make to yourself have an enduring effect even after you have ended your relaxation exercise. Some examples are:

- I can trust my body.
- I can notice my body's signals even if they are faint.
- It is natural to empty the body of things it doesn't need.
- When I void, I can relax, letting go of waste and tension.
- No matter what I am doing, I can hear and respond to the sensations of my body.

- It will make a difference to my body to eat the foods that help me stay healthy.

PROFESSIONAL HELP

Internal Medicine, Gastroenterology, Urology, and Gynecology

If you're having symptoms involving your stomach, gut, or bowel, see your internist or gastroenterologist for diagnosis and determination of the extent of any tissue damage. Some conditions may require prescription medication or surgery. If your symptoms involve problems with urination or sexual functioning, start with your internist, urologist, or gynecologist for diagnosis and a treatment plan. You need to know if your problems are primarily physical in nature such as an obstruction, interruption of blood supply, or some other physical problem that may require medication or surgery.

If you or your physician thinks stress is contributing to your symptoms, a consultation with a behavioral medicine specialist is in order. A team approach works best. The self-regulation techniques we describe can be a very helpful element in the treatment of your symptoms, but use them as part of a total package of treatment.

Behavioral Medicine Specialist

A specialist in behavioral medicine is generally a psychologist or physician trained in the diagnosis and behavioral treatment of physical symptoms and complaints. These techniques should be familiar to them. Many hospitals and medical centers have departments of behavioral medicine or can refer you to a practitioner in your neighborhood. Some behavioral medicine specialists are also trained in hypnotherapy. You can also write or call the Society for Behavioral Medicine, 103 South Adams Street, Rockville, MD 20850, (301) 251-2790.

Hypnotherapy

A qualified hypnotherapist will have credentials in a mental health field such as psychology, psychiatry, or social work as well as certification in hypnosis. Experience in working with people with physical problems is essential as well. You can contact the American Society for Clinical Hypnosis at 2200 East Devon Ave., Suite 291, Des Plaines, IL 60018-4534, (708) 297-3317, or the Society for Clinical and Experimental Hypnosis, 128A Kings Park Drive, Liverpool, NY 13090, (315) 652-7299.

14 IF YOUR HEART RUNS HOT OR COLD

When Anne felt her heart pounding, her hands sweating, and started to feel dizzy, it was her sympathetic nervous system (SNS) overreacting. It is difficult to disregard SNS symptoms. Anne could not ignore her difficulty in breathing or her palpitations. To her, these symptoms meant something was dreadfully wrong. Chest pain associated with SNS arousal is also frightening, because it may mean heart attack. And a painful migraine headache is not something you can wish away.

The SNS is the second part of your autonomic nervous system. Under normal conditions, it works in concert with the PNS to manage the internal affairs of your body. As part of its housekeeping chores, it regulates your blood pressure by controlling your heart rate and the contractions of your blood vessels. In stressful situations, it plays a major role in creating the physiological arousal involved in mobilizing your physical resources.

In normal times, the SNS exerts its effects on the body by secreting small amounts of a neurotransmitter called noradrenaline directly onto the organs it is stimulating. However, in times of stress, the SNS calls upon the adrenal glands to secrete into the bloodstream additional noradrenaline, and a more powerful neurotransmitter, adrenaline. These substances affect the whole body, not just a single organ.

These neurotransmitters circulating in your bloodstream provide a double dose of noradrenaline, accompanied by the extra "kick" of adrenaline. The physiological arousal created by SNS stimulation directly to a particular organ is rather short-lived. But the arousal created by adrenaline circulating through your bloodstream can persist for hours. When your adrenal glands get involved in your physiological reactions, your stress, to paraphrase Yogi Berra, ain't over when it's over.

Hormones also play a part in your chemical recipe for panic. Hormones (particularly cortisol from the outer shell of the adrenal glands) increase organ sensitivity to adrenaline and noradrenaline. This, too, raises your level of physiological arousal. For instance, adrenocorticotrophic hormone (ACTH) is released by your pituitary gland into your bloodstream, where it travels to your adrenal glands. Once there, it stimulates the cells forming the outer layers of the adrenal glands, the adrenal cortex, to release a number of "stress" hormones, including cortisol, into your bloodstream.

One of cortisol's many functions is to increase the sensitivity of organs such as your heart and blood vessels to the stimulating effects of noradrenaline and adrenaline. Your cardiovascular system becomes *sensitized*. When you experience acute, episodic stress, your cortisol-sensitized heart and blood vessels require less and less noradrenaline and adrenaline to climb to higher and higher levels of activity and to stay there for longer and longer periods of time. This is one reason why people who suffer one panic attack are likely to have repeated panicky feelings in the following weeks.

If your levels of arousal climb into the danger zone only occasionally, you're more likely to develop symptoms involving your muscular system and your PNS. If it reaches the danger zone in the repeated bursts of arousal found in acute episodic stress, however, you may also develop symptoms involving your SNS, such as panic attacks or cardiovascular symptoms of rapid heartbeat or migraine headaches. Your particular pattern of symptoms also depends on your genetic makeup, any previous illness or injury, etc.

SNS symptoms due to stress can involve all or part of your cardiovascular system. Stress-related high blood pressure, for instance, is associated with your heart and/ or blood vessels. Or, stress may affect only your heart and cause palpitations or irregular heartbeat. Other conditions such as Reynaud's disease or similar phenomena, on the other hand, provoke spasms in the small arteries supplying blood to your hands and/or feet. In a similar way, stress-related migraine headaches are associated with spasms in the small arteries supplying blood to the brain.

MIGRAINE HEADACHE

Of all the SNS symptoms of stress, migraine headache is the most difficult to ignore. They not only disrupt people's lives, they can be very painful. The most dramatic case of migraine headache we have seen involved Viola, who stood almost six feet tall and weighed 240 pounds. She had migrated to Boston from rural Georgia after high school and had been living here nearly sixteen years. Estranged from Chris, the drug addict father of her four children, she worked as a forklift operator in a warehouse. She didn't think it was "fair" that she had such a hard life, and she was angry about it.

When her migraines would start, usually following a psychotherapy session, Viola would become angry because, on top of everything else, she had to suffer these paralyzing headaches. Viola took medication and analgesics to dull the pain, but they didn't help. She would get angrier, and the headaches would get worse.

Frequently Viola ended up in the emergency room of the nearest hospital, enraged, with a pounding headache, and demanding immediate relief. Tending toward the histrionic, she would fling tables and chairs about the emergency room to emphasize her pain. On one occasion, Viola destroyed an emergency room and had to be forcibly subdued and tranquilized.

During the course of her psychotherapy for depression, Viola became aware of a volcanic rage at her sexually abusive father and older brother. Having fled Georgia to avoid them, Viola nonetheless attached herself to a series of men who were "even worse," and ended up living with Chris.

Viola's recollections of abuse triggered high-level, recurrent, episodic physiological arousal. The SNS and emotional symptoms she experienced would follow shortly thereafter.

As we began our work, we showed Viola how her recollections affected her physiologically. We taught her how to feel safer and to make her reactions to her memories less intense by looking at them in a different way.

We helped Viola associate looking to the past with looking in the rearview mirror of her car. We convinced her that an occasional glance in the mirror was fine to keep track of what was behind her but that she had to focus on what was ahead of her and where she was going. We pointed out to Viola that every time she looked at her rearview mirror, she was throwing her life in reverse. She had to choose whether she wanted to go backward or forward with her life. The memories could return but this method made them seem smaller and farther away. When Viola used this technique, she found she could control her level of arousal by deliberately switching to the future when her memories threatened to overwhelm her. She could focus on her current and future life, on what was here and now, especially the knowledge that she was now safe and secure.

We also taught her how to reduce her level of physiological arousal by relaxing with progressive muscle relaxation techniques and with calming visual images (refer to chapter 19 and appendix 1). Using photoelectric plethysmographic (PPG) biofeedback (discussed later in this chapter), Viola gained remarkable control over her blood vessels and could reduce the vascular spasms involved in her migraines. She extended her control of her blood vessels by monitoring her hand temperature and deliberately warming her hands when they got cold.

Cognitive techniques and self-regulatory skills enabled Viola to control her levels of physiological arousal. The frequency and intensity of her headaches dropped off dramatically and she stopped taking analgesics and opiates for her headache pain.

When her father died, Viola had a major setback after not having had a migraine for several months. After the funeral, she confronted her brother Jason about his abuse of her. The family rallied to Jason's defense and denounced her as a "liar and a troublemaker." Furious, Viola spent the night at a motel alternating between rage and calm as she used the techniques she had learned.

At the airport the next day, Viola thought obsessively about her earlier abuse, how much she hated Jason, how glad she was that her father was dead, how much she resented her mother for never being there for her when she was a child, and how angry she was at God for having assigned her such a woeful lot in life. Her hands turned ice cold. Viola knew she was on the verge of a migraine.

As the plane took off, the migraine struck full force. Viola tried using her self-regulation skills, but the migraine overwhelmed them. She reverted to her emergency room behavior and began screaming and thrashing about, demanding that she be immediately taken to a hospital. Viola was so violent that the pilot returned the plane to the airport. Viola was taken by ambulance to a hospital for treatment of her migraine. Placed on medication, and with a good night's sleep, Viola calmed down. The next morning she took another flight home.

Viola was embarrassed by her failure to control her migraines. We pointed out to her that it takes time and practice. She would have setbacks but she should not worry about it when they happened. The setbacks were just a reminder that she would need to continue daily practice even when she went weeks without a headache. She would need to work even harder during special times of stress.

Continuing with her psychotherapy, Viola set new goals for herself and began taking night school courses. She now works as a paralegal in a local law firm and is considering attending law school. She hasn't had a "real" headache for a long time, and says she seldom looks in her rearview mirror anymore.

Migraine headaches are usually a two-stage process, both equally debilitating. First come the icy cold hands, then the neurological signs of visual problems, difficulty with speech, nausea, and feelings of numbness. Next come the unrelenting, pounding headache and extreme sensitivity to light and sound.

No one really knows exactly how a migraine works, but we do know that the symptoms of the first stage are the result of constriction and spasm of blood vessels supplying the brain. As vessels constrict and go into spasm, there is a reduction in the blood supply to the brain, creating a disturbance called ischemia in specific brain areas. These localized ischemic conditions interfere with brain function and lead to the neurological symptoms of the first stage. It's like a temporary ministroke. Migraineurs are, in fact, more susceptible to strokes than are people who do not have migraines.

The pounding headache stage is a rebound condition where the blood vessels of the brain, particularly in the ischemic areas, dilate and become swollen as they attempt to bring blood to ischemic brain areas to repair any damage. Every time the heart beats there is a surge of blood through distended and swollen blood vessels, creating the pounding pain of the second stage.

Some migraine medications try to relieve the pounding headache by introducing a substance such as caffeine or Cafergot, which will constrict the dilated vessels. The problem with such vasoconstrictive substances is that they often create rebound vasoconstriction and spasm, leading to another headache.

Anything that encourages a biochemical environment for the brain that includes excess noradrenaline or adrenaline can precipitate migraines. These include:

- stress
- caffeine
- allergic reactions (particularly to some foods; see appendix I for dietary considerations in preventing migraines)

- hypoglycemia (low blood sugar)
- fatigue

Migraines can be prevented by avoiding the biochemical environments that trigger them. Once they start, the quicker you can calm the body to reduce noradrenaline and adrenaline levels, the better. Later in this chapter we'll provide a number of techniques for doing this.

HYPERTENSION

An increase in blood pressure is a necessary piece of your "fight or flight" response to stress. It ensures an adequate blood supply to your muscles and brain. Stress creates high blood pressure through its influence on your SNS and by stimulating your kidneys to conserve sodium. Your SNS elevates your blood pressure by stimulating your heart to beat faster and harder and to push out more blood with each heartbeat. It also causes your blood vessels to constrict, thereby increasing resistance to the flow of blood. Your kidneys get into the act by indirectly increasing your blood volume. Stress is a triple threat when it comes to hypertension.

When your heart beats faster and harder and squeezes out more blood per contraction, there is an increase in the blood output of your heart. When your blood vessels constrict, there is an increase in the resistance to blood flow. These are the two primary elements in short-term increases in blood pressure in response to stress. In fact, they multiply each other (cardiac output × total peripheral resistance = mean arterial blood pressure). As you can see, only one has to increase for your blood pressure to go up.

Your kidneys have an automatic mechanism for conserving sodium that kicks in as part of your "fight or flight" reaction to stress. Under nonstress conditions, your kidneys regulate the amount of sodium in your body. The more sodium you take in, the more sodium you excrete in urine. If you continue taking in the same amount of sodium and are under continuing stress, the concentration of sodium in your blood increases because your kidneys are conserving it as their contribution to your "fight or flight" reaction.

As the concentration of sodium in your bloodstream increases, it starts to draw water via the process of osmosis. As more water is drawn into the bloodstream, blood volume increases. As there is only so much room in your vascular system, pressure starts climbing as volume increases.

The clients we see at the Biobehavioral Institute for stress-related hypertension have one, two, or all three of the mechanisms contributing to their high blood pressure. Those who have a heavy contribution from the cardiac-output side learn to self-regulate their cardiac output as well as manage their stress better. Those whose major contribution comes from the resistance side of the equation learn to deal with stress better and relax the muscles in their blood vessels to reduce vascular constriction. Clients who have high blood pressure as a consequence of sodium conservation learn to manage stress better, exercise more (sweating is a good way to reduce sodium levels), and cut back on their sodium intake.

It is not unusual, however, to see people who have more than one component involved in their hypertensive reactions to stress. Ben, whom we discussed in chapter 9, "Beating Environmental Stress," had all three elements of his "fight or flight" response involved in his hypertension. Once he got his major stress under control, cut back on caffeine, learned to slow his heart rate and relax his blood vessels, and started exercising more vigorously, in addition to playing fetch with his dog, his blood pressure got down to a range he and his physician were happy with and stayed there without medication.

SELF-REGULATORY TECHNIQUES FOR MANAGING SNS SYMPTOMS OF STRESS

The techniques we describe in this section will lessen the discomfort, distress, and pain of your SNS symptoms, but they cannot substitute for competent medical care. If you're having SNS symptoms, discuss with your physician how you might use these techniques to alleviate your symptoms. Since many of them involve relaxation, they tend to lower your metabolic rate and general level of physiological arousal. Consequently, they may interact with prescription medications you may be taking. If you are taking a medication for a seizure, cardiovascular, diabetic, or endocrine disorder, be sure to have your physician monitor your medications as you practice relaxation.

You can use some of the techniques by yourself, but you may need help with others. For more information on these techniques and how to use them, see chapter 19.

Self-Monitoring

Keep a daily symptom diary noting the frequency and severity of your symptoms (rate them from 1 to 5, with 5 being the most severe). Notice the relationship of your symptoms to specific events or emotional upsets in your life. Once you've pinpointed particular triggers, try to avoid them or make a special effort to stay relaxed and not let them bother you when you have to deal with them.

Diet

Keep track of what you eat and when you eat it in relation to your SNS symptoms. If there are particular foods that seem to trigger your symptoms, eliminate them from your diet for a few weeks and see what happens to your symptoms. Caffeine, alcohol, and nicotine are notorious triggers for migraines, hypertension, erratic heart rate, and Reynaud's disease (refer to chapter 3 for considerations of caffeine).

Caffeine acts as a vasoconstrictor. It is found in coffee, tea, and cola drinks as well as many medications, including those used to treat migraines. Excess caffeine can also precipitate the symptoms of panic even in people who rarely feel anxious. People who have physical SNS signs of anxiety are often more sensitive to caffeine and can tolerate only minimal amounts. If you have many SNS symptoms, read the section on caffeine care-fully.

You could be allergic to a number of foods that serve as triggers for your symptoms without knowing it. Check the list of foods in appendix I for others that may have allergenic effects on your cardiovascular system.

Deep Breathing

Several items in the SNS section are frequently asso-ciated with hyperventilation brought on by rapid, shal-low breathing: dizziness, palpitations, rapid heartbeat, tightness in the chest, and shortness of breath. Shallow breathing makes your heart speed up when you breathe in and slow down when you breathe out. Shallow breath-ing tends to be more rapid than deep breathing and tends to make your blood "stickier" for oxygen than it should be. As a consequence, your blood picks up oxygen very well in your lungs, but doesn't want to give it up to body tissue where it's needed. Your blood vessels dilate and your heart beats faster and harder to supply tissue with enough "sticky" blood to satisfy its oxygen needs.

If you hyperventilate, first you need to balance the ratio of carbon dioxide and oxygen in your bloodstream. Do this by cupping your hands over your nose and mouth and rebreathing your exhaled breath, which has a higher concentration of carbon dioxide. You could also breathe into a paper bag, but you may not have one with you. Or, just hold your breath for thirty seconds. Just breathing slowly through your nose may have the same effect. When you feel better, resume deep diaphragmatic breathing.

There are few self-regulatory exercises as calming as deep breathing. In addition to its general calming effect, deep breathing will improve the efficiency of your car-diovascular system in delivering vital oxygen to your body tissue including your brain. Try the "one, two, three" deep breathing exercise we teach our clients. In a seated position, place your elbows on your knees, lean forward, and place your chin in your hands. Now, breathing through your nose, take three deep breaths, holding each for a slow count of three. Lean back and continue to breathe slowly and deeply through your nose as you let yourself calm down and relax.

Read the section of chapter 19 on deep breathing to teach yourself the habit of breathing correctly.

Progressive Muscle Relaxation (PMR)

PMR is a powerful technique for releasing muscle tension and for becoming aware of your body. It is particularly helpful for cardiovascular problems such as migraine headache and hypertension. As breathing slows and the muscles relax, the blood vessels tend to relax and expand as well, expanding the amount of space in the cardiovascular system and lowering blood pressure. More blood can then go to the brain. A relaxed capillary can also carry more blood to the fingertips and toes, thus warming the extremities. People who have panic attacks often report that they find PMR tedious and not especially helpful. The breathing exercises seem more helpful.

Electromyographic (EMG), Photoelectric Plethysmographic (PPG), and Temperature Biofeedback

Biofeedback is particularly helpful and is a treatment of choice for circulatory disorders such as Reynaud's disease (cold hands and feet), migraine, certain types of hypertension, and certain types of tachycardia. You can obtain the name of a biofeedback specialist in your region by contacting the Association for Applied Psychophysiology and Biofeedback, 10200 W. 44th Ave., Suite 304, Wheat Ridge, CO 80033, (303) 420-2902.

Biofeedback is best done with the help of a professional, but you can do it at home with home biofeedback training instruments. Start with electromyographic (EMG) biofeedback to develop skill in controlling muscle tension. In EMG biofeedback, muscle-tension levels are amplified and displayed so that you can see just how tense particular muscles are. Given that feedback, most people can learn to reduce muscle tension to very low levels.

After you've learned to regulate your muscle tension, go on to photoelectric plethysmographic (PPG) or temperature biofeedback, which measures blood circulation. This feedback will teach you to increase circulation by relaxing muscles in the walls of your blood vessels.

Temperature training may require professional help at first but can easily be transferred to your everyday life. You can feel whether your hands are cool or cold by placing them on your face. When your hands are cool, use your skills to warm them up. There are a variety of inexpensive temperature-sensitive biofeedback devices available for home use such as "stress cards," "stress dots," thermometers, and temperature-sensitive or "mood" rings. These can be purchased at drugstores and bookstores or ordered through your therapist, behavioral medicine practitioner or from the Biobehavioral Institute (see order form at the back of the book.) They work through chemicals embedded in the card that change color with changes in temperature. They are fairly accurate and give you another source of information as to how your body is functioning.

Many people with panic disorder do not find biofeedback helpful. Breathing exercises and working with imagery seem more helpful to them.

Meditation

Meditation has been found to be a reliable treatment for certain types of hypertension. It can also help you to cope with the thoughts that contribute to migraine and hyperarousal symptoms. People who have trouble sitting still tend not to use formal meditation techniques. A short form of meditation or the practice of mindfulness might be more suitable for them (see chapter 19).

Autogenic Imagery

As you relax with PMR (see appendix I and order form), imagine pictures of warmth and relaxation for your particular symptom. Viola, for example, used images of warm, soothing water running over her hands to promote relaxation of the blood vessels of her hands and feet. Another client was able to relax his blood vessels and slow his heart by simply saying out loud to himself, "My hands are getting warmer and warmer. I can feel my pulse in my fingertips, slow, strong, and steady." Another image he liked was, "My fingers are like radiators with warm steam circulating through them."

Suggested autogenic phrases:

- My heartbeat is steady and regular.
- My skin is becoming cool and dry.
- I can let the muscles of my chest loosen and relax.

If you are more prone to panic symptoms, like Anne, you may have vivid negative images of catastrophe, heart attacks, and ambulances or passing out as part of your symptoms. These images tend to escalate other symptoms. For you, imagery work means first recognizing panic-producing images, then substituting panic-reducing images, such as a picture of yourself coping with the unpleasant feelings, relaxing into the feelings.

Refocusing Attention

Another strategy for coping with panic symptoms such as palpitations or sweaty palms is redirection or attention away from the symptoms. Focusing on the present rather than "what if . . ." thoughts tends to lessen symptoms.

Assertion Skills Training

Assertiveness can forestall many stress situations that escalate SNS symptoms. Limiting the demands that others place on you by learning to say no prevents resentment from building up. Knowing that you can talk yourself out of most situations helps counteract feelings of being trapped or out of control. You no longer have a reason to be overaroused, so your body can repair itself.

Exercise

Gradually increasing exercise will increase efficiency of your cardiovascular system and ease the workload on your heart. A regular aerobic exercise program can help lower your blood pressure. It can also make you less vulnerable to migraine headaches.

If you have SNS symptoms associated with panic attacks, you might initially fear the heart pounding, sweating, and shortness of breath brought on by aerobic exercise. However, if your physician has told you these symptoms don't indicate any cardiac problems, you will benefit from exercise. Knowing that your body is aerobically fit decreases worry about cardiovascular symptoms. If you regularly get your heart rate up to 140 or 160 beats per minute during exercise, you won't worry if it hits 100 beats per minute from stress.

You may need to consult an exercise specialist or physical therapist to get an effective exercise program under way. It's important not to overdo, but at the same time you don't want to underdo.

PROFESSIONAL HELP

Internal Medicine, Neurology, Nephrology, and Cardiology

If you're having symptoms involving your heart or blood vessels, see your internist for diagnosis and medical treatment. Neurologists diagnose and treat migraine and other vascular headaches, nephrologists specialize in the kidneys and certain types of hypertension, and cardiologists deal with the entire cardiovascular system, but particularly with the heart. Some SNS conditions may require medical treatment and prescription medication. The self-regulation techniques we describe will help, but use them as part of a total package of treatment.

Behavioral Medicine

A specialist in behavioral medicine is generally a psychologist or physician trained in behavioral diagnosis and behavioral treatment of physical symptoms and medical problems. Check to see that they have some specific experience in your disorder. Local hospitals may have behavioral medicine divisions or you can write or call the Society for Behavioral Medicine, 103 South Adams Street, Rockville, MD 20850, (301) 251-2790.

Cognitive-Behavioral Therapy

Cognitive-behavioral therapy will help you identify those thoughts that increase your symptoms and help you develop challenges to those thoughts. You learn to "talk back" to panic-producing or anger-producing thoughts.

15 ANGRY, DEPRESSED, AND ANXIOUS

Emotions are found only in warm-blooded animals. The evolution of emotional behavior goes hand in hand with the evolutionary development of the mammalian nervous system and reaches its greatest complexity at the human level. The brain system responsible for our emotions, the limbic system, is buried deep in our brains and is interconnected with all its other parts and systems, including the more "intelligent" parts and systems. The activity of our limbic systems provides emotional color, excitement, and vitality to our thoughts, words, and behaviors.

Emotions are a vital part of human existence. They give meaning to life. While some emotions are pleasant to experience and we seek them, sometimes avidly, others are unpleasant, so we try to avoid feelings such as irritation, anger, apprehension, fear, sadness, grief, guilt, etc. We forget that they are necessary elements of a well-rounded emotional life. Everyone experiences them at one time or another.

Avoiding unpleasant feelings doesn't make them go away—you only become more vulnerable to them and give them time for incubation and growth. Dealing directly with unpleasant feelings, painful as it may be, makes you stronger and rids you of them.

When your level of physiological arousal reaches your danger zone in frequently recurring episodes of stress, you experience anger, anxiety, and/or depression as symptoms. People who see stress as solely an emotional phenomenon often confuse it with anxiety. As we have shown, stress involves both mind and body. Anxiety is just one of many possible symptoms of stress. There are, as we mentioned earlier, three emotional symptoms of stress: anxiety, anger, and depression. These stress emotions are sometimes difficult to separate, often becoming so entangled that you don't know what you're feeling, except that you're "upset."

When emotions intensify, they feed on one another and can become so powerful that they overwhelm you, bringing on fears of losing control of yourself and "going crazy." One client, Andrea, described herself as a "bubbling caldron of emotions about to boil over. Sometimes I'm angry, sometimes I'm depressed, and sometimes I'm just scared, but most of the time it's all of the above. I'm frightened I'll lose it and really make a mess of my life."

One way to get control over your emotions is to sort them out by labeling them, but it's not easy. Emotions are hard to describe because developmentally they precede language. Children express emotions long before they learn to speak.

It requires more than being articulate to label emotions effectively. People, particularly men, who grew up in families that did not talk about emotions have difficulty labeling their feelings. Some families allow expression of only one or two feelings. For instance, a family with an anxious parent may talk frequently about anxiety and fear, but seldom about anger. Other families are comfortable with love but not anger, or vice versa. One of our clients who suffered from panic attacks felt all emotion as anxiety. She had difficulty separating sadness and anger from anxiety. All her feelings blended together into what she called anxiety.

Humans experience a full range of emotions that often go undefined and undifferentiated. To gain more control, we need to identify, classify, and label the elements that constitute our emotional world. For example,

Alma once worked in the substance abuse unit at a Veterans Administration hospital in San Francisco. The men in the unit had particular difficulty in talking about feelings. They had histories of excessive drinking and drug use to deaden pain. They were also limited by the poverty of their "emotional" vocabularies—they simply didn't have the words and labels to describe their feelings.

As a former schoolteacher, Alma drilled them in vocabulary to repair their language deficits. Instead of saying they were upset or angry, depressed or scared, they learned to use more precise words, such as frustrated, annoyed, irritated, aggravated, indignant, irate, enraged, paranoid, anxious, frightened, and terrified, in describing their emotions.

After they had enriched their emotional vocabularies, they could talk more easily about the connections between their feelings and their substance abuse. Next they started rating the intensity of their emotions on a ten-point scale, assigning specific names to specific numbers. They now had words for differentiating the emotions from one another and for communicating the intensity of their feelings to themselves as well as to other people.

Language can express the most subtle and refined nuances of our emotional experience. Use it to enrich your world of emotional feeling and to gain control when emotions threaten to become overwhelming.

Anne, whose case we've followed throughout the book, illustrates how uncontrolled emotional reactions to stress can create physical reactions that, in turn, release overwhelming emotional reactions. As we indicated earlier, Anne's dilemma was a career/family conflict. Anne felt pressure from her mother to marry and have children; she felt equally strong internal pressure to do well in her career. As she saw it, taking one path ruled out the other.

An only child, Anne had been close with her father, who died of a heart attack when she was 12. Her father had always wanted a son. He called Anne "Andy" and treated her like a boy. He told Anne that she was going to have to prove herself in a "man's world." For Anne, success in business meant she was finally "measuring up" to her father's expectations of "Andy."

Anne's mother thought business success was "nice" but no substitute for a home and children. Anne wanted her mother's approval but was unwilling to give up her career to get it. At the time she came to see us, Anne was convinced that her mother was plotting with her boyfriend, Mark, to pressure her into marriage.

Whenever her career was threatened, Anne felt that she was under a personal attack. It meant "Andy" was a failure, and hadn't "made it in the real world." Whenever the possibility of marriage and children was imminent, she would anxiously anticipate her mother's disapproval. As her career flourished, Anne felt her chances of marriage and children slipping away; whenever she considered marrying Mark, she believed her career would go up in smoke.

Caught between the two paths, and seeing them as mutually incompatible, she felt she had no way out. Anne would get anxious and brace herself against attack, tightening her abdominal muscles as though she were about to receive a body blow. A chest breather (defined in chapter 19), her tight abdominal muscles produced even shallower breathing.

Anne's physiological arousal increased her body's need for oxygen. To satisfy her increased oxygen requirements, she had to get more air into her lungs by breathing either more deeply or more rapidly. Since the tension of her abdominal musculature made deep breathing difficult, she was forced to breathe ever more rapidly until she hyperventilated.

Hyperventilation reduced the carbon dioxide level in her blood, making it "stickier" for oxygen. Hence, her blood would pick up oxygen in her lungs, but because it was still "sticky" it would not surrender oxygen to her body tissues as it normally did.

To get enough oxygen to body tissues, including her brain, the blood vessels in her tissues dilated, making her heart beat faster and harder to maintain blood pressure. Blood vessels in less critical parts of the body, such as fingers and toes, then constricted to further elevate blood pressure and increase blood flow to vital organs. In a desperate response to the tissue demand for more oxygen, Anne would breathe even faster, making things worse.

Anne's perception of these complex physiological events taking place in her body was that she got dizzy and felt faint (from a temporary drop in blood pressure), got a "tingling, pins and needles" feeling in her fingers and toes (from constriction of peripheral blood vessels), felt her heart racing and pounding "like it's going to jump out of my chest," and had pains in her chest that meant (to her) that she was going to have a heart attack and die "just like my father" (from chest muscles overworked by her rapid breathing). Terrified and unable to get her breath, Anne would breathe even faster. This compounded and escalated a mind-body spiral until she was in the throes of a full-blown panic attack.

The first order of business was to prevent Anne from hyperventilating. She started on a program of respiratory retraining—to breathe deeply by relaxing her abdominal muscles and to use her diaphragm to fill her lungs from the bottom up. We gave her taped homework exercises, which included a PMR exercise and diaphragmatic breathing exercises.

Anne had difficulty with the diaphragmatic breathing at first, feeling she couldn't get enough air. She was right. As a chronic chest breather and frequent hyperventilator, Anne had drawn so much CO_2 out of her blood bicarbonate buffer system that it was no longer functioning to prevent uncontrolled swings in the acid/base (pH) balance of her blood.

With her bicarbonate buffer depleted, the increased blood CO_2 levels generated by diaphragmatic breathing drove Anne's blood too far in the acid direction, making it less "sticky" for oxygen. So, although there was plenty of oxygen in the air she breathed, her blood couldn't pick it up effectively.

Before she could get her respiratory system back on track, Anne had to restore her blood bicarbonate buffer to guard against those swings in blood pH that made it either too "sticky" or not "sticky" enough to function efficiently. In most cases, this takes about two weeks of regular deep-breathing practice. Once her buffer system had been restored, Anne became comfortable with diaphragmatic breathing and found it calming and soothing.

As we explored her emotional reactions, Anne realized she had been programmed to exaggerate the minuses in a situation and minimize the pluses. Anything unfavorable was seen as "awful." She managed to see a potential catastrophe lurking around every corner, particularly where career, marriage, and children were concerned. She was an "awfulizer" and "catastrophizer." She was full of, "Yes, but what if's . . ."

We began a program of thought stopping and cognitive restructuring. We helped her change her cognitive style and eliminate the thought patterns that precipitated her attacks. She learned to distance herself from her situation and stay in the moment by observing her emotional state and rating it. She developed considerable skill with PMR and learned to relax at will.

Anne thought there were four primary things she could do to get her emotional and cardiovascular symptoms under control. This is what she wrote on her *Stress Action Plan: Symptoms:*

- Remember to breathe through my nose slowly and evenly. I'll need to practice that.
- Stop the catastrophizing thoughts, the "what if . . ." thoughts.
- Remember to stay in the moment, don't worry about what might happen.
- Make myself a relaxation tape with a special emphasis on diaphragmatic breathing.

SELF-REGULATION TECHNIQUES FOR MANAGING THE EMOTIONAL SYMPTOMS OF STRESS

You have much more control over your emotional state than you probably realize. What and how you think determines in large part what and how you feel; what and how you feel colors what and how you think. Getting control of your thoughts changes the way you feel, and getting control of your feelings alters the way you think. The techniques we describe here help you manage this complex equation.

You can use some of these techniques by yourself, but you may need help with others. Since many techniques involve relaxation, they tend to lower your metabolic rate and general level of physiological arousal. They may interact with prescription medications you may be taking for seizure, cardiovascular, diabetic, or endocrine disorders. Be sure to check with your physician before trying these techniques.

For more information on these techniques and how to use them, see chapter 19, "Calling on the Healer Within."

Emotional Release

You don't want to get rid of emotions, you just want to manage and get them under control. A three-step method of emotional release has helped many of our clients. The first step is to identify exactly what it is you're feeling and label it. As we said before, emotions often defy description, but try. Building a better emotional vocabulary makes it easier. Write down as many adjectives as you can for anger, anxiety, and depression. Use a thesaurus, and get words from friends, family, and co-workers. Sort your words in order of intensity. Learn to examine your emotional state and attach a label that describes it with some degree of accuracy.

Next, experiment with thoughts that increase the intensity of the emotion you're feeling. Then try thoughts that reduce that intensity. Rate the intensity level of your emotions on a 1 to 10 scale. Learn to raise and lower your level with your thoughts.

Learning to release emotions is the third step. This can be done in a number of ways, such as acting them out, talking them out, or thinking them out. Shouting, crying, or acknowledging that you are afraid takes the edge off your feelings, allowing you to think more clearly. You can talk about how you feel with a friend, family member, or counselor. Sometimes, images and thoughts can release your emotions.

We talked earlier about our friend who cries while in a hot bath when she's feeling sad. It's a good way to release depressive syptoms. Some people act out their frustrations and anger by shouting into the wind or beating a pillow. Some clients express their fear and anxiety with pat phrases like, "Oh, my God," or, "Oh, oh."

In releasing your emotions through talking to other people, be sure you don't act out the emotion toward them. Try to stay calm and talk to them rationally about how you feel.

A word of caution: We are not advocating that you express your feelings irresponsibly, just to get them off your chest, nor are we suggesting you wallow in your feelings indefinitely. The intensification and expression of feelings is one aspect of learning to manage strong emotions and getting them under control.

If you can learn how to intensify your emotions, you can also learn how to decrease or to transcend them. When you do, you will feel more in control and can choose the emotional option that fits the specific time and place.

Here are a few rules to remember about releasing feelings:

- Mean what you say, say what you mean, but don't be mean when you say it.
- Don't break things that don't belong to you.
- Don't hit other people.
- Don't hurt yourself (physically or with drugs, food, etc.).
- Use good judgment when in public.

Self-Monitoring

Relate your thoughts to your emotions by keeping track of what you're thinking about when you feel them. Try to make connections between your thoughts and your emotional symptoms. Sort out your irrational thoughts and counter them with rational ones. Irrational thoughts can lead to irrational behavior.

Quiet Time

Set aside quiet time for yourself every day. Do it regularly; don't wait until you're angry, depressed, or anxious. It doesn't have to be a lot of time, twenty to thirty minutes is enough. Pick a place where you can be by yourself, undisturbed.

One of our clients chose his lunch hour as his quiet time and spent it in his car in the company parking lot. Another client insisted she couldn't take quiet time for herself because there was no privacy in her home and she had no other place to go. We recommended her bedroom, but she said her children did not respect closed doors. We suggested she put a lock on the door and use it. She did, and finally got a daily respite from the stress of her life.

Deep Breathing

There are few self-regulatory exercises as calming as deep breathing. Deep breathing improves the efficiency of your cardiovascular system in delivering oxygen to your body, including your brain.

Try the "one, two, three" deep breathing exercise we teach our clients. In a seated position, place your elbows on your knees, lean forward, and place your chin in your hands. Now, breathing through your nose, take three deep breaths, holding each one for a slow count of three. Lean back and continue to breathe slowly and deeply through your nose as you let yourself calm down and relax.

Progressive Muscle Relaxation (PMR)

It's impossible to be relaxed and emotionally tense at the same time. They are mutually exclusive. PMR is a powerful technique not only for releasing muscle tension and becoming aware of your body, but for releasing emotional tension. It involves tensing and relaxing muscles in a progressive series and takes about twenty minutes to complete. It is often taught as an introduction to biofeedback and to self-hypnosis autogenic imagery. PMR instructions are available on audio tape from the Biobehavioral Institute of Boston (see order form at the back of the book). You can make your own tape by using the PMR script in appendix I.

Visual Imagery

As you relax using PMR, conjure up images of emotional release. Try different images until you find one that appeals to you. Often, feelings cannot be put into words. Instead, they come out through our imaginations. We fantasize scenes that never happen—what we wish we could have said to the boss, what we should have done to forestall some tragedy. Sometimes the visual image is the recurrent memory of a real event, a "flashback."

You can change your images either to increase or to decrease the intensity of your feelings. Not long ago we had a client, Ellen, whose son had been killed in a terrorist bombing. Three years later she was still grieving. Imagining the capture and trial of the terrorists helped Ellen cope with her anger, grief, and depression. She visualized being in the courtroom and the violent things she'd do and say if she had the chance. Her family worried whenever she talked about these angry scenes. But we gave Ellen permission to work through her grief and anger in this way, with the caution to remember the difference between fantasy and actual behavior.

You can use visual imagery when you are ready to let go of your anger, anxiety, and depression. One client, tired of being upset with her landlord, imagined putting her anger in a black balloon and letting it float away. It got smaller and smaller as it soared into the sky.

PROFESSIONAL HELP AND ASSISTANCE

Behavioral Medicine

A specialist in behavioral medicine is generally a psychologist or physician trained in the diagnosis and behavioral treatment of stress-related emotional and physical symptoms and complaints. Many hospitals and medical centers have departments of behavioral medicine or can refer you to a practitioner in your neighborhood. You can also contact the Society for Behavioral Medicine, 103 South Adams Street, Rockville, MD 20850, (301) 251-2790.

Psychotherapy

If the previously described techniques don't work, your anxiety, anger, and depression may be rooted in more complex psychological problems and you may need psychotherapy. Psychologists, psychiatrists, and social workers are professional psychotherapists. They may come from different schools of thought ranging from doctrinaire Freudian psychoanalysis to cognitive behavioral therapy. Whatever the approach, it has to feel right to you and you have to trust your therapist. If the approach doesn't make sense, or if you don't feel comfortable with the therapist, try another one. You can get referrals from your physician, state professional organizations, and mental health centers, or try the Yellow Pages.

Make your first session a trial interview. Find out something about the therapist's approach, orientation, training, background, and experience with problems like yours. Ask questions about the therapist as a person. While a therapist may prefer not to discuss personal details, general questions about attitudes or experience help you to evaluate their abilities.

Counseling

In addition to psychotherapists, professionals such as ministers, priests, and rabbis offer counseling. Counseling is generally much more short term than psychotherapy and is limited to specific problems and issues. Counselors are more likely to offer advice and assistance in direct problem solving.

Bibliotherapy

There are many excellent books on anger, anxiety, and depression. Look in the psychology section of your bookstore or your local library, and see appendix II for our recommended readings.

16 TOO STRESSED TO THINK STRAIGHT

Human beings are thinking animals. Your capacity for complex thought makes you what you are. In classical psychology, thought, or cognition, is seen as a process consisting of several steps: sensation, perception, apperception, association, and memory. Among the many things your brain does, it conducts these complex cognitive processes, with different parts of the brain being more or less responsible for particular elements. Stress disrupts the functioning of those parts of your brain necessary for cognitive activity, just as it alters the functioning of the sections involved in emotion. When it does, it interferes with your cognitive or thought processes at a number of levels.

Here's what happens. Adrenaline from your adrenal glands stimulates a section of your nervous system buried deep in the brain, your ascending reticular activation system (ARAS). Your ARAS, in turn, activates and energizes your brain, causing its neurons to fire two to three times faster than normal. This increase in brain activity not only creates emotional intensity for you, it makes you think faster. The greater your perceived burden of pressure, the greater the physiological arousal, the greater the stimulation of the ARAS, and the greater the increase in brain activity. At high levels of arousal, your brain becomes hyperactive and so do you.

Brain hyperactivity has profound effects on how you think. Your thoughts race, with scattered fragments of incomplete ideas whirling about in your mind, your memory is impaired, and your judgment deteriorates. You make hasty decisions that lead to impulsive, ill-advised actions; in turn, you create more problems and stress for yourself.

And, the problem compounds itself. You get so used to your hyperactive brain and the thought and behavior patterns it generates, you think it's normal. You may seek stimulating drugs, situations, or activities to whip it up when it starts to flag. Under conditions of recurrent stimulation, your ARAS becomes increasingly sensitive, requiring less and less adrenaline to exert its electrifying effect on your brain.

Your overstimulated brain creates problems for you when it comes time to slow down. You may seek "chemical help" to dampen its activity. A drink before dinner or late at night is a ritualized chemical relaxation. Muffling brain activity, we think, contributes significantly to the popularity of prescription and over-the-counter sleeping medications.

Dennis's hyperactive brain made his life unnecessarily difficult. A 29-year-old cop, he got into trouble because of ill-advised and impulsive behavior on the job caused by his hyperactive brain. Dennis had "roughed up" a drug suspect when the man, who turned out to be a respected civic leader, objected to being searched. After an internal police investigation, Dennis's lawyer cited job stress as a factor in the incident. He was found guilty of using undue force in the "roughing up" incident, was suspended without pay for ninety days, and then was transferred to a desk job where he could not carry a sidearm. The police board followed a physician's recommendation and referred him to our clinic.

Dennis described his overarousal and its effect on his thoughts and behaviors in graphic terms: "I get so wired I can't think straight. I forget things. I get antsy and jumpy and do dumb things. I shouldn't have hit Mr. Frommes [the drug suspect] but I was tired of taking crap from druggies. I just blew it."

Dennis's five years on the police force had been studded with excitement, trauma, citations, reprimands, and stress. There had been numerous high-speed chases, a "shootout" with robbery suspects in which he had been slightly wounded, and a major patrol-car accident. Dennis had been cited for heroism, but he had also been reprimanded on several occasions for insubordinate behavior. Dennis had been "mouthy" with other officers and with his superiors. When he came to see us, he had been told either to "clean up his act" or to turn in his badge. His transfer from the more exciting patrol-car assignment was galling, and he was embarrassed that he had been placed on the "bow-and-arrow squad" without a sidearm. He decided he needed to get his life and himself under control because he loved being a cop.

Beside his job travails, Dennis had domestic problems. He had violent quarrels with his wife, Sandi, and had beaten her on several occasions. Remorseful, at one point, he had placed his gun in his mouth and "almost pulled the trigger." He was also abusive to his children. Sandi repeatedly threatened divorce and had retained legal counsel on two occasions.

Dennis had become almost addicted to the hyperactivity of his brain. He loved excitement and the feeling of physiological arousal. It made him feel "alive." We discussed his use of stimulants and depressants and found that he was "playing uppers and downers" with caffeine and alcohol. Coffee in the morning got him "perking" and repeated doses throughout the day kept him "on his toes." On his way home, he would stop for a beer or two to "relax after being wired all day." In the evening at home he would shift to scotch whiskey to "mellow out." When Sandi berated him for not helping her with the children and other household chores, which she did often, Dennis would curse and sometimes physically abuse her.

We were not particularly optimistic about helping Dennis. A number of character issues stood in the way. Dennis was very "macho," was unable to grasp the idea of self-regulation and self-control, and was ashamed of seeing a "shrink." He surprised everyone, including himself, by doing very well in a relatively short period of time.

Dennis started with PMR (described in chapter 19) and took to it immediately. He said it worked "better than scotch" for him. He went on a caffeine withdrawal program and started going to Alcoholics Anonymous. Marital therapy showed him how to repair the damage to his marriage. Family sessions enabled him to reclaim his children's love. Cognitive-behavioral sessions helped Dennis explore how some of his deep-seated convictions and beliefs led to the irrational thinking underlying much of his "macho" behavior.

Recurrent episodic stress symptoms, such as Dennis's, are more difficult to treat than acute stress symptoms, partly because of acquired organ sensitivity. They generally require eight to ten months of concentrated attention. Dennis had his problem under control in four months. After six months he was off the "bow-and-arrow squad," and four years later was promoted to sergeant. He's still married to Sandi, and his oldest son was recently named to the all-state, all-scholastic football team.

When your brain is running at breakneck speed, it's difficult to concentrate on any one thing. Remember, you can attend only to seven concerns, plus or minus two. It's hard to concentrate on what's going on inside your head, and it's even more problematic to take in new information. It's arduous to set priorities and select which seven items you're going to pay attention to at any given time.

When Dennis's brain was racing, he reverted to his primary cognitive style, a "macho" outlook on the world, one filled with "druggies" and "street slime" that he could subdue and bring to justice by brute force if necessary. Dennis couldn't handle any new information that might enable him to see life from a different perspective, making it almost impossible for him to understand his wife's viewpoint and to maintain communication between them.

Dennis's experience showed him that once his brain slowed down he could think, plan, set priorities, and take in new information. He then saw what he needed to do rather clearly, and he did it. He was, of course, highly motivated, since his job, marriage, and life were threatened.

SELF-REGULATORY TECHNIQUES FOR MANAGING COGNITIVE SYMPTOMS OF STRESS

The techniques we describe here help slow down your brain and get your thoughts and behaviors under better control. Used regularly, they'll reduce your impulsivity and improve your concentration, memory, and judgment. You'll also find you have more energy. Under normal conditions, your brain, which weighs about 2 percent of your body weight, burns about 20 percent of your body's energy. Hyperactive brain states raise your brain energy expenditures.

You can use some of these techniques by yourself, but you may need help with others. Since many of these techniques involve relaxation, they tend to lower your metabolic rate and general level of physiological arousal. They may interact with prescription medications you may be taking for seizure, cardiovascular, diabetic, or endocrine disorders. Check with your physician before using these techniques.

For more information on these techniques and how to use them, read chapter 19.

Self-Monitoring

Keep track of the times you have cognitive symptoms such as difficulty falling asleep, concentrating or remembering things, and when you use poor judgment or indulge in impulsive behavior. Notice the situation, your thoughts and reactions. Write down some of the more persistent thoughts. Ask yourself if they are realistic or rational. Then look for a more positive way of thinking that will calm you down.

Also, keep track of caffeine, alcohol, or medications that may be affecting your thought processes. Be aware of extreme changes in blood sugar associated with high-sugar foods or infrequent meals and stick to a regular schedule of meals. If you experience feelings of shakiness or have other physical sensations which concern you, consult your physician.

Meditation

The regular practice of meditation helps you notice and identify your thoughts, while it clears your mind. It is difficult to meditate when your mind is racing. Practice during non-stress times prepares you to cope when you're under pressure.

Quiet Time

Dennis found that taking quiet time helped him slow down and think about things clearly and rationally. He would often park his police cruiser on a quiet side street, go through his relaxation exercise, and "zone out." On weekends, he would take his quiet time sitting out on his patio listening to the birds.

Deep Breathing

Deep breathing, relaxation, and quiet time go hand in hand. Even though they can be done separately, they have a synergistic effect that is calming and soothing. Take a look at our comments in chapter 15 on deep breathing and try our one, two, three deep-breathing exercise.

Progressive Muscle Relaxation (PMR)

PMR is a powerful technique for releasing muscle tension and for becoming aware of your body. It involves tensing and relaxing muscles in a progressive series and is often taught as an introduction to biofeedback and to self-hypnosis autogenic imagery. You may have some problems with PMR if you're struggling with a hyperactive brain. Don't get upset if distracting thoughts intrude and disturb your relaxation. Just let them drift away. PMR instructions are available on audio tape from the

Biobehavioral Institute of Boston (see order form at the back of the book). You can make your own tape using the PMR script in appendix I.

Autogenic Imagery

As you relax with PMR, begin to imagine thoughts gradually slowing, like ripples on a pool that becomes quiet and still. Imagine yourself looking at a black velvet curtain as you relax. Imagine yourself relaxing at the beach on vacation without a care in the world. Dennis imagined himself floating on a raft on warm, quiet water. Try different images until you find one that appeals to you and works. Refer to appendix I for further instruction.

PROFESSIONAL HELP

Behavioral Medicine

A specialist in behavioral medicine is generally a psychologist or physician trained in the diagnosis and behavioral treatment of physical and mental stress disorders. Many hospitals and medical centers have departments of behavioral medicine or can refer you to a practitioner in your neighborhood. You may also contact the Society for Behavioral Medicine, 103 South Adams Street, Rockville, MD 20850, (301) 251-2790.

Psychotherapy

Psychotherapy is required when individuals can't handle their complex problems. Psychotherapists include psychologists, psychiatrists, and social workers. There are numerous schools of thought in psychotherapy, ranging from doctrinaire Freudian psychoanalysis to cognitive-behavioral therapy. Whatever the approach, it must feel right to you and you must trust and have confidence in your therapist. If you don't, move on. Obtain referrals from your physician, state professional organizations, and mental health centers, or try the Yellow Pages.

Your first session should be a trial interview. Discuss the therapist's approach, orientation, training, background, and experience with problems like yours. Ask questions about the therapist as a person. While a therapist may prefer not to discuss personal details, general questions about attitudes or experience help you to evaluate their abilities. If he or she doesn't feel right, try someone else.

Counseling

Professionals such as ministers, priests, and rabbis offer counseling, which is generally much more short term than psychotherapy and is generally limited to specific problems and issues. Counselors usually offer advice and assistance in solving problems.

17 HORMONES IN DISARRAY

Your endocrine system is highly responsive to stress and is responsible for the mobilization of your body's resources to deal with stress. Acting on signals from your brain, your hypothalamus alerts your pituitary gland, which then releases stress hormones into your bloodstream. These blood-borne stress hormones travel to specific endocrine glands located elsewhere in your body, where they stimulate these glands to add more stress hormones into your bloodstream.

The most significant of these hormones are adrenocorticotrophic hormone (ACTH), released by your pituitary, and the cortisol that ACTH releases from the outer layers of your adrenal glands. Cortisol plays a primary role in your stress reactions, which in the short term is beneficial. It increases the glucose from your liver and stimulates insulin from your pancreas to supply the quick energy needed for a "fight or flight" response. Cortisol boosts the activity of your immune system and the excitability of your brain and sympathetic nervous system. It also protects against inflammation and fights off allergies.

While a number of hormones are released in relatively large amounts in times of stress, others are slowed to very low levels of production and release. Sex hormones, for instance, are inhibited by stress, leading to lowered sexual desire in both men and women, and to menstrual irregularities in women. Growth-hormone production and release diminishes, causing slow or arrested growth and development in children.

Your hormonal system is a delicately balanced clockwork of numerous interacting bits of biochemistry. Stress disrupts this normal balance by putting it on a wartime footing. If this goes on too long, or if your hormonal system can't synthesize key substances, the system stops functioning normally. Stress symptoms then appear.

However, this takes one to five years of fairly chronic stress. Once this happens, it takes time for your endocrine system to repair itself. There are no quick fixes. Your body has marvelous healing powers, but you must provide it with a healthful diet, rest, and peace of mind.

Many endocrine problems, such as diabetes, are related to genetic predispositions. Uncontrolled stress activates hormones which then may throw your system further out of balance and escalate the need for medical care and medication. However, successful medical treatment depends on your ability to follow a recommended regimen, whether diet, exercise, or medication.

Robert, a 58-year-old postal worker, had diabetes for many years but had maintained his health. This changed when his eyes began giving him trouble, he had pains in his feet, and he had almost fainted twice. When Robert's doctor examined him, his blood sugar was far too high. On a previous visit, it had been too low. Robert confessed that he really hadn't been keeping track of his blood sugar levels or his diet. In his life, Robert said, "I had given up so much, I just didn't want to have to give up desserts too." As he talked, Robert became angrier and angrier, at his father, at his deceased mother, and physicians he felt had treated him badly in the past.

Over the next few months Robert saw several more physicians: a specialist in diabetes, an ophthalmologist for his eyes, and a new internist. As he searched for someone to make him feel better, he overlooked the one person who could be the most help—himself. If Robert could have let go of his anger, he could have cared for his body in a way that would have prevented its gradual deterioration.

An alteration in endocrine status changes your ability to manage stress. When Robert's blood sugar was not in the normal range, his mood swings were more dramatic. He would create havoc with his family and friends, thereby alienating his supportive network and increasing his stress.

In working with Robert, we had him monitor his moods in relation to his blood sugar. When he saw the connection for himself, he began to let go of anger and take better care of himself. With his physician's help, he was able to stabilize his endocrine status and keep it that way.

While both men and women have similar difficulties with diabetes and arthritis, men tend to have fewer endocrine problems than do women, who must deal with monthly hormonal changes and other reproductive events. Birth control pills may have side effects. Infertility workups may mean taking doses of strong hormones at different points in the menstrual cycle. Gynecological surgery may disrupt normal hormonal patterns. Menopause may mean years of hot flashes, mood swings, and decreased ability to manage stress.

While there is limited research on hormonal influences on women's adaptation to stress, we do know that there are many individual differences. A hysterectomy may mean relief from discomfort to one woman and the onset of difficulties for another. A growing sensitivity to these factors will make it easier to cope with them if they happen to you.

THE CASE OF THE FLOODED SIDE YARD

Endocrine difficulties are usually in response to chronic stress, situations that pile up over a period of months. For example, some time ago, while we were at a party in her home, our friend Marian asked us if the crippling arthritic pain in her fingers might be caused by the stress of "what the college did to our side yard." As it turned out, her problems with a neighboring college were just the tip of an iceberg of stress and trauma.

Designed by Frederick Law Olmstead, America's greatest landscape architect, the grounds were beautifully planned and planted. Marian had particularly enjoyed the vista her side yard presented. Flanked by a 150-year-old stone wall, the one and a half acres of lush lawn were dotted with giant evergreens and rimmed by 100-year-old hardwoods. Marian told us that just looking at her grounds made her feel "peaceful."

Adjacent to her stone wall was a meadow, owned by a local college, that was uncared for and overgrown with wildflowers. The college had decided to convert it into a playing field and tennis courts. To do so, the college moved in dirt to raise the level of their field and improve its drainage. As a result, the dirt covered Marian's stone wall and changed the natural drainage system. Marian's side yard was flooded by runoff from the field. Her lawn became a lake. The aged evergreens and hardwoods died. Marian was furious and demanded that her property be restored.

Meeting after meeting was held with the college, promise after promise was broken, solution after solution failed. Marian sued. An attorney herself, she was intimately involved in the proceedings. Every time she thought about the "rape of that beautiful piece of land," which was often, she was freshly enraged. Marian's problem with her land was only the most recent in a series of stressful situations.

Three years earlier, Marian and her family had moved from the South and bought the estate. The house was huge, as were the grounds. Pregnant with her third child, Marian cleaned, scraped, painted, chopped, and weeded herself to exhaustion. She finally hired a housekeeper to help with the house and her two children, ages 4 and 1.

She got little help from her husband, Aaron, a high-risk venture capitalist who was always preoccupied with business. Marian resented Aaron's indifference. She felt isolated, alone, overworked, and underappreciated, a prisoner, as she called it, in a "fancy labor camp."

Two months prior to the birth of her third child, Marian's charismatic eldest brother, Sterling, a tragic hero to the end, burned to death when he crash-landed his private plane. Marian's family was grief-stricken, but she was devastated. Sterling had been special to her. Charming, exciting, somewhat eccentric, and brilliantly gifted, his life had played out like a Greek tragedy capped by the drama of his death.

Marian's relationship with Sterling had been intense. Carelessly, perhaps unknowingly, he had wounded her feelings repeatedly over the years with his teasing and ridicule. He continued his torture from the grave by making her executor of his estate. She spent the next two years sorting out his tangled affairs and settling accounts with a contentious ex-wife. Every day seemed to bring fresh reminders of his death and her loss.

Two months after Sterling's death, her third son, Theodore Sterling, "Teddy," was born. Teddy was a colicky baby, and difficult as a toddler. He and his older brother fought constantly. To add to these family woes, Aaron was having problems in business. He became morose and needed continual affection from Marian. She told us, "There's just not enough of me to go around. I feel like I'm letting everyone down. When do *I* get some attention and some appreciation?"

Her burden increased even further when Aaron took a tremendous business loss. They managed to keep their lovely home with its spacious grounds but had to cut back drastically on everything. Marian went back to work as a lawyer. A short time later, her father had a stroke, paralyzing his right side and making speech difficult. Always the "responsible one," Marian continued to struggle with Sterling's estate, the house, the grounds, her children, Aaron's morose despondence, her job, and her parents. It was against this background of constant crisis that the lush greenery of her side yard turned into a stagnant pond.

Stress had become a chronic feature of Marian's existence. Besides her arthritic pain, she also had headaches, muscular aches and pains, and frequent colds and flus, and she was often anxious, irritable, and agitated.

Marian decided that being sick all the time wasn't worth it. She took matters into her own hands. She quit fighting some problems. She delegated to her lawyers the lawsuit against the college. Marian stopped worrying about the details in the settlement of Sterling's estate. And, she realized that some people would never be grateful for all the work she did.

She actively sought emotional support from her friends. She cultivated co-workers who truly appreciated her dedication and ideas. She talked with those members of her family who were generally supportive and avoided those who made her feel worse.

At home, she set out clear expectations for her sons' chores and responsibilities. She also made arrangements with a college student to exchange a spare room for yard work and supervision of the boys.

In addition, Marian started to pay more attention to her own needs. She began a program of consistent exercise, attended communications and self-discovery workshops, and discovered the power of PMR and relaxation tapes.

The tapes helped greatly. "I'm a tape junkie!" Marian said. She has audio tapes for sleeping, for concentration, for exercise, for building confidence, and for making better speeches. The tapes help her relax and focus on the positive. Now, when Marian wakes up at night, she uses a tape to help her go back to sleep, instead of lying awake worrying about the difficulties she faces the next day.

Marian's arthritic hand pain went away within a matter of weeks, but her irritability, insomnia, headaches, and muscle aches and pains continued for a year or so after she started taking active steps to manage the stress in her life. It takes time to recover fully from a chronic stress on the endocrine system.

The stress in Marian's life did not disappear. Aaron continued to have his financial ups and downs, her sons still squabbled and bickered, the lawsuit with the college dragged on and on, and the side yard remained a muddy, stagnant lake.

But Marian's attitude changed. She said, "I work hard, but I only do what I can do. I quit getting bent out of shape by what I 'ought' to do. I just stay relaxed now, do the best I can, then let it go."

Recently she won a major settlement from the college and with it is restoring her side yard. She's brought in a landscape architect and together they've designed a side yard even more beautiful than Olmstead's. Marian can hardly wait to see it green and blooming. "It will be so beautiful when we're through, I'll forget all about how it used to look and be able to start enjoying it again." The last time we saw her, she had looked very much at peace.

Marian managed to reclaim her life on her own, without professional advice. She didn't even see a physician for her arthritic pain. For her, the steps she took to change her outlook and situation just made sense. The strategies Marian used to reduce her arthritic pain are useful for dealing with symptoms of other endocrine problems.

SELF-REGULATORY TECHNIQUES FOR MANAGING ENDOCRINE SYMPTOMS OF STRESS

The techniques we describe in this section lessen the discomfort, distress, and pain of endocrine symptoms, but they are not a substitute for competent medical care. If you're having endocrine symptoms, before you try these techniques see your physician or endocrinologist to rule out systemic disease or malignancies. Discuss the potential role of stress in your disorder. Since many of these techniques involve relaxation, they tend to lower your metabolic rate and general level of physiological arousal. They may interact with any prescription medications you are taking. If you are taking a medication for a seizure, cardiovascular, diabetic, or endocrine disorder, be sure to have your physician monitor your medications regularly as you begin to use these techniques. Used as a synergistic element in an overall medical treatment plan, they are extremely powerful tools.

Endocrine problems seem to be particularly helped by meditation, self-hypnosis, and autogenic imagery. These techniques deepen relaxation and then expand your awareness of healing possibilities. During these moments, you call on your deepest healing resources, your spiritual beliefs, and your trust in your body's ability to balance itself.

You can use some of these techniques by yourself, but you may need help with others. For more about these techniques and how to use them, see chapter 19.

Self-Monitoring

Keep a daily record of your endocrine symptoms and their severity. Notice what makes you feel better and what makes you feel worse. Look at the time of day when things are particularly bad for you. What's going on then? Is it just the time of day, or is it what happens at that time of day? Does it make you feel better to talk to some people but not to others? Because endocrine symptoms take a while to develop, they require a longer time to recede. However, you may have daily or weekly fluctuations that you can track. A diary covering several months will help you see your progress.

Quiet Time

Quiet time for yourself every day is essential to long-term restoration of the body's balance. Longer periods of quiet on weekends are also important, as are periodic vacations. Endocrine symptoms can be serious and lead to complications. Use the quiet time for deep relaxation and autogenic imagery.

Deep Breathing

For endocrine problems, slow deep breathing should be used in conjunction with deep relaxation, meditation, imagery, and affirmations. It can also be used for on-the-spot calming during difficult moments.

Progressive Muscle Relaxation (PMR)

PMR is a powerful technique for calming the body and mind. Use it in conjunction with autogenic imagery and affirmations for help with stress situations and physical recovery. The emphasis should be on very deep relaxation and calming. Initially, practice should be two or three times daily, for at least twenty minutes.

Electromyographic (EMG) Biofeedback

EMG biofeedback can be used to enhance PMR and to deepen the sense of relaxation described in chapter 19. Taking one's blood sugar level is a type of biological feedback that may tell you how you're doing. Otherwise, there are few direct ways to monitor endocrine changes outside of a laboratory.

Meditation

Some people find a deeper sense of calm through meditation rather than through PMR. Both techniques create similar effects and can be used in similar ways. If you do what seems most suitable to you, you are more likely to continue, and, in the end, that's what is most important.

Self-Hypnosis

Self-hypnosis is another way of creating deep relaxation, awareness, and receptivity to suggestions of healing and recovery. The deeper state of auto-suggestion achieved with hypnosis allows positive imagery to have a greater effect.

Autogenic Imagery

As you relax with PMR, meditation, or self-hypnosis, allow images of warmth, comfort, and relaxation to emerge. One favorite is the image of lying on a beach and feeling the warm sun on your body and feeling your body getting progressively heavier as you relax. Another technique is to imagine being carried deeper into yourself, as if on an escalator that slowly takes you down to deeper levels of awareness and relaxation. Religious or spiritual images of a healing power soothing your body and soul may also be reassuring and comforting. Try different images until you find one that appeals to you and works.

Further description and exercises for autogenic imagery and PMR can be found in appendix I. You can also order PMR tapes from the Biobehavioral Institute. (See order form at the back of the book.)

Affirmations

Before ending your relaxation exercise, tell yourself several affirmations regarding your health and well-being. These should be specific to your particular condition. Phrase each one positively, reflecting your intention to care for your body as best you can.

PROFESSIONAL HELP AND ASSISTANCE

Internal Medicine, Endocrinology, Urology, and Gynecology

Some endocrine symptoms and conditions may be indicative of more serious problems or may require prescription medication or surgery. Start your program by seeing your internist, endocrinologist, urologist, or gynecologist. The self-regulation techniques we described will help, but use them as part of a total package of treatment. Ask for details about healthy endocrine functioning to use in your positive images about your body.

Behavioral Medicine

A behavioral medicine specialist will be familiar with integrating these self-regulation techniques with your other medical care. She or he can make an audio tape to facilitate your imagery and deepening of your relaxation or meditation. You can contact the Society for Behavioral Medicine, 103 South Adams Street, Rockville, MD 20850, (301) 251-2790, for specialists in your area.

Bibliotherapy

There are many excellent books available on hormonal dysfunctions. Books on premenstrual syndrome, arthritis, menopause, and diabetes can be found in most bookstores and libraries and in appendix II.

18 SICK OF STRESS

Your immune system operates as a microscopic army fighting a silent, relentless, and endless war against invading microorganisms and renegade cells turned cancerous. Like a corps of bodyguards, it protects us against infections and malignancies by destroying, deactivating, or eliminating the enemy. It searches relentlessly day and night for strangers and either lynches them or rides them out of town on a rail.

There are two parts to the immune system—humoral and cellular. The humoral part floats through the body's fluids. It is composed mainly of antibodies that fight bacterial and viral invasions. The cellular part fights viruses that get inside the cells of your body, transplanted tissue, fungi, protozoa, and cancer cells. When the humoral part breaks down, you are easy prey for infections such as colds and flus. When the cellular part breaks down, you are at risk for developing cancer, among other things.

Stress powerfully influences the ability of your immune system. Day in and day out, your immune system works quietly, efficiently, and independently to keep you healthy. If it's overreactive, it may attack normal body tissue and you may develop allergies and autoimmune diseases.

The cortisol and adrenaline that fuel the physiological arousal of the stress reaction have a negative influence on the immune system. Numerous scientific studies show that stress can make the immune system either under- or overreact. Stress precipitates and/or exacerbates many infectious, malignant, allergic, and autoimmune diseases.

One recent study demonstrated that stress increases susceptibility to the common cold. People with and without high levels of stress were exposed to the same cold viruses through a nasal spray. Those with high stress showed symptoms at a significantly higher rate than did the low-stress people.[1] Other studies have linked stress with cancer, infectious diseases, allergic disorders, and other autoimmune disorders.[2] A reactivation of the herpes virus is often caused by forms of stress, either physical exhaustion or emotional distress.[3] For many infected individuals, the symptoms of AIDS caused by the Human Immunodeficiency Virus (HIV) seem to worsen as stress increases.

Stress reduction strategies increase the efficiency of the immune system and alleviate the symptoms of disease. Nowhere have the effects of stress reduction techniques on the immune system been shown as dramatically as in the behavioral treatment of malignant disease.

STAR WARS

We have seen a number of cancer patients, but none stands out as vividly in our memory as Loren. Referred to us for pain management by his oncologist, 41-year-old Loren had a rapidly growing tumor (spinal glioma) in his spinal cord and was experiencing severe pain from pressure on his spinal nerve tracts. To relieve his pain, Loren's physicians were contemplating severing his spinal cord above the tumor. Of course, this would leave him a paraplegic, putting him in a wheelchair for what was left of his life. Behavioral pain management was seen as a last resort.

We started Loren on relaxation and self-hypnosis to ease his pain. This program worked almost immediately. Loren had a real knack for it. He had read about some of the almost miraculous remissions through behavioral treatment of cancer patients. Loren wanted to know if we could try a similar approach. We agreed.

We began by addressing Loren's stress problems, other than his cancer. We didn't find much at first, but as we talked we were increasingly aware of his emotional isolation from other people, including his family. Loren's parents had been cold, distant, and detached from him and his brother Jay. Loren couldn't recall ever having been kissed or hugged by either of his parents, and didn't think his brother could either. Both parents were dead. Loren seldom saw Jay, who lived less than a mile away. A "loner," he rarely spoke to anyone. He and his wife, Rebecca, had a good relationship, but she complained about his being "undemonstrative."

Loren worked as the comptroller for a small, high-tech firm where he was viewed as an "invaluable employee." He worked long hours and never "wasted time" socializing on the job. His employer kept him on full pay and brought work to his home "so Loren would have something to keep his mind off his illness." Loren managed to get as much done at home as he normally would have at the office. He never asked for help with anything.

Heather, the Biobehavioral Institute therapist who was working with us, and Loren discussed an idea she had for helping him. Both thought *Star Wars* was the greatest movie ever filmed. Building on their common interest, Heather devised a program of guided imagery to directly combat Loren's tumor.

Although they both had seen the movie many times, Heather rented the videotape and played it during their sessions. She started calling Darth Vader's spaceship "tumor" and had Loren imagine he was Luke Skywalker attacking that ship called "tumor" to destroy it. As they played the famous sequence over and over, Heather had Loren fantasize that he was blasting the spaceship/tumor to bits with his lasers and torpedoes.

Next, she had Loren place himself in a trance through self-hypnosis. He had to imagine himself flying down his spinal canal in a starfighter searching for the spaceship, finding it, and attacking it. Heather made an audio tape of that session and sent it home with Loren to practice.

The next week, Heather elaborated on the imagery and included among the starfighters herself, Loren's wife, Rebecca, and his brother, Jay, who were helping Loren destroy the spaceship/tumor. He had some problem accepting even the image of help, but liked it when he got used to it.

Loren's pain eased. At his next radiological examination, the tumor had decreased slightly in density and size. Loren and Rebecca were overjoyed. They invited Jay and his family to dinner to celebrate. This was the first time Loren had sat down at the table with his brother in fifteen years. He liked it. So did his brother. They began to talk about their upbringing and what they had missed. It was the beginning of a closeness between them they had never felt before.

Loren continued to see Heather and, although his tumor was still there, his pain diminished to the point where he walked without a cane and returned to work. Several months later, he came into the clinic limping, in obvious pain, and holding a cane. When he saw the stricken look on Heather's face he explained that he was just stiff and sore from cross-country skiing over the weekend.

Heather's career took her to another state and Loren continued with another therapist in our clinic. And though the cancer finally killed Loren after three and a half years, he led a normal, pain-free life during that time because of guided imagery and therapy.

SELF-REGULATORY TECHNIQUES FOR MANAGING IMMUNE SYMPTOMS OF STRESS

The techniques we describe in this section lessen the discomfort, distress, and pain of immune symptoms but are in no way a substitute for competent medical care. If you've been having frequent colds, bouts of flu, or infections, see your physician first and discuss using these techniques to reduce your distress and pain. Used as a synergistic element in an overall medical treatment plan, they can be extremely powerful tools.

You can use some of these techniques by yourself, but you may need help with others. Since many of these techniques involve relaxation, they tend to lower your metabolic rate and general level of physiological arousal.

They may interact with any prescription medications you are taking. If you are taking medication for a seizure, cardiovascular, diabetic, or endocrine disorder, be sure to have your physician monitor your medication as you try them.

Immune problems seem to be particularly helped by meditation, self-hypnosis, and antogenic imagery. These techniques deepen relaxation and then expand your awareness of healing possibilities. During these moments, you call on your deepest healing resources, spiritual beliefs, and trust in your body's ability to ward off infection. For more information on these techniques and how to use them, see chapter 19.

Self-Monitoring

Keep a daily record of your immune symptoms and what's going on in your life. Notice any connections between the demands and pressures you're dealing with and those deviling colds and bouts of flu. What helps fight them off, and what sabotages your immune system further? If you have chronic symptoms, the daily journal helps you notice progress or setbacks over many weeks.

Quiet Time

Just like war-weary soldiers, your immune system needs rest to regain its fighting edge. Be sure to set aside quiet time for yourself every day. For serious problems, you need to rest two or three times daily. You may also need extra quiet time on the weekends. Use this for deep relaxation and imagery.

Deep Breathing

Deep breathing is a way to enhance relaxation and meditation. It can provide relaxation periods throughout the day.

Progressive Muscle Relaxation (PMR)

PMR is a key step in working with immune problems. The emphasis should be on deepening your level of relaxation with regular practice. Use it in conjunction with meditation, self-hypnosis, and autogenic imagery. There is a PMR exercise in appendix I which can be read into a tape recorder for playback. Tapes are also available for purchase through the Biobehavioral Institute. (See order form at the back of the book.)

Meditation

Some people prefer meditation as a method of quieting and concentration. The spiritual aspects of meditation may be reassuring and calming and may reinforce your belief that you are receiving help for your problem.

Self-Hypnosis

Self-hypnosis is another way to deepen your relaxation and to enhance suggestibility and the impact of imagery. Use it with your imagery and affirmations.

Autogenic Imagery

To develop useful imagery about your disorder, ask your physician or read about the specifics of your illness, what is wrong, and, especially, what needs to happen inside your body to restore its health. The clearer your picture of your body, the better. The more you understand about and believe in healing, the more effective your imagery will be.

When you are in a deep state of relaxed awareness from PMR, meditation, or self-hypnosis, concentrate on your special images.

Affirmations

Write down several positive statements about the future of your health. Post them around your house. At the end of your relaxation exercise, say each one quietly to yourself, allowing yourself to believe the words you are saying.

PROFESSIONAL HELP AND ASSISTANCE

Internal Medicine and Allergology

If you have an infectious, malignant, allergic, or auto-immune disease, you are probably already in treatment with a physician. Take this book along with you the next time you visit your physician to see how our approach and the techniques we describe might be integrated into your overall medical treatment plan.

Behavioral Medicine

A specialist in behavioral medicine can help you understand how these ideas specifically apply to you. You can discuss any difficulties or creative ideas you have. He or she can also make an audio tape to guide you in your relaxation. Contact the Society for Behavioral Medicine, 103 South Adams Street, Rockville, MD 20850, (301) 251-2790, or your local hospital for specialists in your area.

Bibliotherapy

Good self-help books on the immune system are plentiful. We've listed a few in appendix II. Use them as a start and go from there. Your local bookstore and library will be glad to help you find what you need.

NOTES

1. Cohen, S., Tyrrell, D.A.J., and Smith, A. P. (1992), "Psychological Stress and Susceptibility to the Common Cold," *New England Journal of Medicine* 325, 606–612.

2. Locke, S. E., and Hornig-Rehan, M. (1983), *Mind and Immunity: Behavioral Immunology*, Institute for the Advancement of Health, New York, NY.

3. Langston, D. P. (1983), *Living with Herpes*, New York, Doubleday.

19 CALLING ON THE HEALER WITHIN

In most cases, the best medicine is no medicine. You have within you miraculous healing powers tested and proven over the entire course of human existence. However, those marvelous capacities for self-healing have limitations. There are certain physical and mental illnesses that need substantial outside help.

A compound fracture, for instance, requires the assistance of traditional medicine to set the bone properly and to cleanse and dress the wound. Once blood loss and the risk of infection have been minimized and the ends of the broken bone brought together, your internal healing powers come into play. Manic depressive illness and schizophrenia are mental conditions that fare better with the assistance of traditional medicine than if left alone.

However, the marvelous advances medical science has made in support of the natural healer have lulled many people into a false sense of security. The illusion persists that one can do whatever one likes; when your mind and body can no longer tolerate such abuse, modern medicine magically makes you new.

Unfortunately, medical interventions often create more problems than they cure. Modern medicine has particular difficulty with what Hans Selye, inventor of the term *stress*, called the "diseases of adaptation."[1] These stress-related complaints, which account for up to

90 percent of all doctors' office visits, are often responsive to natural healing. Medicine should be the ally of our natural healing powers, not our master.

To enjoy health and happiness, you have to take responsibility for yourself, your life, and your health. Getting stress tough and staying stress smart is the first step. It's the proverbial ounce of prevention that obviates the pound of cure. But modern life is modern life and it's next to impossible to escape stress-related illnesses and complaints entirely. When they catch up with you, learn how to call on your own healing powers by using the self-regulation techniques we mentioned earlier and describe more fully below.

SELF-REGULATION TECHNIQUES

Self-regulation is the deliberate adjustment of your physical, mental, and emotional state to fit the circumstances of the moment. You've done it many times. Remember as a child how often your parents told you to "Hurry up!" "Calm down!" "Not so loud!" "Think carefully!" "Go to sleep." "If you can't behave yourself, you'll have to go to your room." Even, "Stop crying!"

You've been self-regulating for years. You get yourself "psyched up" for challenging events such as presentations, making deadlines, interviewing for new jobs, etc. On the other hand, you've probably also told yourself to "slow down," "take it easy," "cool down," "don't worry," and so on. You might even have used chemicals to regulate your level of physiological arousal to fit your needs of the moment.

Dennis, the policeman discussed in chapter 16, played "uppers and downers" with caffeine and alcohol to regulate chemically his level of physiological arousal. Several cups of coffee kept his level up throughout the day, and several alcoholic drinks lowered it at night. Cocaine and barbiturates are more malignant examples of the same process.

The self-regulation techniques we discuss in this chapter can be used for calming down, for reducing your level of physiological arousal, and for backing down from your danger zone. Read through our descriptions of them, try them out, and see which ones, or combinations, work best for you.

Caution: Since these techniques involve changing your level of physiological arousal, they can affect your reactions to medication. If you are on psychotropic medication of any kind, or medication for hypertension, diabetes, heart condition, or epilepsy, it is imperative that you check with the prescribing physician before you start using these techniques.

SELF-MONITORING AND YOUR TENSION TACHOMETER

Think back over the last few days. Remember when you felt relaxed and calm, and when you felt agitated, tense, or "wired." Note these ups and downs as you go through your day. You'll see that you move from one state of feeling to another. Notice how your level of physiological arousal increases as you get more tense and decreases as you calm down. Become aware of which activities and thoughts help you feel calmer and which bring more tension. Begin to notice, also, your usual, or baseline, level of tension.

Imagine a gauge that enables you to keep track of your level of physiological arousal, something like the tachometer in an automobile—tension tachometer, if you will, that tells you how "revved up" you are at any point in time. Take a look at the tension tachometer below to see what we mean.

The higher your RPMs, the more wear and tear on body and mind. Your natural healing powers repair the damage of driving yourself at high RPMs, but you have to slow down to let them work. Physiologically, we're talking about two different kinds of metabolism. High RPM metabolism is called catabolic metabolism; healing metabolism is called anabolic metabolism.

Notice that the zone for anabolic metabolism, the healing zone, runs from about 1.25 to about 3.80 RPMs. Above 3.80, you shift into catabolic metabolism and start tearing down what you built up during your anabolic time. The more you rev your engine, the more wear and

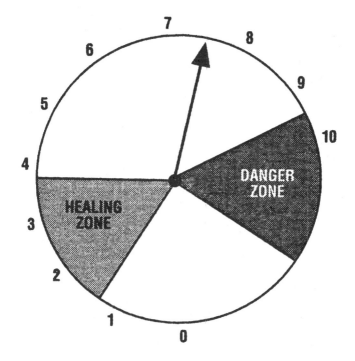

TENSION TACHOMETER

tear you cause. The more you tear down, the more you
need to build up. This natural process of tearing down
and building up goes on every day.

If you spend too much time in the high zones and not
enough time in the healing zone, you wear out and break
down. If you run into the danger zone, you'll wear out
and break down quickly. To repair the devastation of
catabolic metabolism, you have to spend time in your
healing zone.

It's helpful to keep a record of how much time you
spend in high RPM activity and how much time you
spend in low RPM activity. It's also a good idea to keep
track of how your high RPM activity influences your
stress symptoms. Keep a written record. Make four columns on a small sheet of paper that will fit in your purse
or your shirt pocket.

Mark column 1 off in hourly intervals. Every hour, estimate your RPMs and write it down in column 2. In column 3, put a plus if you're having symptoms, a minus if you're not. In column 4, make a note of what's going on at the time.

After a few days of keeping track of your tension RPMs, you'll see how high your baseline level of arousal is, what activities or situations push it up or lower it, and how your symptoms are connected to your level of arousal.

Some people have a naturally low level of arousal. These people remain cool under fire, handle emergencies with aplomb, and can fall asleep at any opportunity. They often work in high-pressure or dangerous jobs because they can tolerate high levels of stress. We rarely see these folks in treatment, unless some particularly bad episode has put them into their danger zones for extended periods.

Others rarely relax, maintaining a constant level of tension that only goes higher under stress. The most extreme case we ever saw in treatment was a woman, Hilda, 37, who couldn't close her eyes or even rest her head against a chair. She had to be alert at all times. Hilda told us that she would not even go to sleep before her husband did. Hilda had gone to her physician with many physical complaints. She found it impossible to do our standard relaxation exercise because it felt "weird" to her to be that relaxed. She had to feel safe while she was trying out the new sensations. In her case, we modified the exercise, suggesting she sit up and keep her eyes open while relaxing her muscles.

As you experiment with the following strategies for physical, mental, and emotional self-regulation, become aware of the difference between being tense and being relaxed, of being in a high versus a low RPM zone. With practice, you'll know automatically how tense you are and when to relax and lower your arousal level. You won't have to wait for a particular symptom to tell you that you are stressed.

PHYSICAL STRATEGIES FOR LOWERING YOUR RPMS

There are a number of physical strategies for lowering your level of physiological arousal. Some are simple and easy to perform and some are more complex and difficult. We advise that you start with the easy ones and work up to the more complex and difficult ones.

Deep Breathing

The easiest way to slow yourself down is to deepen your breathing. Deep or diaphragmatic breathing is central to most forms of relaxation and meditation. It improves the distribution of oxygen to tissues and is a powerful means of shifting your body into an anabolic metabolic state and recharging yourself.

While it is deceptively simple, regular, deep breathing is found in almost all forms of physical relaxation. The Eastern meditation techniques that have healing powers all have correct posture and deep breathing as fundamental elements.

Your lungs are like an accordion. There is a set of muscles at each end of the rib cage that helps pull air into the lungs. If you just use the muscles at the top, you can't get much air in with each breath. If you use the large diaphragm muscle at the bottom, lower organs are pushed aside to make room for air in the lungs and you get a lot more air into your lungs with each breath.

Most of us use both sets of muscles to breathe, but some people are primarily chest breathers and don't use their diaphragms for breathing. They pull only on one end of their lungs. These folks, like Anne, are prone to hyperventilation, with all its ramifications, and particularly if they have small chest cavities. The primary determinant is the distance between the front and back walls of your chest.

Before we go any further, it might be instructive for you to find out if you're a chest breather. First, let most of the air out of your lungs. Count to three. At three, inhale as quickly and deeply as you can. Hold it right there. Did you breathe mostly through your mouth? Did your shoulders go up? Does it feel tight around your neck and throat? Does it feel as if the upper part of your lungs are especially full? If so, you probably tend to breathe more with the upper part of your lungs.

If, however, when you breathed quickly, your belt or waistband got tight, your stomach pushed out, and you felt fullness in the lower part of your chest, your diaphragm was doing most of the work. Try the quick breath a couple more times, noticing more closely your automatic pattern.

If you are a diaphragmatic breather, your chances of developing a hyperventilation syndrome such as Anne's are rather remote. Unless, of course, your pattern of breathing changes in times of stress. If it does and you run into frequent stress situations, you may still be at risk.

If you do have a hyperventilation episode, it can be stopped just by rebreathing the air you have exhaled. Exhaled air has a higher concentration of carbon dioxide and quickly restores your blood to its proper balance. Cupping your hands over your mouth and nose traps exhaled air for rebreathing. Breathing into a paper bag does the same trick, but it's a little obvious in public. You can also stop a hyperventilation episode by holding your breath for twenty seconds, until more carbon dioxide builds up in your lungs. Another method is to concentrate on slowly breathing in and out through your nose, thus restoring a proper rhythm. It is difficult to hyperventilate if your only air passage is your nose.

Hyperventilation is likely if:

- You breathe through your mouth.
- You wear tight belts or undergarments that squeeze the diaphragm.
- You have a small rib cage.
- Your shoulder posture squeezes your chest cavity.
- You tend to "chest breathe," i.e., pull air into your lungs with the muscles of your chest and neck, rather than with your diaphragm.

How to Breathe Diaphragmatically

Lie on your back with a small pillow under your head. Lying in a reclining chair will work as well. You want to be comfortable, with your head supported so that you can see your hands clasped across your lower chest, with your little fingers just above your navel. Begin by taking a slow deep breath. Allow your stomach to rise as you breathe in, noticing the rising of your hands as well. As you breathe out, your hands should sink slightly. With each breath in, your fingers might slide apart slightly, and glide together as you exhale. Notice the full feeling in the lower part of your chest cavity as you breathe. Continue breathing this way for ten or fifteen minutes, allowing yourself to relax as you exhale.

If you are still unsure if you are breathing with your diaphragm, try sitting in a straight chair, leaning over with your elbows on your knees, and your chin in your hands. This posture immobilizes the upper chest and neck muscles, forcing you to breathe only with the diaphragm.

With regular practice, several times a day, you can develop the habit of breathing mostly with your diaphragm. If your tendency or habit is to breathe quickly, or with your upper chest and neck muscles, it may take longer, generally about two weeks of daily awareness and practice.

Progressive Muscle Relaxation

Progressive muscle relaxation (PMR) training consists of learning to first tense and then relax different muscles throughout the body, at the same time paying close attention to the feelings associated with tension and relaxation. In addition to learning to relax, you eventually recognize the feelings of tension in your muscles so you can pinpoint and release tension as it develops.

Like a rubber band that has been stretched and then loosened, muscles relax even more after they have been tightened. After you have released most of the muscle tension, your muscles continue to relax even more as you move on to other muscle groups.

Learning PMR is like learning any other motor skill. It just takes practice. Don't expect to relax totally the first few times you try. In the beginning, you have to learn how the sensations of tension and relaxation differ. Allow yourself the luxury of a quiet time. As you progress, you will notice when you are even more relaxed than before. As you practice regularly, you will become relaxed in a shorter time. Then you can shorten the exercise time by skipping the tensing of certain muscles and moving directly to the relaxation phase.

PMR puts you in the healing zone by reducing your level of arousal. With relaxation, muscle fibers loosen and smooth out, releasing pressure on your tendons where they are attached to the bone. As your muscles relax, the small blood vessels of your body also relax and expand, improving circulation to your organs. Your hand temperature slowly rises as your circulation improves, and your heart rate and respiration slow. The transmission of pain signals is muted. The glandular activity of your skin is reduced. Stomach and bowel activity normalizes.

Caution: If you are currently on medication for a thyroid condition, hypertension, diabetes, anxiety, pain control, or cardiac regulation, coordinate your muscle relaxation practice in consultation with your physician. Some individuals find they need less medication after several weeks of practice. *Do not make changes in your medication without consulting your physician.* Taking either too much or too little medication for those conditions can be risky.

While most people like the sensations of relaxing, some people experience sensations of floating or feel they have lost sensation in their limbs. Others report peculiar or unfamiliar sensations as the tension leaves their muscles. Sometimes strong feelings arise during the exercise. Should you feel uncomfortable at any time during the PMR, slowly open your eyes, move or stretch a bit, and regain your bearings. You can continue the exercise with your eyes open until you feel like closing them again.

Deep Muscle Relaxation and Stress Inoculation

Deep muscle relaxation is another powerful way to deal with stress symptoms. In 1939, Edmund Jacobson demonstrated that muscle relaxation lowered blood pressure in three of his patients.[2] Since then, hundreds of researchers have explored its effects on treatment of anxiety, hypertension, insomnia, headache, addictions, diabetes, back and other muscle pain, gastrointestinal disorders, nausea from chemotherapy, and chronic pain from illness. Repeated studies have found that deep relaxation is the key element in symptom improvement for many individuals.

Once you have mastered the skill of developing a deep state of relaxation, you can use it to inoculate yourself against specific stress situations. At the end of the exercise, when you're deeply relaxed, imagine yourself in what is for you a stressful situation. Imagine staying deeply relaxed in this situation and dealing with it calmly and thoughtfully. The practice will carry over into the real situation. It's a powerful technique for dealing effectively with unavoidable stress situations.

You can also think about special problems in your life during this quiet time. Some people use this time to think about the future or to reflect on the past.

Read more about imagery and how to use it in conjunction with muscle relaxation in appendix I.

Other Relaxation Methods

Progressive muscle relaxation exercises are the best training for the awareness and prevention of tension. But other relaxation methods add variety. Moist heat such as a hot bath or shower, a warm face cloth, or a heating pad dilates small blood vessels, improving circulation. The warmth also relaxes muscle fibers.

Facial or body massage also improves circulation and loosens muscles. One client with headaches reported several hours of relief after having a facial at her beauty salon. A body massage may relieve tension for a short period of time. However, if you are in the habit of holding tension in your muscles, your tightness will return. PMR training helps you to recognize tension as it builds and to let it out often during the day.

You may find that yoga and other physical disciplines, such as Tai Chi, complement your deep relaxation practice. Yoga relaxes muscles by slow, continuous stretching and then relaxing. The exercises focus on different parts of the body in sequence. This develops elasticity of the muscles, improves circulation, and increases mobilization of the joints. Yoga training usually includes proper posture and breathing as well. In addition, a group experience may be more motivating and interesting as a variation to your other relaxation practices. Most communities have yoga classes available.

Look for other opportunities to work your muscles and then relax them. Bending and stretching exercises help minimize the strain of long hours at a desk or computer terminal. Regular rhythmic exercise not only helps make you stress tough, it's a way of releasing tension created by stress.

Maximize your opportunities to relax. Become consciously aware of letting go of residual tension after muscles have been worked hard. Physical exercise can be used as a calming device as well as a strengthening and aerobic exercise. Muscles relax even further after they have worked and become fatigued. Relax completely after exercise for fifteen or twenty minutes. Take natural opportunities for this: sitting in a hot tub after skiing, taking a sauna or warm bath after your workout, letting all muscles relax between weight-training repetitions, lying down on the floor or bed.

Develop the habit of mentally scanning your body for muscle tightness. Wherever you find muscle tension, release it. Follow up with a mental reminder to keep that muscle relaxed.

Tension can develop unnecessarily. When driving a car, you need tension in your right leg for the accelerator and some tension in your arms and shoulders for steering. Yet, many times, unused muscles become tense as well, leading to overall fatigue. People pleasers, who frequently deal with others by smiling, find face and jaw tension developing into muscle contraction headaches as the tension in the face and jaw spreads to other muscles of the head, neck, and upper back.

Autogenic Training

Autogenic means "self-generation" or "self-regulation." This term was used by Drs. Johannes Schult and Wolfgang Luthe[3] to describe a way of talking to yourself to suggest an internal state of being that adjusts your physical body for optimal functioning. Autogenic phrases help the body return to homeostasis, the mechanism that automatically regulates body functions.

After you have learned progressive muscle relaxation, autogenic phrases can be used as a quicker way to relax. They can also be used to regulate more automatic (autonomic) functions such as cardiovascular and gastrointestinal functions, which are regulated more indirectly than muscle tension. For more detailed information, see the autogenic exercises described in appendix I.

Biofeedback

Under most circumstances, you're probably unaware of the subtle internal adjustments your body makes to meet the demands of your daily activities. They take place below the level of your conscious awareness because you've practiced these adjustments so often that you do it by habit, or because your body has automatic mechanisms for dealing with demands as they arise.

The coordinated tensing and relaxing of muscle groups required to pick up a pencil is a highly practiced motor act you perform every day without thinking about it or knowing how you do it. The increase in heart rate, blood flow, and respiration that takes place when you run happens automatically in response to increased metabolic demands. These normal patterns of activity can, however, be disrupted by physical injury, disease, or through the strains involved with excessive stress in your life.

Biofeedback involves the use of sensitive electronic instruments to detect subtle changes in muscle tension, heart rate, skin temperature, perspiration, and a variety of other physiological activities. If this information is then displayed or "fed back" to us, we can be made aware of these changing bodily processes. By observing yourself through this process of biofeedback, you can learn to modify these activities in a short period of time.

For instance, you can, through biofeedback training, learn to control your heart so that it doesn't pump any harder or faster than is absolutely necessary. Thus, when you're tense and under stress, you can slow down your heart so that you run a lesser risk of suffering a "stress related" heart attack. The more you learn to relax and not overwork your body, the longer your body will last. Biofeedback is a tool that helps you learn to relax in specific ways.

These techniques are currently being applied in the treatment of a variety of disorders such as tension headache, migraine headache, and high blood pressure, and in training stroke and accident victims to regain control of their bodies.

You can do biofeedback at home and get a good bit of benefit from it. Home biofeedback instrumentation is offered in a number of mail order catalogs and some of the systems are fairly good. The best home biofeedback training instruments, though, are available from Thought Technology.[4]

However, biofeedback is best done with the help of a professional. One organization you can call to get the name of a local clinic which uses biofeedback is the Association for Applied Psychophysiology and Biofeedback, 10200 W. 44th Avenue, Suite 304, Wheat Ridge, CO 80033, (303) 420-2902. Pick a biofeedback therapist who has earned the highest degree in his particular field and has been certified either by the Biofeedback Certification of America or the Biobehavioral Institute. Pick one who has good equipment where the displays make sense to you and are easily understood. Ask the therapist what kind of equipment he has. We use the DAVICON computerized system, the Medac System 3, at the Biobehavioral Institute and have been pleased with the results.[5]

CALMING THE MIND

Just as you rated muscle tension on a scale of 1 to 10, you can rate your mental tension. Think of your mind as an empty space when it is truly quiet. Your thoughts are quiet and serene, with little or no conscious awareness (arousal level of 1). There may be occasional stray thoughts drifting through this space, which can leave as easily as they came. As you drift up toward alertness, you are conscious of your surroundings, yet you still feel quiet and relaxed (arousal level of 2). Imagine relaxing on the beach watching the sunset.

At 3, you may be talking with a friend or doing minor tasks or recreational activities in a relaxed frame of mind. As your arousal increases to 4 or 5, you may be engaged in routine tasks that take effort and thought but have minor tension associated with them. When your arousal level moves above 5, your tension level is increasing because you're worried about the *outcome* of your task. When your mind seems busy with repetitive worries or fears, or depressed by dark thoughts, your tension level may climb above 6 or 7.

Take a few moments to reflect on the last couple of days. Have you had periods when your thoughts were quiet, peaceful, relaxed? Have you had moments when thoughts were swirling fast and furious, some thoughts appearing over and over again? Assign a number to your level of mental tension today. Note the fluctuations in your thought patterns, their speed, content, and variety. As you notice your thoughts more, you will be better able to direct them.

Your awareness can fluctuate through memories of the past, awareness of the present, and anticipation of the future. Consciousness may seem like a voice talking inside your head. We call this "self-talk." Consciousness may also be visual images, such as the faces of friends. They may be tactile or "body" memories, like the feeling of cold water in a pool or of a painful injury. Even distinctive smells or tastes can be remembered or imagined. Take a moment to imagine sucking a slice of lemon. Can you feel your mouth react?

How you feel at any given moment is greatly influenced by the content of your thoughts and awareness. Regulating consciousness is a major part of stress management. There are several strategies for regulating mental processes. Some are simple and easy to learn, although sometimes difficult to practice on a regular basis. Others are complex and address fundamental beliefs and assumptions you may have developed over your lifetime and require a special effort on your part to correct, possibly including professional help. We will discuss the strategies in turn.

Distracting Yourself

Engaging in mental activity that disengages you from stress is a common form of relieving mental tension. Distracting mental activities include watching television, playing cards, doing a crossword puzzle, or reading the daily newspaper, magazines, light literature, or playing sports. One executive we saw found that playing squash relaxed him mentally. He was unable to think about his business problems when the ball was bouncing toward him at eighty miles an hour. These activities change your focus of attention from demanding tasks or stressful issues to light or repetitive tasks that require little effort and push away worrisome thoughts. While the stressful situation doesn't change, your mind has a rest from worrying about it.

Thought Stopping

Sometimes you need something stronger than distraction to interrupt a negative train of thought. You need emergency brakes. If you are about to lose your temper because your child has bugged you once too often, count to ten. If you are about to say something hurtful, critical, or threatening, don't. Zip your lip. When you find yourself anxiously reviewing all the bad things that could happen to you, say, *"Stop!"* loudly to yourself. You can give yourself a firm reminder to control your inner turmoil and its effects. This method is simple but it works, giving you time to come down from a tension level of 7 or 8 to a level where you can think more clearly.

Affirmations, Spiritual or Philosophical Recitations

Affirmations are statements that reinforce an idea or belief. In training your mind to think more positively, frequently repeating a positive statement cues other positive thoughts, just as listening to a song over and over tends to bring that tune into your mind when the music is no longer playing.

Our clients often question whether such repetition of an idea can really make a difference, or ask, "Isn't it some form of brainwashing?" It isn't. Actually, it is somewhat like learning a new language. To acquire a new language you first listen to others say the words over and over. You then begin to practice the new words exactly as you heard them. Daily listening and repetition slowly builds vocabulary. Eventually, with practice, you can become fluent in the new language.

Just as you learned to speak and think in your mother tongue as a child, you also learned to think in positive or negative ways using that language. If your parents spoke critically and judgmentally, you tend to think and speak in similar ways. As you might change an accent to make it more pleasing, you can change the accent of your thoughts to make yourself feel better about yourself and the world around you.

The memorization of spiritual passages, poetic verses, or ancient sayings has guided thought for centuries. Children are taught to memorize the Ten Commandments, the Declaration of Independence, and the Golden Rule as guides for living and getting along with others. Affirmations continue that tradition. In selecting affirmations for use in managing stress you can borrow from literature, religious texts, the words of a spiritual leader, or create your own, tailor-made for you.

For example, when we were writing this book, Alma posted a note near her computer keyboard: *You can write this book.* She added a smiling face as well. If you tend to worry, you might use the phrase, "Things will work out somehow." If you have self-doubt, you might try, "I am a wonderful human being." The following are some other phrases our clients have found helpful.

- God loves me.
- I feel part of the earth's spirit.
- I accept my body as it is.
- I can relax.
- I can transcend sorrow.
- Make new friends, but keep the old; one is silver and the other gold.
- Every cloud has a silver lining.
- I can learn from my pain.
- I can eat moderately.

You don't have to believe fully in your statement. An affirmation is a statement of hope as well as intention. Choose affirmations you can believe in somewhat, or believe occasionally. Repetition will increase your belief in the statement. Affirmations utilize the phenomenon of "self-fulfilling prophecy." The more we expect something to happen, the more likely it is to happen.

We are not promoting magical thinking here. Saying over and over, "I will win the lottery," doesn't increase your chances unless it inspires you to buy more and more lottery tickets. Saying, "It will stop raining," doesn't change the weather. However, saying, "I can handle all kinds of weather," encourages you to find an umbrella.

Rather than list possible affirmations here, we refer you to the many books available that have inspirational thoughts. Some calendars also have a "thought for the day," so that when you check your schedule you can also take a moment to reflect.

As you read or think about affirmations that will support your *action plan*, write down those that would be helpful in maintaining your plan. Keep a notebook, index cards, or stick-it pads handy for writing them down. Post your affirmations in convenient spots—your mirror, near the telephone, on the refrigerator—where you will be reminded of the thought. Throughout the day, gently repeat your statement and consider how it may be true.

If you notice "yes, but . . ." thoughts, recognize them as unhelpful and let them go. This inner struggle may continue for a while. Stay with it until you feel better.

Meditation

Most spiritual practice includes some form of meditation. Prayers of all religions are a way to focus attention through recitation of spiritual phrases, directing your attention to God, or to a certain inner state of peace, love, or understanding. By reciting prayers with themes of hope, joy, thanksgiving, or forgiveness, our hearts are more likely to be filled with those feelings.

Some people find listening to music helpful in meditating. We do not mean having music in the background while your mind is busy with the daily grind. Instead, really listen to the music, follow each note and musical phrase, and let your soul be uplifted by the sounds. Singing or playing music may have similar effects. One client who had to have frequent blood tests was terrified of needles. She hummed spiritual hymns during the procedure, and she never felt the pain.

The natural world has a pace and quality that can bring us to greater awareness. A walk on the beach, watching the sunset, birdwatching, hiking, fly-fishing with no intent to catch anything—these can also be forms of meditation. The contemplation of nature is a time-honored form of meditation.

Alma was lucky to grow up in the South in a house with a big yard. The natural world was ever present. The house had no air-conditioning, so windows were usually open, even during thunderstorms. At night she could hear crickets. In the morning she could listen to mockingbirds singing, and blue jays scolding.

Alma's father loved to fish. He and Alma would go several times a week, not just to catch fish but to sit by the lake and watch the birds, turtles, and an occasional alligator. They would sit together without talking, sharing the evening sunset.

You can build on the forms of meditation and expand them through regular practice. Learning to extend your meditation practice can yield even greater benefits of awareness of your body, your moods, and your perceptions of the world. As a consequence, you can then direct your life toward greater peace and sensitivity.

Formal Meditation

There are two types of formal meditation. In the first, you focus or narrow your attention to one point of sensation. In the second, you open your awareness to all external and internal stimuli without judgment, like a blotter absorbs ink.

Focusing attention on one point is the easier of the two. For a focal point, choose something that is meaningful or appealing to you. That focus may be an external visual point, such as a candle, religious picture, altar, or scene from nature. The focus can also be internal, such as your breathing or recitation of certain phrases. The important idea is that you find something that fits your personal style and background.

A quiet, comfortable environment is the best place to practice meditation. Once you are more experienced, you can practice anywhere. You may want to arrange a special place in your home for your meditation. If you attend church, temple, or synagogue, you may want to meditate at your place of worship once or twice a week. In good weather, try practicing outdoors. Twice-daily practice for twenty minutes gives you the most benefit.

We recommend a balanced upright posture when meditating. Lying down may cause you to fall asleep. Some people prefer sitting in a straight-backed chair with their feet on the floor; others like sitting cross-legged on the floor. Another position is to kneel on the floor or on a cushion, sitting back on the heels. You may keep your head either balanced comfortably upright or let your chin drop onto your chest.

Begin to focus your attention in a passive way, not trying to accomplish anything. Gently keep your awareness focused. Do not rush. Do not judge your progress. You will not stay exclusively focused at all times. When your thoughts wander or you feel worry or confusion intruding into your thoughts, gently return your awareness to your focal point, either your breathing, the visual image, or the recitation.

At the end of your meditation, take your time to return to your normal state of alertness. Move or stretch a bit before getting up. If your body has slowed its metabolic rate during the meditation, allow a few moments for heart rate and blood pressure to return to normal.

In the second type of meditation, rather than narrowing your focus to a particular image, the object is to be aware of experiences, thoughts, and feelings as they enter your consciousness. Meditate on whatever comes into your mind. This is called insight meditation. If something new comes in, just be aware of that. Let all experience in without judgment and follow your train of thought wherever it leads you.

Notice your thoughts, feelings, and perceptions. While sitting quietly, become aware of any thoughts that enter your mind. If you begin to think about food, silently recognize, "I am thinking about food." If you are thinking about an argument and begin to feel angry, say to yourself, "I am thinking about that argument. I feel angry." Do not judge your thoughts as good or bad.

As your meditation practice becomes more habitual, it can be done while sitting, walking, or working. You are developing mindfulness, or the awareness of what you are doing, feeling, and thinking, throughout the day.

For physical health benefits, mindfulness of the body can be extended into everyday practice. An example would be taking a long breath when you feel anxious, awareness of breathing gently for three minutes before each meal, or the twice-daily, twenty-minute practice of following the breath. Other meditations on the body can be done while walking, being aware of your feet touching the earth, feeling the air on your face, or feeling the muscles of your body move.

Many people combine exercise with meditation. While jogging, do not think of what you will do later when you return home. Use the time while jogging to focus your attention on the sensations of your body. Develop your awareness of your physical self. If it is a bright day, feel the sensation of brightness on your eyes. If it is rainy, cold, or warm, notice what that feels like.

Cognitive Restructuring

How we think determines what we feel and how we behave. It is not the situation that makes us happy or unhappy but our perspective of it. It is the meaning of an event or situation. Daniel Defoe in his masterwork *Robinson Crusoe* demonstrated how cognitive restructuring works. Alone on the island, Crusoe made a list of the good and bad parts of his experience. On one side he wrote that God must be punishing him. On the other side he wrote that he was alive. God may have a special purpose for him. He then wrote that he was all alone. But, on the other hand, he noted he had the time to think that he always wished for. With this thinking, Crusoe survived.

Practice looking at situations and problems from several different angles. Stay flexible in your thinking. Sometimes thinking of a situation in a different way leads you to see it differently, feel differently about it, and behave differently.

Hypnosis

Hypnosis is a temporary condition of altered attention that is induced by the repetition of certain phrases designed to narrow your focus and then to suggest a particular behavior, memory, or physical phenomenon. While in a hypnotic trance, the individual is more amenable to suggestions, within certain limitations.

Hypnosis is yet another dimension of consciousness, similar to deep relaxation and meditation. While it is sometimes called an altered state of consciousness, hypnosis is similar to the normal fluctuations in awareness that we all experience to one degree or another, such as when we daydream during a boring school lecture.

People's responses to hypnosis vary greatly. About 10 percent of adults are not susceptible to becoming hypnotized. Susceptibility is associated with high intelligence, a tendency to daydream, a capacity for vivid imagery, and a positive attitude to the idea of being hypnotized. In children, susceptibility increases with the mastery of language and reaches its peak at 8 to 10 years of age, thereafter declining to adult levels.

The following effects have been demonstrated with careful experimental investigation but may not occur in every individual: initiation or inhibition of muscle contraction; increased tolerance of fatigue and discomfort of the muscles; increased strength; changes in stomach secretions; greater pain tolerance; enhanced capacity to recall previous experiences, especially emotional or traumatic memories; improved recall of meaningful learned material; skin changes; age regression, or the memory and behavioral traits of a younger person.

Conditions treated with some success include addictions, asthma, excessive appetite, eczema, irritable bladder, stress incontinence, menstrual disturbance, headaches, dental pain and alleviation of dental anxiety, and alleviation of anxiety. Hypnosis has been used in habit control, such as smoking and eating patterns.

In the practice of medicine and psychotherapy, subjects are taught self-hypnosis so that they can use their skill to care for themselves. Most commonly, an audio tape is made of the session, allowing the subject to practice at home.

If you are interested in pursuing hypnosis as a possible treatment, contact the American Society for Clinical Hypnosis at 2200 E. Devon Ave., Suite 291, Des Plaines, IL 60018-4534, (708) 297-3317, or the Society for Clinical and Experimental Hypnosis, 128A Kings Drive, Liverpool, NY 13090, (315) 652-7299, for practitioners in your area. You may also inquire among behavioral medicine specialists for a therapist with training and experience in these methods. As with choosing any specialist, select one who has good credentials in his or her field of expertise.

COMBINING TECHNIQUES

We have found that combining self-regulation techniques has an additive effect—that is, each technique builds on another. For example, general relaxation training may not be sufficient to correct a specific muscle spasm or circulation problem without a specific type of biofeedback. Practicing physical relaxation without calming the mind yields only temporary benefit. You need to find the right combination of strategies for you, your personality, your symptoms, and your resources.

Now that you're aware of some of the self-regulation techniques available for symptomatic relief, go on to fill out your *Stress Action Plan: Symptoms.*

At the end of this chapter, you'll learn about the barriers you will face in carrying out your *Action Plans.* Read section IV, "If at First You Don't Succeed, You're Human," to find out what they are, how they came to be, and what you can do about them.

NOTES

1. Selye, Hans (1974), *Stress Without Distress*, New York, Lippincott.

2. Jacobson, E. (1938), *Progressive Relaxation*, Chicago, Chicago University Press.

3. Linden, W. (1990), *Autogenic Training: A Clinical Guide*, New York, Guilford Press.

4. Thought Technology, 2180 Belgrave Ave., Montreal, Quebec, H4A 2L8, Canada, 1-(800)-361-3651

5. DAVICON, 755 Middlesex Turnpike, Billerica, MA 01821, 1-(800)-DAVICON

ANNE'S STRESS ACTION PLAN: SYMPTOMS

DIRECTIONS: Review your *Stress Audit: Symptoms* section. Write down a symptom rated 4 or 5 you'd like to work on, describe it in terms of when, where, how it's a problem, what makes it better, what makes it worse. Stop. Read chapter 11 and the following pertinent chapters, write down some actions that might help. Stop. Read chapter 20, write down your barriers to change. Stop. Read chapter 21 and write down your supports for change. *Implement* your plan by trying out the easiest and least expensive treatment action you've written down. *Evaluate* the success of that action and try the next if necessary.

SYMPTOM: Shortness of breath

SYSTEM: Sympathetic Nervous System

DESCRIPTION OF SYMPTOM: (Anne's description of her symptom and how it affects her)
Whenever I get real upset and nervous like when I have a fight with Mark or my boss, I start having trouble breathing. Then I start to hyperventilate trying to get my breath. I feel strange and dizzy. It just gets worse and worse and I get so scared I think I'm going crazy. My heart starts racing like crazy and I start getting numb. Sometimes I get pains in my chest and I think it's my heart going bad and that I'm going to die any minute. What's worse is that I worry so much about it happening that sometimes I think I make it happen.

POSSIBLE ACTIONS: (Anne's application of chapters 14 and 15 to her symptoms)

BARRIERS TO CHANGE: (Anne's application of chapter 20 to her life)

SUPPORTS FOR CHANGE: (Anne's application of chapter 21 to her life)

STRESS ACTION PLAN: SYMPTOMS

DIRECTIONS: Review your *Stress Audit: Symptoms* section. Write down a symptom rated 4 or 5 you'd like to work on, describe it in terms of when, where, how it's a problem, what makes it better, what makes it worse. Stop. Read chapter 11 and the following pertinent chapters, write down some actions that might help. Stop. Read chapter 20, write down your barriers to change. Stop. Read chapter 21 and write down your supports for change. *Implement* your plan by trying out the easiest and least expensive treatment action you've written down. *Evaluate* the success of that action and try the next if necessary.

SYMPTOM: **SYSTEM:**

DESCRIPTION OF SYMPTOM   (When, where, and how it's a problem. What makes it better or worse):_____

_____

_____

POSSIBLE ACTIONS: _____

_____

_____

_____

BARRIERS TO CHANGE   (personal, social, financial, practical, etc.):_____

_____

_____

SUPPORTS FOR CHANGE: _____

_____

_____

IV

IF AT FIRST YOU DON'T SUCCEED, YOU'RE HUMAN

20 ENEMIES OF CHANGE

Carrying out your *Stress Action Plans* means that you have to make changes in how you do things, how you take care of yourself, and how you interact with other people. To succeed, you need to know a few principles of behavior modification.

- *Change is inescapably stressful.*
    Change, no matter how positive, is stressful. The rule is to make a few changes at a time. Some people believe they have to conquer stress quickly, so they try to change everything at once. That never works. It just creates more stress.

- *Don't make too many changes at once.*
    We've asked you to do only three *Stress Action Plans*, limited to one item each, because change *is* so stressful and difficult. But one small change sets a myriad of other changes in motion for you and for other people.

- *Don't expect change to happen quickly.*
    As you implement your *Stress Action Plans*, don't expect your life to improve overnight. If you do, you'll be disappointed. Lasting change takes time, and lasting change is what you're after. Remember—"slow and steady wins the race."

• *Make only necessary changes.*

Another problem with making too many changes at once is that you may alter some aspects of your life unnecessarily. You already have many well-established, habitual ways of caring for yourself. Most of them work. Keep those. It's the others that are causing stress.

Remember all those items you circled 1 or 2 or skipped entirely when you were taking the *Stress Audit*? You *don't* need to change them. As the old saying goes, "If it ain't broke, don't fix it."

BARRIERS TO CHANGE

Internal Barriers to Change

Most of the resistance to change comes from within yourself. Understanding those resistances to change makes it easier for you to overcome them and decreases the likelihood that you'll blame yourself when you experience a setback.

Behavioral Law of Inertia

In physics, the Law of Inertia states, "Objects at rest tend to stay at rest unless acted upon by an outside force; objects in motion tend to stay in motion unless acted upon by an outside force." The same law applies to behavior. It takes effort, or force, to initiate a behavior; and it takes effort, or force, to extinguish a behavior.

To create behavioral change, you must recognize what you're up against. You have to initiate new, desirable behaviors *and* stop old, undesirable ones. This is more difficult when we must stop one behavior before we can start another. Much of the time, getting started is the biggest problem.

Behavioral Law of Effect

Another internal barrier is the Behavioral Law of Effect, which states, "The effects of our behaviors determine whether we will repeat them." If some activity has a good result, we tend to repeat it; if it has a bad result, we don't. A very good result will have a greater effect than just a good one. Whether a result is good or bad, obviously, is a subjective determination. That's where your perceptions come into play again.

We have all asked ourselves, "Why do I keep on doing something that's not good for me?" The problem is we can't always tell what pays off and what doesn't. Remember Debby, who had difficulty giving up cigarettes because they reminded her of her father? Her payoff was that smoking cigarettes brought back memories of her father and made it seem like he was still alive. Once Debby understood this, she quit rather easily. The link with her father was illusory; the payoff was the memory of him in life.

Sometimes we get confused and can't decide whether the outcome of a behavior is good or bad. When this happens, behavioral inertia takes over. We keep doing what we've always done, whether it helps us or hurts us, whether it pays off or not.

As you implement your *Stress Action Plans*, keep track of how well you're carrying them out. If you're moving toward your goal, reinforce it by rewarding yourself; if you're not making progress, try something else within the action steps available to you.

Habit

You've learned to take care of yourself from what you've been told, read, and observed. You've developed patterns of eating, sleeping, and social interaction that became habits. Along the way, you also acquired habits of thinking, feeling, and expressing that determine how you communicate with yourself and others.

Habits are useful because they conserve energy and effort. The sooner we reduce behaviors to habit, the less we have to think about them. We're on "automatic pilot." When we develop adaptive habits, our lives run smoothly and easily with little stress or friction. When we develop maladaptive habits, life gets rough.

Habits are by nature highly resistant to change because they incorporate the laws both of behavioral inertia and of behavioral effect. The biggest internal barrier to carrying out your *Action Plans* is stopping bad habits and starting good ones. The bad ones are difficult to alter because it requires energy to change them, and there's a payoff in saving the energy. The good ones are hard to start because it requires energy to get them going and there isn't a payoff for doing so, at least in the beginning.

Fear

Another problem you face is fear of change itself. We cling to the comfortably familiar because it is known. We avoid the unknown because it's disquieting in its uncertainty. That's where the *Stress Audit* helps. It pinpoints what you need to work on, and what you need to do, based on proven scientific principles and our years of clinical experience.

Often our clients procrastinate because they fear they will be judged by how well they are carrying out their *Action Plans*. It's a form of performance stress. They feel they can't do anything unless it's perfect. Again, there's the specter of narcissism. We ask them again and again, "When will good enough be good enough for you?"

Sheldon was a macho young man with a panoply of stress symptoms, including muscular aches and pains, heartburn, irregular heart rate, and insomnia. A gregarious extrovert, Shel loved to party. Eating and drinking came right after sex as his favorite indoor activities. Shel was dissatisfied with his sales job, but he drove himself hard to support his high-flying lifestyle. When he took his fiancée, Robin, out at night, he always got involved with business or "networking." Robin was furious because she felt they never had time to themselves. They quarreled bitterly about Robin's demands and her lack of appreciation of his hard work.

A former high-school athlete, Shel was forty pounds overweight and had lost much of the muscle tone of his younger days. We tried to get him started on an exercise program to reduce his susceptibility to stress, but he wouldn't go to a health club "looking like a fat mess."

Whenever he exercised at home, Shel tried to pick up where he had left off in high school. Invariably, he was bitterly disappointed that he no longer had his former strength or stamina. Instead of fifty pushups, he could do only five. He tried jogging and could make it only half a block. Working out made him so aware of his poor physical condition that he couldn't continue. Narcissism stood in his way.

We tried several tacks with Shel. We put him on an exercise program to get in good enough shape to work out. We sent him to an exercise physiologist and enlisted Robin's help for a modest program of weight lifting. As Shel started building muscle tone, a glimmer of self-pride shone through. The partying continued, but his food and alcohol intake dropped sharply. As his physical condition improved and he "looked halfway decent," Shel started working out at his health club again. He gave up coffee and cigarettes entirely. In a few months, his symptoms dwindled away, his sales increased, and the quarreling with Robin dropped off dramatically.

The problem with Shel was getting started, by-passing his narcissism so that he could admit his lack of perfection and begin working on being good enough. Once Shel overcame his behavioral inertia and began lifting weights, the Behavioral Law of Effect kicked in. Shel got the payoff of increased stamina and strength and a sense of physical well-being. This payoff encouraged him to stop abusing himself with alcohol, nicotine, and caffeine. His new well-being reinforced his behavior to the point that it became as habitual as his earlier, more destructive behavior had been.

External Barriers to Change

Your Nearest and Dearest

As hard as it is to accept, your friends and family, who are governed by the same behavioral laws, are major barriers to changing your life. You have a particular place and identity within your family and among your friends. They expect you always to "be yourself." If you change, they too must change, if the relationship is to continue. As long as they don't have to alter their behaviors too much they'll go along with you; but if they have to readjust their thinking or change a lot, they will sabotage you by setting up barriers to keep you from changing. They may also view your changes as an imposition on them. They will be angry and resentful toward you for making life difficult for them. This may be hard for you to handle emotionally.

Remember Joe, the plumber, and his wife, Betty? They underwent considerable change to maintain their marriage and to deal with Joe's impotence. As they worked on their problems, there were many emotional outbursts. Yet, for the first time in their relationship they were fighting in the open.

Their childen couldn't handle this new behavior. They had never seen their parents express anger toward each other. Their oldest son, Les, called one day and accused us of pushing his parents into divorce. Les angrily told us that his parents had never quarreled before seeing us. Now they were "fighting all the time."

We reassured him that his parents were closer than ever. As we talked, it became apparent that Les was confused. He wanted his parents to be the way they had been. His mother was talking directly to his father now. Les's role as intermediary had all but disappeared. He was having a hard time adjusting to the reality that he wasn't as important in keeping the family together as he had been.

Even well-intentioned friends and relatives can erect formidable barriers to prevent you from changing your behavior. Parents, children, brothers, sisters, lovers, spouses, and buddies all want you to stay the way you've always been. Shel's pals, for instance, expected him to continue drinking and partying with them as he always had. They did their best to discourage his new, healthy habits. They liked him just the way he was.

Try to understand what your nearest and dearest are going through and forgive them. Try to get them to understand why you need to change your life and why it's important for you.

Lack of Resources

One common excuse for not changing is that you don't have enough of whatever it takes to try new behaviors. You don't have enough *time* to listen to a tape or go through a relaxation exercise; there are no realistic *opportunities* for you to build a social network; you can't *afford* to be assertive because your boss may fire you; you don't have the *money* to make your living arrangements more comfortable; and so on. Sometimes these are excuses, sometimes they're not.

When you find yourself blocked from making changes by lack of resources, you have to determine whether it's a convenient excuse or whether it's real. If it's an excuse, own up to it, deal with the real internal barrier to change, and carry out your *Stress Action Plans.*

One young woman named Stacey wanted to lose weight and thought an exercise program would help. We concurred and helped her set up a plan. Stacey couldn't jog or take aerobics because the jarring might hurt her knees. She didn't swim. She had never played tennis, softball, or racquetball. She could ride a bicycle, but her bike had had a flat tire for over a year.

It took three weeks for Stacey to figure out how to get the flat fixed. When she did, the weather was too cold for her to ride. We talked her into getting a stand to turn her bike into a stationary bike. That worked. Stacey exercised daily. By spring she had lost the weight. That summer she went on a cycling tour of Nova Scotia.

If you're creating a lack of resources as an excuse, be honest with yourself. If the lack is real, however, alter your plans accordingly. Sometimes, it takes real ingenuity to carry out an *Action Plan* when resources are limited. Be creative.

OVERCOMING BARRIERS TO CHANGE

If your *Stress Action Plan* is realistic, you can overcome almost any barrier preventing its implementation. Lasting behavioral change follows a step-by-step process. You've already taken some of these steps. In this section, we will outline additional techniques to help you.

Awareness

The first step in dealing with a problem is becoming aware of its existence. You need to know what's wrong and what to do to correct it. Then you need to plan before you take corrective action. You made your first step in getting control of your stress problems when you took the *Stress Audit*. You refined your awareness when you described your selected problems in greater detail on your *Stress Action Plans*. The specifics of your problems and of some of your behaviors were brought into sharper focus.

Decision

Once you became aware of the specific behaviors causing you problems, you decided which ones you wanted to change and which new behaviors you wanted to initiate. Writing them down on your *Action Plans* helped focus your attention on what you needed to do and how you could do it.

Commitment

As Robert Burns said in the eighteenth century, "The best laid schemes o' mice and men gang aft a-gley." No matter how good your *Stress Action Plans*, nothing changes unless you're seriously committed to carrying them out. You do only what you really want to do.

You won't make changes because someone else wants you to. You may respond to escape nagging, but you'll go back to your old behavior as soon as it stops. If you're having trouble putting your plans into action, check your level of commitment. If it's not something you're invested in, you're going to have difficulty doing it.

Setting Modest Goals

Set modest goals. Many people trap themselves with all-or-none thinking and try to deal with everything at once. When they do, they are on the way to disappointment and failure.

By trying to go too far too fast they end up going nowhere. They feel confused, dispirited, angry, and frustrated because nothing has changed. Remember, one of the cardinal characteristics of a good *Action Plan* is that it doesn't have to solve all your problems immediately.

Action

Even with a good plan, serious commitment, and modest goals, you still have to overcome your behavioral inertia, fear of the unknown, and the desires to be perfect and to procrastinate. In short, you've got to get off your duff and do it.

When you get started, if you're interrupted or have to take time out, don't worry. Above all, don't write off your first attempt as a failure. Look at it as practice. Even if it takes several starts to get your *Plans* rolling, do it. Practice makes perfect. And persistent starting is the key.

Lyle was addicted to nicotine at an early age. He'd quit smoking when he had to participate in sports, but after the season finished, he always relapsed. Lyle quit so often that he became an expert at it. When he finally quit for good, it was easy. "Redeye" Smith, his friend and co-worker at the print shop, dared him to stop. Lyle flipped away the cigarette he was smoking, and he was through. That was more than 30 years ago, and he hasn't touched nicotine since. Persistent stopping was the key.

Contingency Management

Once you get your *Action Plan* started you need to keep it rolling. As we pointed out earlier, a behavior has to pay off for you to continue it. If you make the payoff something that won't be realized soon, you'll become discouraged and stop before you reach your goals.

To keep motivated, give yourself little rewards along the way. You'll feel that your changes are paying off, and you'll have a reason for continuing with your *Action Plan*. Set subgoals and make deals with yourself that when you reach one you'll reward yourself according to the magnitude of the goal. Attainment of subgoals may earn small rewards like going to a movie or buying a dress; major goals earn bigger ones such as going on a vacation or buying an expensive coat. You can also give yourself mental rewards. You can reflect on how well you've done and give yourself a pat on the back. You can take pride and pleasure in having overcome barriers and changes in your behavior. State these ideas aloud to yourself. Say things like, "I've really done a good job of changing things around and I'm really proud of myself." Sounds a little corny, but such self-talk works. Try it.

New Goals

Once you've reached your original goals, keep on going. You'll be in better shape to make additional changes and to set new goals for yourself. Use the skills you developed in reaching your first set of goals to move on to new ones.

ANNE'S BARRIERS TO CHANGE AND HOW SHE OVERCAME THEM

We've been following Anne's case through this book to guide you in tailoring your own stress management program. Anne's barriers to change and her solutions to them are particularly instructive.

Anne decided that the most important step to make herself less susceptible to stress was to get more sleep. As you saw in chapter 3, she had specific ideas and plans for changing her behavior.

Her first plan involved going to bed early. She would turn off her TV at 10:00 P.M. There were to be no exceptions.

Anne faced immediate barriers to her carrying out this one element of her *Action Plan*. She and Mark liked late night TV shows and didn't want to miss them. When she told Mark they couldn't stay up to watch *Northern Exposure* together, he said, "But you know how we love to talk about whether Maggie and Joel are going to make it." After several days of icy silence, Mark stopped pouting and agreed to Anne's compromise. They would tape *Northern Exposure* each Monday night and watch it on the weekend.

She also decided she'd have no meals later than 8:00 P.M. and no caffeine or alcohol after 6:00 P.M. Again, Mark was a barrier because he liked eating out and enjoyed long, lingering dinners followed by coffee and cognac. Anne was concerned that he would feel rejected and be angry with her. When she told Mark, he agreed to no late dinners during the week. Friday and Saturday would be their special nights.

The third part of Anne's plan was that after 9:30 P.M. she would not make phone calls and would let her answering machine handle all incoming calls. Her biggest barrier to this element of her *Action Plan?* Fear. Her mother liked to call her in the evening and spend hours on the phone. Anne thought that if she altered this pattern, her mother would be angry at her.

Anne overcame this barrier by talking to her mother as she had with Mark. She explained why she had to have ground rules for evening telephone calls and why she had to get her sleep. Her mother agreed.

The rest of Anne's plan involved changing her evening routines and her waking hour. Organizing things the night before, taking a hot bath before 10:00 P.M., doing PMR after going to bed, and rising at 7:00 A.M. on weekdays and 9:00 A.M. on weekends helped Anne overcome behavioral inertia. Once she managed to do that, the payoff in extra time and increased effectiveness helped consolidate her new behaviors into new, healthy habits.

Anne's Sources of Stress Barriers to Change

Anne decided that a source of stress she wanted to work on was the trouble she was having with her boss, Charlie, who she thought was disorganized, insensitive, and dictatorial. He was driving her to distraction and she wanted him to stop.

Anne sat down with Charlie and calmly told him what the problem was and how it affected her and her work. After this discussion Anne felt they could negotiate a clear, written job description.

What were the internal barriers to taking this course

of action? Anne was afraid of what might happen if she spoke up to Charlie. First, her co-workers might get mad at her for "making waves." There could also be a major blow-up between Charlie and herself. Or, she could be fired.

As we all must do at times, Anne gathered her courage and talked to her boss in a candid and forthright way. Her fears proved groundless. She and Charlie negotiated a clear, written job description that eliminated a major portion of her stress.

Anne's Symptoms of Stress Barriers to Change

In setting up her *Action Plan* to deal with her symptoms of stress, Anne pursued a plan of self-regulation to eliminate her panic attacks. She decided to learn deep breathing and a thought-stopping program to alter her catastrophic thought patterns. Anne practiced staying in the moment and not worrying about what might happen. In addition, she made herself a relaxation tape.

Predictably, Anne ran into a number of barriers. She was fearful of the unknown, thinking she would get too excited and panicky to remember what to do when she suffered an attack. Anne doubted that she could ever learn to self-regulate effectively. She had to deal with behavioral inertia in changing her chest breathing to diaphragmatic breathing. Last, she didn't think she had the time to do all these exercises.

It took some hand holding and moral support from Mark and her mother, and backup from us, to get Anne to execute these aspects of her *Action Plan*. In about three weeks Anne started to establish healthy new habits. She had a couple of setbacks, but she used her newfound skills to weather them without going to the emergency room. The reinforcement of gaining control over her body kept Anne on track with her *Action Plan*.

TECHNIQUES FOR STAYING ON TRACK

Self-Monitoring

Keeping a record of your progress is a powerful aid to staying on track. It's a constant reminder of what you're trying to do for yourself and how well you're doing it. It can reinforce your behavior by showing you how far you've come. For instance, keeping a record of your stress symptoms over several weeks reminds you of what it was like when you started.

Keeping records also helps you avoid distorting your progress. Luke, for instance, kept daily records of his perceived muscle tension levels and his headache pain. He was struck by the difference between his recollection of what his tension and pain had been and what his records indicated. We graphed out his muscle tension and pain records to demonstrate that when his muscle tension levels went down, the frequency and severity of his headaches went down as well. The demonstration kept him on track until his headaches disappeared entirely.

Making Agreements with Others

You'll keep agreements with others more often than you'll keep them with yourself because of social pressure. For example, tell friends and family about your *Action Plan* goals and your timetables for meeting them. This sets up expectations and creates social pressures for you to follow through on your pronouncements. Remember Lyle's behavior when "Redeye" Smith dared him to quit smoking. It worked for Lyle; it will work for you.

Reminders

Amid our busy lives, we can often forget our best intentions. Posting reminders to relax near the telephone can prompt you to take a thirty-second relaxation break after every phone call. A reminder on the bathroom mirror helps you remember to start your day on the right foot. A brief reading of a Twelve Step book, a religious

verse, or a morning meditation can help you keep a relaxed attitude all day.

Anne used reminders a lot to help her keep on track,
particularly in the beginning. She stuck little notes all
over her house. She stuck one on the telephone to remind
her not to make or take calls after 9:30 P.M. She stuck
one to her TV to remind her to turn it off at 10:00 P.M.
The wall next to her bed had a checklist that reminded
her to have everything ready for the next day, to do her
PMR, and what time to set her alarm. After she and Charlie had written her job description, she framed a copy
and hung it on the wall over her desk to keep her on
track at work.

Setting Higher Goals

Nothing succeeds like success. After you've had some
success in achieving your initial goals, go on to deal with
the tougher ones. You'll find that the skills you developed
in reaching the more modest goals transfer directly to
pursuing the more difficult and complex goals you set
for yourself.

WRITE THE BARRIERS SECTION OF YOUR *STRESS ACTION PLANS*

Now that you've completed this chapter and have
some idea what to expect in terms of barriers to change,
go back and fill out the "Barriers to Change" portion of
all three *Stress Action Plans*. Be thoughtful and specific
as you complete them. Then, read the next chapter for
tips on how to integrate outside support into your programs of behavior change.

ANNE'S STRESS ACTION PLAN: SUSCEPTIBILITY

DIRECTIONS: Review your *Stress Audit: Susceptibility* section. Write down an item you rated as never being true of you, describe the problem, set a reasonable goal for change. Stop. Read pertinent section of chapter 3, write down some possible actions that might help. Stop. Read chapter 20, write down your barriers to change. Stop. Read chapter 21, write down your supports for change. *Implement* your plan. *Evaluate* results. *Adjust* your plan.

SUSCEPTIBILITY ITEM: I never get seven to eight hours of sleep at least four nights per week.

DESCRIPTION OF PROBLEM: (Anne's description of her own situation)
I can hardly keep my eyes open after lunch. Sometimes, I'm so tired I just put my head down on my desk and take a nap. It's difficult to get up in the morning and I generally oversleep a couple days a week. I'm late to work so often that it's become a joke, except to my boss. I have to get more sleep, but I have trouble getting to bed at night. I watch TV with Mark and get wrapped up in it, or Mom or Mark calls and I talk for hours. If I eat late or drink alcohol or coffee I have trouble getting to sleep and then staying asleep. Because I'm too tired to get things done at work, I often bring work home and stay up late trying to get caught up.

REASONABLE GOAL: (Anne sets personal goal) Get eight hours of sleep five nights per week.

POSSIBLE ACTIONS: (Anne's application of "Sleep" portions of chapter 3 to her life)
1) Turn TV off at 10:00 P.M. whether Mark's here or not. No exceptions.
2) Make no phone calls after 9:30 P.M. Let answering machine take calls after 9:30 P.M. and return them when appropriate.
3) No meals later than 8:00 P.M. No caffeine or alcohol after 6:00 P.M.
4) Organize things for next day before 9:00 P.M.
5) Take hot bath by 10:00 P.M. In bed by 10:30 P.M.
6) Do progressive muscle relaxation (PMR) exercise after going to bed.
7) Up at 7:00 A.M. weekdays. Up no later than 9:00 A.M. on weekends. No exceptions.

BARRIERS TO CHANGE: (Anne's application of chapter 20 to her life)
1) I like some late night TV shows. I can tape them, but Mark likes to watch TV at my place. He may get upset if don't watch it with him or if I turn it off at 10:00 P.M.
2) Mom will be hurt if I don't take her phone calls or if I don't spend a long time talking with her. Mark also likes to talk for hours when he calls. He'll get mad at me too.

3) If I'm working against a deadline, I have to finish on time even if it means staying up late to get it done. I'll be disappointed in myself and my boss will be mad at me if we miss a deadline.

4) Mark will feel rejected and hurt if I don't go out to dinner with him when he wants me to. Dinner with Mark is always long, with coffee and cognac. He won't like it if I insist on an early dinner or skip the coffee and cognac.

SUPPORTS FOR CHANGE: (Anne's application of chapter 21 to her life)

ANNE'S STRESS ACTION PLAN: SOURCES

DIRECTIONS: Review your *Stress Audit: Sources* section. Write down an item you rated 4 or 5 you'd like to work on, describe the situation and problem. Stop. Read the chapter dealing with that problem, write down some specific actions to take. Stop. Read chapter 20, write down your barriers to change. Stop. Read chapter 21 and write down your supports for change. *Implement* your first choice of action. *Evaluate* results. *Adjust* your plan.

ITEM: Trouble with the boss.

DESCRIPTION OF SITUATION AND PROBLEM: (Anne's description of her own situation)

Charlie, my boss, jerks me around all the time. One minute I'm told to do one thing, the next he wants me doing something else. Then he gets mad and screams at me if everything doesn't get done right on time. He goes ballistic. He interferes with my getting things done when he changes his mind all the time. His disorganization really impacts on my efficiency and could affect my professional career in marketing. Sometimes the tension gets so thick between us you could cut it with a knife.

POSSIBLE ACTIONS: (Anne's application of chapter 4's options to her life)

Alter: (Anne's application of "Alter" portions of chapter 4 to her life)

1) Sit down with Charlie (during a quiet time when we've been getting along well) and have a real heart-to-heart talk about how we work together.

2) Negotiate a clear, written job description with Charlie and then make sure we both keep to it. No unilateral renegotiations.

3) Take my problem with Charlie upstairs to the president of the company and be prepared to fight it out head to head with Charlie.

Avoid: (Anne's application of "Avoid" portion of chapter 4 to her life)
1) Request a transfer to another division.
2) Take the job I've been offered with our top competitor.
3) Just quit and marry Mark.

Accept: (Anne's application of "Accept" portion of chapter 4 to her life)
1) Get so good at relaxing that I can relax anytime, anyplace, and just relax when things get tense.
2) Understand that Charlie has his problems too and doesn't handle pressure well.
3) Quit personalizing things so much.

BARRIERS TO CHANGE: (Anne's application of chapter 20 to her life)
1) People will get mad at me if I make waves.
2) Things could really explode between Charlie and me and make things even worse.
3) I'll get fired.

SUPPORTS FOR CHANGE: (Anne's application of chapter 21 to her life)

ANNE'S STRESS ACTION PLAN: SYMPTOMS

DIRECTIONS: Review your *Stress Audit: Symptoms* section. Write down a symptom rated 4 or 5 you'd like to work on, describe it in terms of when, where, how it's a problem, what makes it better, what makes it worse. Stop. Read chapter 11 and the following pertinent chapters, write down some actions that might help. Stop. Read chapter 20, write down your barriers to change. Stop. Read chapter 21 and write down your supports for change. *Implement* your plan by trying out the easiest and least expensive treatment action you've written down. *Evaluate* the success of that action and try the next if necessary.

SYMPTOM: Shortness of breath

SYSTEM: Sympathetic Nervous System

DESCRIPTION OF SYMPTOM: (Anne's description of her symptom and how it affects her)
Whenever I get real upset and nervous, like when I have a fight with Mark or my boss, I start having trouble breathing. Then I start to hyperventilate trying to get my breath. I feel strange and dizzy. It just gets worse and worse and I get so scared I think I'm going crazy. My heart starts racing like crazy and I start getting numb. Sometimes I get pains

in my chest and I think it's my heart going bad and that I'm going to die any minute. What's worse is that I worry so much about it happening that sometimes I think I make it happen.

POSSIBLE ACTIONS: (Anne's application of chapters 14 and 15 to her symptoms)
1) Remember to breathe through my nose slowly and evenly. I'll need to practice that. (chapter 14 and appendix I)
2) Stop the catastrophizing thoughts, the "what if . . ." thoughts. (chapter 15 and appendix I)
3) Remember to stay in the moment, don't worry about what might happen. (chapter 15 and appendix I)
4) Make myself a relaxation tape with a special emphasis on diaphragmatic breathing. (chapter 14 and appendix I)

BARRIERS TO CHANGE: (Anne's application of chapter 20 to her life)
1) I get too excited and panicky to remember what to do.
2) Self-doubt: I'm not sure this will work for me. Maybe I really need medication.
3) Old habits: I'm not used to the feel of deep breathing, it feels funny to breathe that way.
4) Time: I don't know when I can make time to do the exercises.

SUPPORTS FOR CHANGE: (Anne's application of chapter 21 to her life)

21 FRIENDS AND ALLIES

Armed with your *Stress Action Plans*, you now should have a clearer idea of what you would like to do about your stress and the difficulties you'll face. You can make some changes without assistance. But, if you're stuck, or overwhelmed, numerous resources are available.

Family, friends, co-workers, social and spiritual organizations, self-help groups, and a variety of professionals are all potential sources of help. Each one offers something different. You have to be clear about what to expect from them and recognize their limitations if you are to make the most of their assistance.

We've talked a lot about support systems throughout this book because they're important. Human beings have clustered together for assistance, support, and comfort since the beginning of time. Not having a support system increases your susceptibility to stress and creates stress for you.

Support systems received a lot of consideration when we constructed the *Stress Audit*. We included specific items in the *Susceptibility* section, such as: I have a network of friends and acquaintances; I have someone to talk with about personal issues; I regularly attend club or social events; I have a relative within fifty miles on whom I can rely. In chapters 6, "Managing Family Stress," and 8, "Dealing with Social Stress," we discussed your family and social network both as sources of support and as sources of stress.

Support comes in many forms: emotional help can be a hug or verbal reassurance; practical help can be going to the grocery store when you're sick; financial aid can be a loan from a relative, credit union, or bank when you're down on your luck. During particularly difficult times, you may need substantial support from several different sources.

You may feel shy or uncertain about calling on sources of support. But do it. Support makes a job more fun and less difficult and often is the difference between success and discouragement. Ask for help if you need it, want it, feel stuck, are curious about how someone else would handle your situation, or have tried to make changes with little success on your own. Don't wait until you are in a crisis.

Asking for or receiving help does not mean that you hand your problem over to someone else to solve. Social support is no substitute for having a strong sense of self-efficacy. The best support enhances your sense of mastery.

As with every other part of your *Stress Action Plan*, tailor your supports to your needs. Use your *Action Plan* as a guide. Be careful about too much help as you carry out your *Action Plans*. Sources of support can conflict and create confusion, resulting in no action.

Let's look at how different people who needed support found it. In Anne's case, she had three stress problems—lack of sleep, problems at work, and "heart attacks." For her sleep and work problems she turned to her mother and Mark. She looked to co-workers for help with her boss. For panic, she sought support from Mark when she did her relaxation homework.

Another client, Sabrina, a working, single woman with two children, Alexander and Mallory, who was seeing us for mild depression, also illustrates how to use support systems. Sabrina's depression had been induced by a seemingly minor incident—her baby-sitter had quit with only a week's notice. Without a sitter to cover the hours between when elementary school was over and Sabrina came home from work, her already shaky coordination of work, children, school, and home could fall apart.

Changes in child-care arrangements had always made Sabrina anxious because of the range of personalities, personal problems, and capabilities among sitters. As she worried, Sabrina reexperienced the depression she'd felt following her divorce two years earlier. Sabrina started on an "if only" train of thought. She was glad not to be married to her ex-husband, Fred, anymore, but: "If only things could have worked out"; "If only I weren't a single mother"; "If only Fred hadn't moved to the next town he'd be closer and more available for little emergencies like this. At least he helped out when he lived closer." Her "if only" thoughts just made her feel more hopeless, helpless, and depressed.

With our assistance, Sabrina realized that she could dissipate her depression if she sought help. Sabrina assessed her support system. She listed all her options. If she had to, she could borrow money and keep on the young women from the nanny agency while she interviewed potential sitters. Her sister, Charlene, who lived close to Alexander and Mallory's school, could take the children some afternoons. But tension had existed between Sabrina and Charlene ever since they'd had a fight the past Christmas. Any other friends to tap? we asked. Sabrina said she had baby-sat Kip, Alexander's best friend, a couple of times. Maybe Kip's mother would reciprocate for a short while? Sabrina thought of additional support if her plans didn't work. A fellow church member might know of an older woman or a high school student who could come over for a few weeks. She remembered the 12-year-old girl in the apartment upstairs. Maybe she could fill in until something permanent was arranged?

Then Sabrina became even more inventive—she could talk with her boss about taking time off during the week. She could work on weekends while the children were with Fred.

After all this planning Sabrina was ready to act. First, she called her best friend from work, who had gone through a similar situation two months earlier, to share her frustration and get some encouragement. Next, she called the local paper to place a classified ad for child-care assistance. Then she called Charlene, who to Sabrina's surprise was glad to hear from her and immediately said yes to some temporary baby-sitting. Finally, she asked Alexander and Mallory to be more cooperative and helpful. If they would take care of their rooms a little better and give her a hand with the dishes, she would have more free time to interview sitters. With a hug for their mother, they agreed.

In responding to her stress overload, Sabrina handled her emotional reactions, overcame her negative thoughts, assessed her resources, and reached out for help and support. Sabrina hired a new baby-sitter, whom the children loved, within two weeks of making her *Action Plan*. And, of course, her depression vanished as quickly as it appeared.

Another client, Murray, a 33-year-old middle manager, had a much harder time asking for and accepting help when he lost his job. His layoff was particularly destructive. He had been at his company for five years and thought his job was secure. The firing happened late on a Friday afternoon. He was given only time enough to collect his personal belongings, say goodbye to his staff, and pick up six months' severance pay.

At first Murray didn't even want to tell his wife, Margaret. He was so upset that he had a few drinks on the way home. That night he did tell her, but he made her promise not to tell anyone else—not the kids, not her folks, no one—until he had a new job. That way, people would think he had changed jobs.

Murray's decision deprived him and Margaret of the emotional support of friends and family. Without it, friction increased between them. Murray tended to keep his anger and worry to himself. His silence upset Margaret, who needed to talk to keep her fears at bay.

Keeping Murray's secret also cut them off from his support network. Friends were concerned about his moodiness. Their children were puzzled by their parents' increased irritability and anxiety about money.

Margaret finally put her foot down after six weeks. Murray told his family and close friends. To his surprise, they were sympathetic. They weren't ashamed of his "failure," as he'd thought they would be. Now he could use them to job hunt. It took a while, but Murray was back at work before his severance pay ran out.

Reaching out for help involves several steps. You have to acknowledge that you need help, identify the type of assistance or support you need, and enlist that help in a meaningful way.

BARRIERS TO REACHING OUT FOR HELP

If you need support in carrying out your *Action Plans* and are having trouble requesting it, take a few minutes to ask yourself some questions. What thoughts do you have about asking for help? What do you expect others' reactions to be to your requests? Are you imagining what others might think of you if you have to ask for help? Are you afraid of confiding in someone else? If so, why? Will you feel foolish, vulnerable, or obligated if you ask for support?

If such thoughts and fears are preventing you from asking for help, ask yourself how rational they are. How many of them are just "dumb" ideas? How much of the problem is pride? Dump thoughts that are just "dumb" and swallow your pride. Face the fact that you need help and support, and ask for it.

You may not have a good support network. If you have moved recently, or made significant changes in your life, the support system you had may no longer exist. If you are recently divorced, or someone close to you has died or moved, your system may have changed. Rebuilding or repairing support systems takes time.

It also takes certain skills. If you grew up in a close community where everyone knew everyone else, you may not know how to build a new support system. It may feel awkward and artificial to reach out. Do it anyway. You'll get used to it.

You may have grown up in a family that discouraged involvement with "outsiders." One young woman, Linda, had a father who would not ask simple favors of his neighbors, such as help in pulling his boat out of the water in the winter. He would wait for his son to come help him. Linda's father criticized her for accepting invitations to dinner at neighbors' homes, cautioning her against incurring obligations. As an adult, she had difficulty even accepting rides to social functions.

Some families don't support one another. If you grew up in a family where confidences were not kept, and there was an atmosphere of criticism, you may be reluctant to confide in others, even your close friends. Such experiences may make it difficult for you to build a support system.

Shyness also affects your ability to make connections with other people. Anxiety about how you appear to others may make you avoid social settings where you might meet new people who could become part of your support system. You may have such problems with assertiveness that they affect your ability to make clear requests of others.

Even if you have a good and longstanding community of people who care about you, you may not be using the support available to you effectively. The most common reason why people do not ask others for what they need is the fear of rejection. "What if I ask and they say no?" Sensitivity to rejection inhibits people from seeking emotional support, much less material help or financial assistance.

Anxiety about exposing personal vulnerability is another common reason not to seek help. Some men can't ask for directions because being lost feels like a sign of weakness. If your relationships with others are generally ones of competition rather than connection, you may be uncomfortable with letting others know that you want and need help.

EXPRESSING STRONG FEELINGS IN A SAFE PLACE

In sharing feelings with a neutral and safe person, such as a counselor, group member, or trusted friend, you can talk freely about frustrating or difficult situations without having to censor yourself or worry about harming your relationships with others. Later, when you're thinking more clearly, you can choose what you will actually do or say to handle the situation.

Take our client Elizabeth. She was furious at her father and never wanted to see him again. But he had written her a card inviting her to Thanksgiving dinner. She didn't know what to do.

A few words about Elizabeth's background before we discuss her final decision. Elizabeth's parents had divorced during her teenage years after many years of a difficult marriage. But the fighting didn't end with the divorce. Her father would periodically call on the phone to denounce her mother. In addition, her father provided only minimal child support and refused to pay for Elizabeth's college education.

Lack of funds made college difficult for Elizabeth. She had to take out loans and work part-time while she went to school. None of her friends did and she resented it. Years later, she was still paying back her college loans.

Elizabeth eventually discovered that her father had secreted large amounts of money in a foreign bank account. He had lied about his financial status at the time of the divorce to avoid sharing his wealth with her and her mother. Elizabeth was furious when she found out. She vowed never to visit him again.

Five years passed. Then the Thanksgiving invitation arrived. What should she do? Elizabeth knew that if she were to reopen her relationship with her father, she would have to express her anger to him. She wanted to talk to someone about how to approach her father, but whom? Her mother wouldn't be objective, and this was too personal a matter to discuss with her co-workers. However, she did have a good friend, Patty, whose parents had also divorced. She too was still dealing with its aftershocks. Elizabeth called her on the phone. After Patty heard Elizabeth's story, she volunteered to listen to Elizabeth talk about her father. Patty also suggested that, before their meeting, she buy a book, *Making Peace with Your Parents*, and fill out the resentments writing exercise in it.[1]

A few days later they got together in Patty's apartment. As they worked together, Elizabeth felt for the first time in her life that she could air her feelings. Using her "resents" list, Elizabeth said out loud all the names she wanted to call her father. As her fury grew, her voice became louder and louder. The apartment walls almost shook; Patty's cat dived under the couch to escape the verbal onslaught. But Patty patiently listened. As she neared the end of the list, with the last profanity escaping her mouth, Elizabeth started to laugh. Her anger was spent. A catharsis had been achieved. The two friends embraced.

Elizabeth decided she'd go to Thanksgiving dinner. She now believed she could talk to her father about her feelings without being bitter. Maybe they could heal the hurt that had divided them.

While you air your frustrations, your support person should not escalate your feelings with his or her opinions, fears, or depressions, but should simply encourage you to speak your mind openly.

VALIDATION

In addition to having someone listen, it helps when someone agrees with your point of view. Many clients feel confused, wondering, "Did I do the right thing? Am I crazy? Would another reasonable human being see things the way I did?" Validation is especially important for people who hold contrary views or are members of minority or less powerful groups.

Rape victims need to talk to someone who understands what it was like, not someone who will blame him or her for being a bad judge of character or in the wrong place at the wrong time. African-Americans need to affirm the positive aspects of black experiences and validate experiences of discrimination. Recently, Robert Bly's book *Iron John* confirmed for many men that it was all right "to cry and show their pain."[2]

UNDERSTANDING AND ACCEPTANCE

Being understood is a basic human need. It is essential for feeling connected to the rest of humanity. People want to know, "Is there anyone else like me or who can understand what it is like to be me?"

Learning that you can tell even one other person about your struggles and weaknesses and find that he or she understands reduces the pressure to be perfect. Understanding and acceptance are antidotes to the shame, guilt, and negative self-perception that we feel when we don't have our lives in order.

CLARIFICATION

Besides ventilation and validation, talking through your situation and emotions brings clarification. Just describing your problem to someone else helps you think more clearly. You may have noticed that thoughts about your stress situation float about in an incomplete, amorphous way, shifting from one association to another, or going around and around in circles on the same theme, endlessly repeating themselves without conclusion.

When you speak to another person, you must find words to describe your feelings, you must fill in background details, and you must explain many circumstances so that the other person understands what you are experiencing. Through this effort you come to understand yourself and your situation more fully.

Philip's case illustrates the power of clarification. In his early thirties, he came to see us because he hadn't been feeling well. Philip had been dating a man, Andrew, whom he greatly admired, but who was jealous of his friends and his community activities. In addition, Andrew often called him late at night when he was exhausted. Philip had other concerns, but he wasn't sure how important they were. Mostly, he felt confused and tired.

Philip also had a difficult and demanding job, coordinating services for AIDS patients and their families. It required unpaid evening and community work. State funding for his position was running out, however, so he was seeking a new position.

Philip had other problems. His parents were elderly and his mother had recently recovered from a brief illness. In addition, Philip had recently purchased and moved into a two-family home that needed a major overhaul.

We gave Philip a *Stress Audit*. As expected, he scored high on the Work, Social, Personal, and Environmental scales. His symptoms were mostly emotional signs of burnout. Although it took a few weeks, Philip finally realized how complex and stressful his life had become and how much he needed to develop a social network to help him with his problems.

He had not resolved all of his concerns when he terminated treatment. At the last visit, he said, "When I first came in, my life was like a messy desk, with everything piled on top in a big jumble, and I didn't know where to start. Now we've sorted the issues out into piles, and I think I can handle it from here." Clarification was all Philip needed to set priorities and effectively address all the problems in his life.

INFORMATION AND FEEDBACK

Among the most important outcomes we get from talking to other people are information and feedback. Sometimes we get caught up in irrational beliefs that promote distorted thinking and maladaptive behaviors. We need someone to talk to us about them. Just as skeptics couldn't believe the world was round until it was proven, it may be hard to let go of your irrational beliefs. Such information can come from professionals, but often it comes from friends, family, or co-workers.

Talking with someone else lets us see ourselves and our situations from a different perspective. By changing our viewpoint of ourselves and our lives, we learn more about ourselves, and we redefine who we are, how we think, and how we feel. Other people don't always think the same way we do. They can help you laugh at your unrealistic fears, correct your misperceptions, and inject a situation with optimism when you have given up hope.

For example, a friend's 4-year-old son, Stuart, was teased by another little boy, Daniel, for having "breasts." Stuart was confused and more than a little upset. Only girls were supposed to have breasts. Nevertheless, he could see that he had round places on his chest where breasts were on women, and they were more prominent than Daniel's. He didn't know what to think.

That evening when he was undressing for bed, Stuart told his father that he had a problem. Embarrassed and unable to articulate his concern, he pointed to his chest. After supportive prompting from his father, he blurted out, "Daniel says I've got breasts like a girl's."

It took a few minutes for his father to determine what Stuart meant. When he did, he told his son, "You just have big chest muscles. Those are your pectoral muscles. You're a big, strong boy to have muscles like that." Taking off his own shirt, he told his son, "See, Daddy has big pecs just like you and he's sure not a girl, is he." Stuart leaped into his father's arms with a grin of relief and gave him the strongest "bear hug" ever.

Within moments the child's fears were put to rest through feedback and information. He might have worried for days about having "breasts" without the information provided by his understanding father.

Motivation

One of the prime contributions of a supportive community is motivation. Sports teams have cheerleaders. Armies have marching bands. Politicians have dedicated volunteers. In your personal support network who are your cheerleaders? At your job, who appreciates your work and values your ideas? At home, with whom do you share your successes? Begin to increase your awareness of positive remarks, praise, and encouragement. Notice how often you tell others when you like something. Be aware of who is encouraging you. Compliments, praise, and other positive reinforcements are free, and they make a real difference to other people.

You can make contracts or deals with friends as a way to increase your motivation. Psychological research has documented that verbal reinforcement from others, making public statements of intention and making agreements with others contribute significantly to behavior change and to the establishment of new habits.

Asking someone to help you with self-management may be as simple as asking him or her to compliment you for not smoking, or to talk with you for five minutes each day about your efforts to quit. Announcing to others your intention to change creates a sense of controlled social pressure. When you make a public commitment you are more likely to stand behind your words. You'll keep agreements with others that you won't keep with yourself. Use the effects of social pressure as a source of support in carrying out your *Action Plans*. It works.

For example, if you want to reduce your weight to lower your vulnerability to stress, get your family on your side. Call a family meeting to explain your problems with stress. Talk about your *Stress Audit* scores and your *Stress Profile*. Discuss your results and tell them why it is so important for your health that you deal with your stress problems. Explain that you need their help to succeed.

You may need to do what Eric did. He had two problems—he was overweight, and he had borderline diabetes. If he lost weight, his diabetes would be easier to control. At one point he lost thirty pounds, but he had difficulty keeping it off. He struggled valiantly to keep his weight down.

His wife, Molly, also worried about Eric's health. She questioned him about his food intake to the point where he felt criticized and accused whenever he ate. Quite firmly, Eric insisted that she stop. Eric clearly told Molly what would be helpful to him—preparing approved diabetic menus and listening to his concerns about managing his appetite. He also informed her of what was not helpful—questioning, criticizing, and predicting illness and death if he gained weight.

When you ask for help from your family or friends, be specific. If you want advice, ask for it; if you just want them to listen, tell them so. Don't let them get confused. You may only want them to listen to you. They may think you want advice. If they give advice, you won't feel helped, only annoyed. If you don't follow their advice, *they* feel annoyed. You could begin by saying, "I've been upset lately, and I wonder if you would listen while I try to sort out my feelings?" Another example: "I'm feeling particularly lonesome since I broke up with Cliff. Do you mind if I call you or we plan to go out more in the next few weeks?" Or: "When I get stressed, I tend to [eat, drink, take drugs, have inappropriate sex]. Could I call you to plan something constructive instead?"

By being specific, you are letting others know what they can do to be supportive. Such limits decrease their anxieties about solving your problems for you. "Can I lean on you during this difficult time? Can I count on you to be there for me?" may be too global and possibly threatening.

A few months into the process of writing this book, Alma found herself putting off rewriting an important section. Several weeks passed and no work got done. She had joined a writers' support group at the beginning of the project and had received a lot of help in earlier meetings. How could she use the group now? She made an announcement to the four other members that she would take two steps before the next meeting: (1) arrange her calendar to free up time to write; (2) read to them whatever she wrote. She did not want their criticism at this point, just their support to get past her writer's block. By announcing to the group what she would do, Alma used social pressure as a motivational tool.

You make social contracts in your daily life, at work and at home, all the time. They're as simple as "I'll meet you at seven" and as complex as prenuptial agreements. We have contracts that are written, reviewed, and notarized by lawyers, memos with "OK" scrawled at the top, verbal contracts, and, trickiest of all, unspoken agreements.

Make your agreements with family and friends simple, clear, and spoken. There'll be fewer opportunities for misunderstanding, disappointment, and conflict. In general, the following principles are helpful in asking for motivational support.

- Make agreements with others for their input.
- The behaviors and rewards should be spelled out.
- The goal must be possible, not a setup for failure.
- Keep the agreement fair.

- Ask for the type of help you need, not the type they usually give you.
- Be specific.
- Share your successes. Ask for positive feedback, praise, or acknowledgment. Tell others what their helpful remarks have meant to you.
- Ask for reminders, not criticism, when relapses occur.
- Avoid asking for penalties or punishment if you relapse. Focus on positive rewards.
- Revise the agreement as needed.

HELP YOURSELF BY HELPING OTHERS

You can also be helped by helping others. Your growing knowledge of stress issues may help increase your awareness of their problems. If you are quitting smoking, they may be inspired to stop some of their unhealthy habits. A commitment to regular tennis matches helps both you and your friend stay fit. Regular phone contact or social activities work both ways. People in Alcoholics Anonymous have noted how helpful it is to their recovery to be a sponsor for someone else. By offering your assistance to someone else, you are helped yourself.

THE KIND OF "SUPPORT" YOU DON'T WANT

Supportive people do not downplay your feelings, blame you for your situation, tell you what to do, ask you to snap out of it, or make you feel bad in any way.

IDENTIFY YOUR RESOURCES

One way to feel ready to reach out for help is to understand the many sources of support available to you. Think about your current situation. Whom do you most often see or talk with? Family, friends, co-workers? If you are married, your partner is probably your greatest source of both emotional and practical support. If you are having relationship difficulties or are not in a committed relationship, that kind of support may come instead from close friends, brothers or sisters, or associates from work or school. Do you belong to any religious, political, social service, or hobby- or work-related organizations? Do you attend a self-help group or see a professional counselor?

There are differences between the kind of help family, friends, and co-workers can give and what community organizations, self-help groups, and professionals can provide. Your relationship with family and friends is based on the pleasure of their company. They are a primary source of help, but there are limits on what they can do for you. This is particularly true if you are dealing with deep emotional problems. They are not therapists. Attempts to make them fill this role won't help you and will only damage your relationship with them.

WHERE TO FIND SUPPORT

The great French observer of American life Alexis de Tocqueville wrote nearly 150 years ago that Americans loved what he called "associations."[3] In these groups they "meet together in large numbers, they converse, they listen to one another, and they are mutually stimulated to all sorts of undertakings." Little has changed since de Tocqueville traveled through this country. You are surrounded by every imaginable group and organization that can be of help, if you only reach out to them.

Your church, temple, or mosque is a good place to start. These spiritual refuges help us celebrate the major transitions of life—marriage, death, birth of a child— while providing a community of like minds, where common values are shared and support is given.

Within most communities there are many other kinds of organizations centered around a common concern, hobby, charitable goal, or interest. The time to participate in such associations is not when you are in crisis, but as part of a long-term plan to establish gratifying associations with others in your life.

Among the more traditional charitable clubs and organizations you might consider are the Elks, Kiwanis, Lions, Odd Fellows, and Optimists, just to name a few.

There are also business clubs, such as your local chamber of commerce, and, if you're eligible, professional clubs and alumni clubs. There are veterans' organizations such as the American Legion, Veterans of Foreign Wars, and so on.

There are numerous hobby clubs, too—gardening, hiking, biking, hunting, dancing, and photography, just to name a few.

Groups exist to promote social and political change. Unions have been instrumental in coping with work stress as well as improving overall conditions for workers. The National Association for the Advancement of Colored People, the Anti-Defamation League, the National Organization for Women, and other groups have organized specifically to assist with ethnic and gender discrimination.

Self-Help

Self-help groups involve more than 15 million people in approximately half a million groups.[4] These groups are voluntary associations of people with similar concerns for the purpose of mutual assistance. Many groups were formed because their needs were not being met by existing institutions. Formal care-giving or political institutions often seem unresponsive, overly technical, impersonal, and costly.

Changes in modern society have meant disruption of close-knit communities where mutual aid was commonplace through kinship networks, religious affiliations, and service organizations. These disrupted networks have been partially replaced through the creation of self-help groups. The range of groups is enormous, including health-related groups and groups for parents, victims of violence, and displaced workers. There are groups for cultural or lifestyle minorities, feminist consciousness-raising groups, teen groups, and men's groups. There are neighborhood safety groups and political-action groups. Perhaps the most visible and largest is Alcoholics Anonymous, with its affiliates Alanon, Alateen, ACOA, and CODA.

Health-related groups generally focus on adjustment to medical illness, prevention of relapse, support for chronic-care patients, and support for behavioral change. Groups assisting in adjustment to medical illness include those who have had mastectomies, cancer, heart attacks, and strokes. Support in adjusting to chronic illness is available through nonprofit foundations such as the Arthritis Foundation. Habit-management groups include those for weight loss, smoking cessation, and control of addictions to drugs, alcohol, gambling, or sex. Recovery, Inc. was created to aid recovery from mental illness.

Groups for coping with family stress include Parents Without Partners, and New Beginnings, which is for widows, widowers, and divorced persons. Parents of children with learning difficulties or physical illness have created support groups. There are organizations for teens, adoptive parents and their children, stepparents, new mothers, play groups, and baby-sitting co-ops.

Crime victims have organized for mutual aid as well as political clout. Neighborhood watch organizations look out for one another's children and property, and in the process they get to know their local police force and one another better. Mothers Against Drunk Driving lobby for stricter laws, educate teen students, and give meaning to their personal losses all at the same time. In the inner city, mothers of children murdered by gang or drug wars have done the same. Support groups for incest survivors, rape victims, and battered women help in the recovery process and in offering emotional support should a case come to trial.

The strength of numbers helps individuals regain a sense of control, which is an essential part of reducing stress. By helping others, they help themselves. They are victims no longer, but active members of their communities.

These groups may not be exactly what you need, but they can give you an idea of the variety of resources available. It is up to you to look around to find what best fits your situation.

ADVANTAGES OF WORKING WITH A GROUP

While the stated goals for each self-help group may differ, many similarities exist. Because groups are usually led by a layperson rather than an authority or expert, participants take a more active role in their own health and recovery. This increased sense of control is in sharp contrast to the passive "patient" stance often found in traditional helping institutions. Groups organized around a common theme reduce feelings of isolation, especially the belief that no one else has ever felt the way you do. In addition to social contact, there is practical help and access to resources. Other members who are further along in adjustment or recovery often model coping behaviors and offer information, encouragement, and hope. A self-help group can't be the answer to all your problems, but it can keep you on track.

There are several ways to find the right community or self-help group for you. If you have a health-related problem, ask your physician, nurse, or medical social worker for information on local resources. School counselors, coaches, teachers, and librarians may have information on resources for patients. Talk to friends for groups they may know. Check church and community organizations for ongoing events. Local bulletin boards may list resources in your area. For other local organizations, look in the listings for Social and Human Services in the Yellow Pages of the phone directory. If your community has a hotline, it can be a good referral source.

Your local newspaper provides a wide range of information about your community. Read the calendar listings for lectures and group meetings. Check it out. Many newspapers have readers' exchange columns where readers ask for information or offer suggestions in dealing with problems. You can also write letters to the editor or list any group you have organized yourself. The news media value your input.

Talk shows are another rapidly growing opportunity for people to exchange views and information. The electronic media have connected people from all over the world in an "electronic town hall" for our "global village."

As you examine what a self-help group offers, use your *Stress Action Plans* to guide you. Look for the kind of help that you need to carry out your plans. If you don't get it after a sincere effort, try another group.

TAILORING YOUR SUPPORT

Just as you tailored your *Action Plan* to deal with your stress points, tailor your support network to your particular personality, lifestyle, and circumstances. Each person needs to find what best suits him or her. We encourage you to examine your circumstances and interests and then expand your network of support, knowing more about how to give and receive help.

Another source of outside help is professional support. Your *Stress Action Plan* provides you with specific ideas about what you need from professionals. In that section, we examine what you can expect from them.

WHEN TO GO TO A PROFESSIONAL

If you have physical symptoms, you should go to a physician to rule out any illness or disease process that may mimic stress symptoms. If no organic cause is identified, ask your physician if your symptoms may be stress related. If the answer is yes, you might try to manage your stress on your own or within your existing support network. However, when you feel stuck with your problem and you've tried other resources, when the problem is too personal or upsetting to share with friends or family, when your family and friends are tired of hearing you talk about the same thing all the time, or when symptoms persist in spite of your best efforts, you need a nonjudgmental, knowledgeable person. What type of professionals might you consider?

- behavioral medicine specialists
- psychologists
- psychiatrists
- physicians
- ministers, priests, and rabbis

- school counselors
- employee assistance personnel
- social workers

IN CONCLUSION

We are hoping that after reading *The Stress Solution* you've learned something about stress, how it works, and how it affects your mind and body. You've found out a lot about yourself and your personal stress patterns. You've taken the *Stress Audit*, plotted your *Stress Profile*, and generated a *Stress Action Plan* for dealing with your susceptibility to stress, your sources of stress, and your symptoms of stress. You now have the tools, the knowledge, and a plan for managing your stress. What happens from now on is up to you.

As you implement your *Action Plans*, draw on your sources of support when you run into trouble. Talk to friends. Talk yourself through. Set up reward systems so that making changes pays off in more ways than one.

Once you get to where you want to be, the challenge is to stay there. Stress is a fact of life and must be dealt with constantly. It gets easier with practice, but you need to be aware of the dangers of backsliding into old habits or developing new ones that are just as bad. There will be setbacks. Be prepared for them.

Keep this book as a reference guide. Take the *Stress Audit* whenever you feel stress is becoming a problem again. You can keep track of changes in your stress patterns by using different colors each time you take the *Audit*. As new issues pop up, or old ones return, make up new *Action Plans*. Use your skills to put these new *Action Plans* to work just as you did the first one. You'll get better and better with practice.

How will you know when you're starting to slip? You'll start getting symptoms again. They may be the same ones as before or they may be new ones. Your mind and body are your best barometers. They'll tell you when stress is becoming a problem again. Next time, however, you'll know what to do to solve it.

N O T E S

1. Bloomfield, H., and Felder, L. (1983), *Making Peace with Your Parents*, New York, Ballantine.

2. Bly, R. (1990), *Iron John*, Reading, MA, Addison-Wesley.

3. de Tocqueville, A. (1945), *Democracy in America*, New York, Vintage.

4. Gartner, A., and Kobasa, S. (1988), "Self-Help," in *Handbook of Behavioral Medicine for Women*, New York, Pergamon Press.

ANNE'S STRESS ACTION PLAN: SUSCEPTIBILITY

DIRECTIONS: Review your *Stress Audit: Susceptibility* section.
Write down an item you rated as never being true of you, describe
the problem, set a reasonable goal for change. Stop. Read pertinent section of chapter 3, write down some possible actions that
might help. Stop. Read chapter 20, write down your barriers to
change. Stop. Read chapter 21, write down your supports for
change. *Implement* your plan. *Evaluate* results. *Adjust* your plan.

SUSCEPTIBILITY ITEM: I never get seven to eight hours of sleep at least
four nights per week.

DESCRIPTION OF PROBLEM: (Anne's description of her own situation)
I can hardly keep my eyes open after lunch. Sometimes I'm so tired I
just put my head down on my desk and take a nap. It's difficult to get
up in the morning and I generally oversleep a couple days a week. I'm
late to work so often that it's become a joke, except to my boss. I have
to get more sleep, but I have trouble getting to bed at night. I watch
television with Mark and get wrapped up in it, or Mom or Mark calls
and I talk for hours. If I eat late or drink alcohol or coffee I have trouble
getting to sleep and then staying asleep. Because I'm too tired to get
things done at work, I often bring work home and stay up late trying to
get caught up.

REASONABLE GOAL: (Anne sets personal goal) Get eight hours of sleep
five nights per week.

POSSIBLE ACTIONS: (Anne's application of "Sleep" portions of chapter
3 to her life)
1) Turn TV off at 10:00 P.M. whether Mark's here or not. No exceptions.
2) Make no phone calls after 9:30 P.M. Let answering machine take
   calls after 9:30 P.M. Return them when appropriate.
3) No meals later than 8:00 P.M. No caffeine or alcohol after 6:00 P.M.
4) Organize things for next day before 9:00 P.M.
5) Take hot bath by 10:00 P.M. In bed by 10:30 P.M.
6) Do progressive muscle relaxation (PMR) exercise after going to
   bed.
7) Up at 7:00 A.M. weekdays. Up no later than 9:00 A.M. on weekends.
   No exceptions.

BARRIERS TO CHANGE: (Anne's application of chapter 20 to her life)
1) I like some late night TV shows. I can tape them, but Mark likes
   to watch TV at my place. He may get upset if I don't watch it with
   him or if I turn it off at 10:00 P.M.

2) Mom will be hurt if I don't take her phone call or if I don't spend a long time talking with her. Mark also likes to talk for hours when he calls. He'll get mad at me too.

3) If I'm working against a deadline, I have to finish on time even if it means staying up late to get it done. I'll be disappointed in myself and my boss will be mad at me if we miss a deadline.

4) Mark will feel rejected and hurt if I don't go out to dinner with him when he wants me to. Dinner with Mark is always long, with coffee and cognac. He won't like it if I insist on an early dinner or skip the coffee and cognac.

SUPPORTS FOR CHANGE: (Anne's application of chapter 21 to her life)

1) Mark is really a sweetheart and will help me. He'll be willing to make some changes too.

2) I'll have a talk with Mom. She'll understand if I phrase things right.

3) My friends will help me stay on track.

4) Dr. Smith will be very supportive and will coach me on PMR and assertiveness if I start having trouble carrying out my plan.

ANNE'S STRESS ACTION PLAN: SOURCES

DIRECTIONS: Review your *Stress Audit: Sources* section. Write down an item you rated 4 or 5 you'd like to work on, describe the situation and problem. Stop. Read the chapter dealing with that problem, write down some specific actions to take. Stop. Read chapter 20, write down your barriers to change. Stop. Read chapter 21 and write down your supports for change. *Implement* your first choice of action. *Evaluate* results. *Adjust* your plan.

ITEM: Trouble with the boss.

DESCRIPTION OF SITUATION AND PROBLEM: (Anne's description of her own situation)

Charlie, my boss, jerks me around all the time. One minute I'm told to do one thing, the next he wants me doing something else. Then he gets mad and screams at me if everything doesn't get done right on time. He goes ballistic. He interferes with my getting things done when he changes his mind all the time. His disorganization really impacts on my efficiency and could affect my professional career in marketing. Sometimes the tension gets so thick between us you could cut it with a knife.

POSSIBLE ACTION: (Anne's application of chapter 4's options to her life)

Alter: (Anne's application of "Alter" portions of chapter 4 to her life)

1) Sit down with Charlie (during a quiet time when we've been getting along well) and have a real heart-to-heart talk about how we work together.

2) Negotiate a clear, written job description with Charlie and then make sure we both keep to it. No unilateral renegotiations.

3) Take my problem with Charlie upstairs to the president of the company and be prepared to fight it out head to head with Charlie.

Avoid: (Anne's application of "Avoid" portion of chapter 4 to her life)

1) Request a transfer to another division.

2) Take the job I've been offered with our top competitor.

3) Just quit and marry Mark.

Accept: (Anne's application of "Accept" portion of chapter 4 to her life)

1) Get so good at relaxing that I can relax anytime, anyplace, and just relax when things get tense.

2) Understand that Charlie has his problems too and doesn't handle pressure well.

3) Quit personalizing things so much.

BARRIERS TO CHANGE: (Anne's application of chapter 20 to her life)

1) People will get mad at me if I make waves.

2) Things could really explode between Charlie and me and make things even worse.

3) I'll get fired.

SUPPORTS FOR CHANGE: (Anne's application of chapter 21 to her life)

1) Mark will support and advise me.

2) Other people at work know about Charlie and will be supportive.

3) Dr. Smith will coach and advise on how I should proceed.

ANNE'S STRESS ACTION PLAN: SYMPTOMS

DIRECTIONS: Review your *Stress Audit: Symptoms* section. Write down a symptom rated 4 or 5 you'd like to work on, describe it in terms of when, where, how it's a problem, what makes it better, what makes it worse. Stop. Read chapter 11 and the following pertinent chapters, write down some actions that might help. Stop. Read chapter 20, write down your barriers to change. Stop. Read chapter 21 and write down your supports for change. *Implement* your plan by trying out the easiest and least expensive treatment action you've written down. *Evaluate* the success of that action and try the next choice if necessary.

SYMPTOM: Shortness of breath

SYSTEM: Sympathetic Nervous System

DESCRIPTION OF SYMPTOM: (Anne's description of her symptom and how it affects her)
Whenever I get real upset and nervous, like when I have a fight with Mark or my boss, I start having trouble breathing. Then I start to hyperventilate trying to get my breath. I feel strange and dizzy. It just gets worse and worse and I get so scared I think I'm going crazy. My heart starts racing like crazy and I start getting numb. Sometimes I get pains in my chest and I think it's my heart going bad and that I'm going to die any minute. What's worse is that I worry so much about it happening that sometimes I think I make it happen.

POSSIBLE ACTIONS: (Anne's application of chapters 14 and 15 to her symptoms)
1) Remember to breathe through my nose slowly and evenly. I'll need to practice that. (chapter 15 and appendix I)
2) Stop the catastrophizing thoughts, the "what if . . ." thoughts. (chapter 15 and appendix I)
3) Remember to stay in the moment, don't worry about what might happen. (chapter 15 and appendix I)
4) Make myself a relaxation tape with a special emphasis on diaphragmatic breathing. (chapter 14 and appendix I)

BARRIERS TO CHANGE: (Anne's application of chapter 20 to her life)
1) I get too excited and panicky to remember what to do.
2) Self-doubt: I'm not sure this will work for me. Maybe I really need medication.
3) Old habits: I'm not used to the feel of deep breathing, it feels funny to breathe that way.
4) Time: I don't know when I can make time to do the exercises.

SUPPORTS FOR CHANGE: (Anne's application of chapter 21 to her life)
1) Make a card for emergencies to remind me what I'm supposed to do, how I'm supposed to think when I have these symptoms. (chapter 7 and appendix I)
2) Tell Mark about the program and call him if I get panicky. I could also call my friend who has had panic attacks too.
3) Read up on hyperventilation, panic disorders, and their treatments. (suggested readings keyed to sources, symptoms, and vulnerabilities, appendix II)
4) If I don't get better soon, I can contact the group for anxiety problems in my area.
5) If I schedule the time to practice the exercises and really stick with them, I should feel better and that will be encouraging.

Appendices

Self-Regulation Techniques

Progressive Muscle Relaxation (PMR)

If possible, select a room that is reasonably quiet and comfortable. Dim or low lighting is preferable. Sit in a comfortable chair or lie down on a couch, bed, or the floor. If you are lying down, you may want to place a rolled-up towel or something similar under the small of your back or your head to make yourself more comfortable. Loosen any tight clothing.

The following is a relaxation scrip that includes muscle relaxation, breathing control, and a calm mental focus. We recommend that you make a tape-recording of this script for your personal use. Read the script into a tape recorder. Be sure to read slowly, following the pauses indicated in the script. They allow silences periodically so that you don't feel hurried during the exercise. The entire exercise should take fifteen to twenty minutes.

Make yourself comfortable and let yourself start to relax. Let your whole body relax gradually, sinking down as you let go of tension. Breathe slowly through your nose. Feel the cool air as you breathe in and the warm air as you breathe out. Let your awareness turn away from your daily cares and concerns. Close your eyes and let your awareness turn inward to the physical sensations of your body. Feel the pressure of your back on the chair or floor. Notice how it feels as you let go of your tension and start to relax. Concentrate on your right hand and forearm. Keeping the rest of your body relaxed, make a tight fist with your right hand. Hold it tight. Notice the pressure on your fingers and thumb. Notice the tightness of the wrist, forearm, and upper arm. Good. Hold it. [four-second pause] Now release. As you let go, notice the change. Slowly let the tension drain out as you relax the muscles of your hand and arm, noticing the difference between being tense [two-second pause] and relaxed. Let your hand and arm continue to relax and become very heavy.

Now let your awareness go to your left hand and forearm. Make a tight fist with your left hand [one-second pause] noticing the tension and tightness. Good. Hold it. [one-second pause] Now let go. Notice the change in sensation as you release. Let your hands and arms continue to relax and become very heavy. You may feel your hands getting warmer and you may feel a pulse beating in your fingertips or tiny sensations of tingling.

Now tighten the muscles of the shoulders and upper back, shrug your shoulders up toward your ears, feeling the tightness across your upper back. Then release, letting your shoulders drop down. Then let them go even a little more, so any residual tension is gone. Now let all the muscles of your arms and shoulders feel comfortable and relaxed.

Press the back of your head against the chair (or floor) and make the muscles in your upper back and neck tight and tense. [six-second pause] Feel the strength and tightness of the muscles as you do this. [five-second pause] Relax again, letting all the tension drain out. Let your head get heavier, and the muscles in your neck looser, so that you can gently move your head from side to side.

Tighten the muscles of your face by first raising your eyebrows as high as you can. Feel the pull on all those little muscles in your scalp. [five-second pause] Gradually let that tension drain out and feel all those little muscles in your scalp relax. Now knit your eyebrows together and get real tension on those forehead muscles.

[four-second pause] And relax, letting your forehead become smooth and relaxed.

Next, tighten the muscles in the middle of your face by shutting your eyes tightly. Feel the tightness throughout your cheeks, face, and eyes. Good. Now let go and let your face relax again.

Let your awareness go to your lower face and jaw. Clench your teeth firmly, pressing your tongue against the roof of your mouth. [four-second pause] Feel the tension in your jaw muscles and in the muscles at your temples. Feel the tension on your tongue and the muscles under your chin. Now gradually let go of the tension, letting your teeth part slightly so your jaw can relax. As your tongue relaxes you'll notice that it seems to get thicker and wider till it almost fills your mouth. Let your face and scalp continue to relax as you go on to the rest of the exercise.

It may be that from time to time you notice thoughts drifting through your mind or your mind wanders. If you notice this, just let the thoughts drift away gently and easily, letting your awareness return to the physical sensations of relaxation in your body. It is sometimes easiest to focus on the rhythm of your breathing as a way of focusing your awareness. Take a few moments now to follow the gentle rhythm of your breath. [pause] Feel the cool air as you breathe in . . . and the air warmer as you breathe out. Notice the turning of the breath . . . the moment between in . . . and out again. Allow your breathing to gradually become longer, slower, and deeper, feeling your stomach rise gently with each breath. [pause]

In a moment, take a slow, deep breath in and hold it. [three-second pause] As you let go, let yourself sink into relaxation. [pause] Continue to breathe gently and evenly.

Let your awareness now move to the muscles of your abdomen. Keeping the rest of your body relaxed, tighten the muscles of your abdomen and torso. Then relax.

Keeping the rest of your body relaxed, tighten the muscles of your legs by pressing your legs against the floor or chair, making the muscles tight and tense. Notice this tension. Feel the tightness in the muscles. Compare the tight, tense muscles in your legs with the relaxed muscles in the rest of your body. Now slowly release that tension and let your legs, thighs, and calves relax all the way. Let the sensations of relaxation spread all the way down to your toes.

Take a moment now to check back over your body to see if tension has crept back into any muscles or if there is residual tension anywhere. If so, let it go. Now your body can relax completely. Just lie there and enjoy that feeling of deep relaxation. Let your body sink down as it gets heavier and heavier. You may feel as though your body is heavy or, the opposite, quite light. You may even feel as though you're floating right up out of your body like a feather on a current of air.

As you lie there and relax, imagine, as vividly as you can, that you're lying on a nice warm beach. You can feel the warm sand on your back. Imagine the warm sun on your body. There's a cool breeze blowing in from the ocean and you can smell the salty sea air. Imagine the sound of the waves as they wash up on the shore, or the call of a seabird. Overhead there are soft white fluffy clouds floating across a bright blue sky. Let yourself become peaceful, relaxed, and warm, and feel comfortable and secure.

Continue to let yourself relax and just let yourself float right up out of your body just like a feather on a current of air. Just floating up—and up—aimlessly and weightlessly—just floating. And now you begin to drift—just drifting. After a while, you may begin to drift slowly downward. Drifting down—and down—and down—until finally you land—just like a feather on a pile of feathers.

In a few moments you'll end the exercise by counting backward from five to one. At five, notice how deeply relaxed you have become, noticing what it feels like so you can become this relaxed again more easily. At four, begin to feel energy returning to your arms and legs. At three, you may want to move or stretch a bit. At two, become aware of the room. Whenever you are ready, at one, open your eyes, feeling refreshed, relaxed, and ready to go on with your day. Five . . . four . . . three . . . two . . . one.

Modifications to the Basic Exercise

If there are parts of your body that are particularly difficult to relax, spend a little more time on the special muscles of that area. If you have headaches, for instance, you may want to tense and relax your shoulder, neck, and face muscles twice in a row before moving on to the rest of your body. If you have circulatory problems, you might spend more time on deep breathing and imagining your hands becoming warmer. For gastrointestinal problems, you might imagine your stomach area feeling cool and relaxed.

Autogenic Imagery

You can use the autogenic exercise in several different positions. This is useful if you are at the office or in a meeting. Sit in an armchair with your head, back, and arms comfortably supported. Sit as relaxed as possible. If there is no head rest, sit upright, with feet on the floor, in a comfortable position. Or you can sit slightly stooped over, with your arms resting on your legs and hands draped between your knees. If you are at home, lie down with your head supported, legs about eight inches apart, toes pointed slightly outward, and arms resting comfortably at the side of your body without touching it.

If you are in private, closing your eyes usually enhances the relaxation effect. If you are in your office, at a meeting, or in a public place, closing your eyes may seem awkward. In that case, pick a spot about ten feet away to look at. Let the spot go slightly out of focus as you do the exercise. You'll still be able to see around you without being unnecessarily distracted.

Simply say the following phrases to yourself:

My arms are heavy and relaxed. (As you say this, let tension flow out of your arms and shoulders.)

My legs are heavy and relaxed. (Let tension drain out of your legs.)

My breathing is gentle and even. (Follow with a few breaths.)

My mind is calm and quiet. (Let your mind rest. Let
your mind be like a quiet pool, with no thoughts rippling
the surface.)

Repeat this process two or three times until you feel
quiet and rested.

If you are working to assist healing of a particular
part of your body, add some special images and phrases
for that area, such as:

My heartbeat is calm and regular.
My hands are warm and full (for migraine).
My forehead is cool and relaxed (for migraine).
My stomach is calm and smooth (for stomach and
intestinal problems).
My throat is cool and soft (Lyle uses this when he has
a sore throat).
My blood vessels are relaxed and dilated (for hyper-
tension).
My white blood cells are vigorous and plentiful (for
immune system problems).

As you practice autogenic imagery, be creative in using your own symbols for how your body heals itself.
Ask your physician for an explanation of your illness or
symptom so that you can use this information to create
an accurate image of wellness and healing. As we have
emphasized before, these methods are used to assist
healing but are not a substitute for consultation with
a physician.

Dietary Consideration in Migraine Headache

It is not unusual to discover that some of an individual's migraines are triggered by substances in their diet.
We recommend that you greatly reduce or eliminate
your consumption of the substances listed below for the
next several weeks and then begin gradually testing
them one at a time to determine whether they trigger
headaches for you.

ABSOLUTELY NO CHOCOLATE OR PEANUT BUTTER

SEASONINGS

Salt (use Morton's "Lite Salt")
Monosodium glutamate (Accent)
Worcestershire sauce & variants
Meat tenderizer
Soy sauce
(Note that all prepared foods are
   heavily salted)

BEVERAGES

Tea
Cola
Champagne
Beer
Red wines (Burgundy, Chianti,
   etc.)
Bourbon
Vodka
Gin
(Drink decaffeinated or instant
   coffee instead of regular coffee)

MEDICATIONS

Some multivitamins
Cold remedies
Hay fever medicines

FOODS

Cheese, aged or strong types
cottage & processed cheeses are
   acceptable
Sour cream
Pickled herring
Liver
Canned figs
Aged beef—supermarket beef is
   acceptable
Hot dogs
Bacon
Ham
Salami
Nuts
Raisins
Citrus fruits—frozen orange juice
   is admissible
Broad bean pods
Chinese foods
Olives
Anchovies
Bologna
Yogurt
Bananas
Sausage

APPENDIX II

Suggested Readings: A Bibliotherapy Resource List

SECTION I. Getting in Touch with Stress

CHAPTER 1:
STRESS POINTS

Benson, H. (1975). *The Relaxation Response.* New York: Avon.

Davis, M., Eshelman, E. R., and McKay, M. (1982). *The Relaxation and Stress Reduction Workbook.* Oakland, CA: New Harbinger.

Girdano, D. A., and Everly, G. S. (1986). *Controlling Stress and Tension: A Holistic Approach.* Englewood Cliffs, NJ: Prentice-Hall.

Tubesing, D. A. (1981). *Kicking Your Stress Habits.* New York: New American Library.

Woolfolk, R. I., and Richardson, F. C. (1978). *Stress, Sanity, and Survival.* New York: New American Library.

CHAPTER 3:
SUSCEPTIBILITY: THE TOUGHER YOU ARE,
THE MORE YOU CAN TAKE

Nutrition, Weight

Bailey, C. (1978). *Fit or Fat.* Boston: Houghton-Mifflin.

Brody, J. (1987). *Jane Brody's Nutrition Book.* New York: Bantam.

Groger, M. (1985). *E.A.T.: Eating Awareness Training.* New York: Summit.

Hall, L., and Cohn, L. (1986). *Bulimia: A Guide to Recovery.* Santa Barbara: Gurze.

Hollis, J. (1985). *Fat Is a Family Affair.* San Francisco: Harper & Row.

Kano, S. (1985). *Making Peace with Food.* Danbury, CT: Amity.

Mallek, H. (1989). *The Woman's Advantage Diet.* New York: Pocket Books.

Orbach, S. (1987). *Fat Is a Feminist Issue II: The Anti-Diet Guide to Permanent Weight Loss.* New York: Berkley.

Rippe, J., and Ward, A. (1990). *Dr. James M. Rippe's Complete Guide to Fitness Walking.* New York: Prentice-Hall.

Roth, G. (1984). *Breaking Free from Compulsive Eating.* New York: Signet.

Stuart, R., and Davis, B. (1978). *Slim Chance in a Fat World.* Champaign, IL: Research Press.

Substance Abuse

Johnson, V. (1980). *I'll Quit Tomorrow.* New York: Harper & Row.

McKean, M. K. (1987). *The Stop Smoking Book.* San Luis Obispo, CA: Impact.

Miller, W. R., and Munoz, R. (1982). *How to Control Your Drinking: A Practical Guide to Responsible Drinking.* Albuquerque, NM: University of New Mexico Press.

Steiner, C. (1971). *Games Alcoholics Play.* New York: Ballantine.

Optimism

Seligman, M. E. P. (1990). *Learned Optimism.* New York: Pocket Books.

Psychotherapy

Engler, J., and Goleman, D. (1992). *Consumer's Guide to Psychotherapy.* New York: Simon & Schuster.

Sleep

Maxmen, J. (1981). *A Good Night's Sleep.* New York: Warner Books.

Social Networking

Rubin, L. (1986). *Just Friends.* New York: Harper Collins.

Time Management

Blanchard, K., and Johnson, S. (1982). *The One Minute Manager.* New York: Morrow.

Fiore, N. (1989). *The NOW Habit.* Los Angeles: Tarcher.

Section II. Sources: Playing Hardball with Stress
CHAPTER 4:
PLANNING A WINNING STRATEGY

Beattie, M. (1987). *Codependent No More: How to Stop Controlling Others and Start Caring for Yourself.* New York: Harper & Row.

CHAPTER 5:
GETTING THE UPPER HAND ON JOB STRESS

Bolles, R. (1978). *What Color Is Your Parachute?* Berkeley, CA: Ten Speed Press.

———. (1974). *The Three Boxes of Life.* Berkeley, CA: Ten Speed Press.

Field, J. (1981). *A Life of One's Own.* Los Angeles: Tarcher.

Figler, H. (1988). *The Complete Job-Search Handbook* (rev. ed.). New York: Henry Holt.

Morin, W. J., and Carbrera, J. C. (1991). *Parting Company: How to Survive the Loss of a Job and Find Another Successfully.* New York: Harcourt, Brace, Jovanovich.

Petras, K., and Petras, R. (1989). *The Only Job Hunting Guide You'll Ever Need: The Most Comprehensive Guide for Job Hunters and Career Switchers.* New York: Poseidon Press.

Sinetar, M. (1989). *Do What You Love, The Money Will Follow: Discovering Your Right Livelihood.* New York: Dell.

Snelling, R., and Snelling, A. (1989). *Jobs! What They Are . . . Where They Are . . . What They Pay* (rev. ed.). New York: Simon & Schuster.

CHAPTER 6:
MANAGING FAMILY STRESS

Bass, E., and David, L. (1988). *The Courage to Heal.* New York: Harper & Row.
Beck, A. T. (1988). *Love Is Never Enough.* New York: Harper & Row.
Bloomfield, H., and Felder, L. (1983). *Making Peace with Your Parents.* New York: Ballantine.
Colgrove, M., Bloomfield, H., and McWilliams, P. (1976). *How to Survive the Loss of a Love.* New York: Bantam.
Faber, A., and Mazlish, E. (1980). *How to Talk So Kids Will Listen and Listen So Kids Will Talk.* New York: Avon.
Garber, S. W., Garber, M., and Spitman, R. (1987). *Good Behavior: Over 1200 Sensible Solutions to Your Child's Problems from Birth to Age Twelve.* New York: Villard.
Gordon, T. (1970). *Parent Effectiveness Training.* New York: Peter H. Wyden.
Kirshenbaum, M., and Foster, C. (1991). *Parent-Teen Breakthrough: The Relationship Approach.* New York: Plume.
Kubler-Ross, E. (1969). *On Death and Dying.* New York: Macmillan.
——. (1975). *Death, The Final Stage of Growth.* Englewood Cliffs, NJ: Prentice-Hall.
Kushner, H. (1981). *When Bad Things Happen to Good People.* New York: Avon.
McEvoy, A. W., and Brookings, J. D. (1984). *If She Is Raped: A Book for Husbands, Fathers, and Male Friends.* Holmes Beach, FL: Learning Publications.
Nowinski, J. (1988). *A Life-Long Love Affair: Keeping Sexual Desire Alive in Your Relationship.* New York: Dodd, Mead, & Co.
Pearsall, P. (1990). *Power of the Family.* New York: Bantam.
Rosellini, G., and Worden, M. (1985). *Of Course You're Angry: A Family Guide to Dealing with the Emotions of Chemical Dependence.* San Francisco: Harper & Row.
Scarf, M. (1987). *Intimate Partners, Patterns in Love and Marriage.* New York: Ballantine.
Schaefer, C. E., and DiGeronimo, T. F. (1991). *Teach Your Child to Behave: Disciplining with Love from 2 to 8 Years.* New York: Penguin.
Sonkin, D., and Durphy, M. (1989). *Learning to Live Without Violence.* Volcano, CA: Volcano Press.
Tannen, D. (1990). *You Just Don't Understand.* New York: Ballantine.
——. (1990). *That's Not What I Meant! How Conversational Style Makes or Breaks Your Relations with Others.* New York: Ballantine.
Turecki, S., with Tonner, L. (1989). *The Difficult Child.* New York: Bantam.
Viorst, J. (1984). *Necessary Losses.* New York: Fawcett.
Wegscheider-Cruse, S. (1980). *Another Chance: Hope and Health for the Alcoholic Family.* Palo Alto, CA: Science & Behavior.
Westbert, G. (1962). *Good Grief.* Philadelphia: Fortress.

CHAPTER 7:
OVERCOMING PERSONAL STRESS

Adams, C., and Fay, J. (1989). *Out of the Shadows: Recovering from Sexual Violence.* Oakland, CA: New Harbinger.

Adderholdt-Elliott, M. (1987). *Perfectionism.* Minneapolis, MN: Free Spirit.

Beattie, M. (1989). *Beyond Codependency: And Getting Better All the Time.* New York: Harper & Row.

Black, C. (1981). *It Will Never Happen to Me.* New York: Ballantine.

Bloomfield, H., and Felder, L. (1985). *Making Peace with Yourself: Turning Weaknesses into Strengths.* New York: Ballantine.

Bradshaw, J. (1988). *Healing the Shame that Binds You.* Deerfield Beach, FL: Health Communications.

Bridges, W. (1980). *Transitions: Making Sense of Life's Changes.* Reading, MA: Addison-Wesley.

Briggs, D. C. (1986). *Celebrate Yourself.* New York: Doubleday.

Burka, J., and Yuen, L. (1983). *Procrastination: Why You Do It, What to Do About It.* Reading, MA: Addison-Wesley.

Chamberlain, J. M. (1978). *Eliminate Your SDBs: Self-Defeating Behaviors.* Provo, UT: Brigham Young University Press.

Ellis, A. (1988). *How to Stubbornly Refuse to Make Yourself Miserable About Anything—Yes, Anything!* Secaucus, NJ: Carol Publishing Group.

Engle, J., and Goldman, D. (1992). *The Consumer's Guide to Psychotherapy.* New York: Simon & Schuster.

Forward, S. (1990). *Toxic Parents.* New York: Bantam.

Harvey, J., and Katz, C. (1986). *If I'm So Successful, Why Do I Feel Like a Fake? The Impostor Phenomenon.* New York: Pocket Books.

Johnson, K. (1985). *If You Are Raped: What Every Woman Needs to Know.* Holmes Beach, FL: Learning Publications.

Lerner, H. G. (1989). *The Dance of Intimacy.* New York: Harper & Row.

Levinson, D. (1978). *Seasons of a Man's Life.* New York: Knopf.

Lew, M. (1988). *Victims No Longer: Men Recovering from Incest and Other Sexual Child Abuse.* New York: Nevraumont.

McConnell, P. (1986). *Adult Children of Alcoholics: A Workbook for Healing.* San Francisco: Harper & Row.

McKay, M., and Fanning, P. (1987). *Self-Esteem: A Proven Program of Cognitive Techniques for Assessing, Improving, and Maintaining Your Self-Esteem.* Oakland, CA: New Harbinger.

Mantell, M. R. (1988). *Don't Sweat the Small Stuff: P.S. It's All Small Stuff!* San Luis Obispo, CA: Impact.

Meryman, R. (1984). *Broken Promises, Broken Dreams.* New York: Berkley.

Miller, A. (1981). *The Drama of the Gifted Child: The Search for the New Self.* New York: Basic Books.

Parrot, A. (1988). *Coping with Date Rape and Acquaintance Rape.* New York: Rosen Group.

Sanford, L. T., and Donovan, M. E. (1984). *Women and Self-Esteem.* New York: Penguin.

Sheehy, G. (1976). *Passages: Predictable Crises of Adult Life.* New York: Dutton.

Silber, S. J. (1981). *The Male: From Infancy to Old Age.* New York: Charles Scribner's Sons.

Stearns, A. K. (1984). *Living Through Personal Crisis*. Chicago: Thomas More.

Woititz, J. G. (1983). *Adult Children of Alcoholics*. Deerfield Beach, FL: Health Communications.

———. (1985). *Struggle for Intimacy*. Deerfield Beach, FL: Health Communications.

CHAPTER 8:
DEALING WITH SOCIAL STRESS

Alberti, R., and Emmons, M. (1974). *Your Perfect Right: A Guide to Assertive Living*. San Luis Obispo, CA: Impact.

Baer, J. (1976). *How to Be an Assertive (Not Aggressive) Woman in Life, Love, and on the Job*. New York: Signet.

Bolton, R. (1986). *People Skills*. New York: Simon & Schuster.

Burns, D. (1985). *Intimate Connections*. New York: Signet.

Butler, P. (1981). *Self-Assertion for Women*. San Francisco: Harper & Row.

Cheek, J., Cheek, B., and Rothstein, L. (1990). *Conquering Shyness*. New York: Dell.

Gabor, D. (1983). *How to Start a Conversation and Make Friends*. New York: Simon & Schuster.

Jakubowski, P., and Lange, A. (1978). *The Assertive Option*. Champaign, IL: Research Press.

McKay, M., Davis, M., and Fanning, P. (1983). *Messages: The Communication Skills Book*. Oakland, CA: New Harbinger Publications.

Phelps, S., and Austin, N. (1987). *The Assertive Woman: A New Look*. San Luis Obispo, CA: Impact.

Smith, M. (1975). *When I Say No, I Feel Guilty: How to Cope, Using the Skills of Systematic Assertive Therapy*. New York: Bantam.

Zimbardo, P. (1977). *Shyness: What It Is, What to Do About It*. New York: Jove.

CHAPTER 10:
CONQUERING FINANCIAL STRESS

Porter, S. (1979). *Sylvia Porter's New Money Book for the 80's*. Garden City, NY: Doubleday.

CHAPTER 11:
THE BODY'S DELICATELY BALANCED ECONOMY

Webster, A. "Psychoneuroimmunology and HIV Disease," *The Wellness Book* by Benson, H., et al. (1992). New York: Birch Lane.

SECTION III. Symptoms: Soothing the Body, Calming the Mind

CHAPTER 12:
YOUR ACHING BACK, HEAD, JAW, ETC.

Goleman, T., and Bennett-Goleman, T. (1986). *The Relaxed Body Book: A High-Energy Anti-Tension Program*. Garden City, NY: Doubleday.

Prudden, B. (1982). *Pain Erasure: The Bonnie Prudden Way*. New York: Ballantine.

Tobias, M., and Stewart, M. (1985). *Stretch and Relax: A Day by Day Workout and Relaxation Program*. Los Angeles: The Body Press.

Travell, J. G. (1983). *Myofascial Pain and Dysfunction: The Trigger Point Manual*. Baltimore: Williams & Wilkens.

CHAPTER 13:
WHEN IT GETS YOU IN THE GUT

Barbach, L. G. (1984). *For Each Other: Sharing Sexual Intimacy*. New York: Signet.

Goldstein, I. (1990). *The Potent Male*. New York: Putnam and Sons.

Williams, W. (1988). *Rekindling Desire*. Oakland, CA: New Harbinger.

CHAPTER 15:
ANGRY, DEPRESSED, AND ANXIOUS

Agras, S. (1985). *Panic: Facing Fears, Phobias, and Anxiety*. New York: W. H. Freeman.

Bach, G., and Wyden, P. (1976). *The Intimate Enemy*. New York: Avon.

Bloomfield, H., and Kory, R. (1980). *Inner Joy: New Strategies for Adding Pleasure to Your Life*. New York: Jove.

Breton, S. (1986). *Don't Panic: A Guide to Overcoming Panic Attacks*. New York: Facts on File.

Burns, D. (1980). *Feeling Good: The New Mood Therapy*. New York: New American Library.

———. (1989). *The Feeling Good Handbook*. New York: Morrow.

Ellis, A. (1985). *Anger: How to Live With and Without It*. Secaucus, NJ: Carol Publishing Group.

Handley, R., and Neff, P. (1987). *Anxiety and Panic Attacks: Their Cause and Cure*. New York: Fawcett.

Harris, T. (1967). *I'm Okay, You're Okay*. New York: Avon.

Lerner, H. G. (1985). *The Dance of Anger*. New York: Harper & Row.

McKay, M., Davis, M., and Fanning, P. (1981). *Thoughts & Feelings: The Art of Cognitive Stress Intervention*. Oakland, CA: New Harbinger.

Travis, C. (1989). *Anger: The Misunderstood Emotion*. New York: Simon & Schuster.

Weekes, C. (1990). *Peace from Nervous Suffering*. New York: New American Library.

Weiner, E. (1986). *The Ostrich Complex: A Personalized Plan of Action for Overcoming the Fears that Hold You Back*. New York: Warner Books.

Weisinger, H. D. (1985). *Dr. Weisinger's Anger Workout Book*. New York: Morrow.

CHAPTER 16:
TOO STRESSED TO THINK STRAIGHT

De Bono, E. (1985). *Six Thinking Hats*. New York: Penguin Books.

———. (1970). *Lateral Thinking*. New York: Harper & Row.

CHAPTER 17:
HORMONES IN DISARRAY

Arthritis Foundation Editors (1986). *Understanding Arthritis.* New York: Scribner's.
Bierman, J. (1990). *Diabetics Book Revised.* Los Angeles: Tarcher, Inc.
Edelwich, J. (1986). *Diabetes: Caring for Your Emotions as Well as Your Health.* Reading, MA: Addison Wesley.
Greenwood, S. (1989). *Menopause Naturally.* Volcano, CA: Volcano Press.
Greer, G. (1992). *The Change: Women, Aging, and the Menopause.* New York: Knopf.
Harkness, C. (1992). *The Infertility Book.* Berkeley: Celestial Arts.
Harrison, M. (1985). *Self-Help for Premenstrual Syndrome.* New York: Random House.
Kilo, C. (1987). *Diabetes: The Facts That Let You Regain Control of Your Life.* New York: Wiley.
Rooney, T. W., and Rooney, P. R. (1990). *The Arthritis Handbook.* New York: Ballantine.
Sheehy, G. (1992). *The Silent Passage.* New York: Random House.
Sobel, D., and Klein, A. C. (1992). *Arthritis: What Works.* New York: St. Martin's.

CHAPTER 18:
SICK OF STRESS

Ader, R. (ed.) (1981). *Psychoneuroimmunology.* New York: Academic Press.
Borysenko, J., and Rothstein, L. (1987). *Minding the Body, Mending the Mind.* Reading, MA: Addison-Wesley.
Cousins, N. (1989). *Head First.* New York: Dutton.
Langston, D. (1983). *Living with Herpes.* New York: Doubleday.
Michaud, E., and Feinstein, A. (1992). *Prevention Magazine's 30-Day Immune Power Program.* Emmaus, PA: Rodale Press.
Morra, M., and Potts, E. (1987). *Choices: Realistic Alternatives in Cancer Treatment.* New York: Avon.
Siegal, B. S. (1988). *Love, Medicine, and Miracles.* New York: Harper & Row.
Simone, C. B. (1992). *Concerned Nutrition.* New York: Avery Publishing Group.

CHAPTER 19:
CALLING ON THE HEALER WITHIN

Alman, B., and Lambrou, P. (1992). *Self-Hypnosis: The Complete Manual for Health and Self Change,* 2nd ed. New York: Brunner/Mazel.
Goleman, D., and Bennett-Goleman, T. (1986). *The Relaxed Body Book: A High-Energy Anti-Tension Program.* Garden City, NY: Doubleday.
Jacobson, E. (1978). *You Must Relax.* New York: McGraw-Hill.
Linden, W. (1990). *Autogenic Training: A Clinical Guide.* New York: Guilford Press.
Samuels, M. (1990). *Healing with the Mind's Eye.* New York: Summit.
Tobias, M., and Stewart, M. (1985). *Stretch and Relax: A Day by Day Workout and Relaxation Program.* Los Angeles: The Body Press.

SECTION IV. If at First You Don't Succeed, You're Human

CHAPTER 20:
ENEMIES OF CHANGE

John-Roger and McWilliams, P. (1991). *DO IT! Let's Get off Our Buts.* Los Angeles: Prelude Press.

CHAPTER 21:
FRIENDS AND ALLIES

Quinnett, P. (1985). *The Troubled People Book: A Comprehensive Guide to Getting Help* (rev. ed.). New York: Continuum.
Yoder, B. (1990). *The Recovery Resources Book.* New York: Simon & Schuster.

APPENDIX III

Psychometric Properties of the *Stress Audit*

TABLE 1

Internal Consistency/Reliability

Hoyt's Estimate of Reliability

SCALE	N OF ITEMS	PAST	FUTURE
Family	30	.89	.90
Individual	25	.85	.88
Social	19	.90	.91
Environment	17	.86	.90
Financial	16	.85	.89
Job	41	.94	.95
Muscular	10	.82	.87
PNS	10	.81	.85
SNS	10	.84	.88
Emotional	10	.91	.92
Cognitive	10	.89	.91
Endocrine	10	.78	.83
Immune	10	.80	.86
Vulnerability	20	.76	
SOURCES	148	.97	.98
SYMPTOMS	70	.96	.97

TABLE 2

Cronbach's Alpha for Composite Scores

SOURCES	148	.87	.89
SYMPTOMS	70	.92	.93

TABLE 3

Test-Retest Reliability Coefficients

SCALE	N OF ITEMS	1 WEEK	2 WEEKS	6 WEEKS
Family	30	.78	.71	.54
Individual	25	.83	.71	.68
Social	19	.87	.63	.65
Environment	17	.76	.70	.61
Financial	16	.65	.82	.65
Job	41	.83	.63	.69
Muscular	10	.73	.65	.66
PNS	10	.78	.76	.62
SNS	10	.79	.63	.54
Emotional	10	.71	.77	.66
Cognitive	10	.80	.53	.66
Endocrine	10	.76	.55	.58
Immune	10	.82	.48	.59
Vulnerability	20	.88	.84	.63
Comb. Sources	148	.92	.75	.72
Comb. Symp.	70	.81	.66	.70
STAI-State			.42	
STAI-Trait			.59	

TABLE 4

Interscale Correlations

	MS	PNS	SNS	EM	COG	END	IM	COMB. SYMPTOMS
Family	.52	.57	.51	.50	.50	.56	.56	.62
Individual	.58	.58	.55	.71	.66	.59	.55	.72
Social	.48	.54	.46	.69	.62	.49	.54	.65
Environment	.52	.61	.55	.47	.50	.59	.70	.65
Financial	.50	.58	.55	.59	.56	.52	.56	.65
Job	.54	.49	.52	.64	.60	.48	.57	.66
Comb. Sources	.62	.64	.61	.71	.68	.62	.67	.77

INDEX

FaxScore
Stress Audit

FaxScore® Evaluation

You can use *FaxScore*® to get your personal Stress Audit professional evaluation. Here's how it works.

First, Remove the Stress Audit test forms on the following pages. Carefully cut the test pages out of the book along the binding and photocopy both halves of each grid onto a single 8½ x 11 sheet of paper. If your copy of the Stress Audit test forms is damaged call *FaxScore*® at (214) 221-3046 to receive another copy of the forms at no charge.

Then, Complete the test using a #2 pencil to mark each response. Marks should completely fill the appropriate box.

To score your Stress Audit using a FAX. You may use a FAX machine to send the Stress Audit test forms to *FaxScore*® and get your results within one hour. To use a FAX complete the credit card information and the return FAX information, place the Stress Audit test forms in your FAX, and call **1-800-934-8877** in the U.S. or Canada. You will receive your results via return FAX and you will also receive a printed copy via First Class mail.

To score your Stress Audit using the mail. If you do not have a FAX machine you can mail the completed forms with payment to

> **FaxScore**
> **P.O. Box 292847**
> **Lewisville, TX 75029-2847**

Your test results will be returned via First Class mail.

The cost for your professional evaluation is $22.95 U.S. Texas residents add 7.25% sales tax or $1.66 for a total of $24.61.

If you need multiple copies of the Stress Audit forms or if you have any questions please call **(214) 221-3046** between 8:00 A.M. and 5:00 P.M. Central Time Monday through Friday.

Please indicate billing preference.

MasterCard ☐   Visa ☐   Payment Enclosed ☐

If you are paying by credit card write card number in the boxes and encode below.

0
1
2
3
4
5
6
7
8
9

For credit card billing only please complete: Expiration Date: _____

Signature: _____

Please PRINT your return address below. Write clearly,
this will appear as your address on the return envelope.

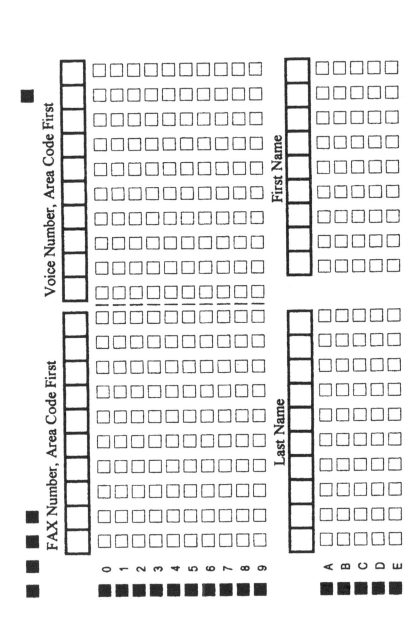

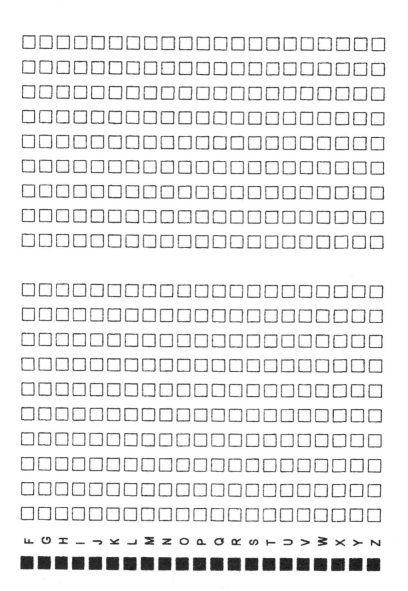

Indicate stress level
1 is lowest, 5 is highest
If not applicable leave blank.

Family

	Stress past 6 months						Stress next 6 months				
	1	2	3	4	5		1	2	3	4	5
Holidays, celebrations, family vacations	☐	☐	☐	☐	☐		☐	☐	☐	☐	☐
Starting marriage/significant relationship	☐	☐	☐	☐	☐		☐	☐	☐	☐	☐
Marital difficulties	☐	☐	☐	☐	☐		☐	☐	☐	☐	☐
Marital separation	☐	☐	☐	☐	☐		☐	☐	☐	☐	☐
Marital reconciliation	☐	☐	☐	☐	☐		☐	☐	☐	☐	☐
Divorce	☐	☐	☐	☐	☐		☐	☐	☐	☐	☐
Death of a spouse	☐	☐	☐	☐	☐		☐	☐	☐	☐	☐
Death of a close relative	☐	☐	☐	☐	☐		☐	☐	☐	☐	☐
Death of a distant relative	☐	☐	☐	☐	☐		☐	☐	☐	☐	☐
Disciplinary problems with children	☐	☐	☐	☐	☐		☐	☐	☐	☐	☐
Alcoholism or drug problems in family	☐	☐	☐	☐	☐		☐	☐	☐	☐	☐
Pregnancy in family	☐	☐	☐	☐	☐		☐	☐	☐	☐	☐
Son or daughter leaving home	☐	☐	☐	☐	☐		☐	☐	☐	☐	☐
Sex difficulties	☐	☐	☐	☐	☐		☐	☐	☐	☐	☐
Difficulties with other family members	☐	☐	☐	☐	☐		☐	☐	☐	☐	☐
Serious illness in family	☐	☐	☐	☐	☐		☐	☐	☐	☐	☐

Divorce or remarriage of parents

Divorce or remarriage of children

Difficulty in meeting family obligations

Family conflict over money

Child care responsibilities

Birth of a child or adoption

Abortion, miscarriage, or stillbirth

Inability to have children

Change in number of arguments with spouse

Family violence

Troubles with in-laws

Wife or husband begins or stops work

Change in number of family get-togethers

Child with special needs

Personal

Vacations or travel

Feeling unattractive

Personal injury or illness

Indicate stress level
1 is lowest, 5 is highest
If not applicable leave blank.

	Stress past 6 months (1 2 3 4 5)		Stress next 6 months (1 2 3 4 5)
Pregnancy	☐☐☐☐☐		☐☐☐☐☐
Noticeable aging	☐☐☐☐☐		☐☐☐☐☐
Started menopause	☐☐☐☐☐		☐☐☐☐☐
Outstanding personal achievement	☐☐☐☐☐		☐☐☐☐☐
Change in personal habits (smoking, bedtime, meals, etc.)	☐☐☐☐☐		☐☐☐☐☐
Problems from being too successful	☐☐☐		☐☐☐
Lack of personal privacy	☐☐☐		☐☐☐
Difficulty in meeting obligations to yourself	☐☐☐		☐☐☐
Failure to meet personal goals	☐☐☐☐☐		☐☐☐☐☐
Not enough time for yourself	☐☐☐☐☐		☐☐☐☐☐
Philosophical or religious preoccupation	☐☐☐☐☐		☐☐☐☐☐
Problems with weight	☐☐☐☐☐		☐☐☐☐☐
Not enough time to get things done	☐☐☐☐☐		☐☐☐☐☐

Minor violations of the law ☐☐☐ ☐☐☐ ☐☐☐ ☐☐☐ ☐☐☐ ■■■
Assaulted or robbed
Involved in lawsuit or other court procedure

Minor violations of the law ☐☐☐☐☐☐ ☐☐☐☐☐☐ ☐☐☐☐☐☐ ☐☐☐☐☐☐ ☐☐☐☐☐☐ ■■■■■■
Jail term
Change in living conditions
Change in residence
Change in recreation
Change in religious activity

Social

Leading a group ☐☐☐☐☐ ☐☐☐☐☐ ☐☐☐☐☐ ☐☐☐☐☐ ☐☐☐☐☐ ■■■■■
Identification as a group leader
Following along with a group
Major responsibility for or to a social group
Feeling excluded from a group

Starting new relationship(s) ☐☐☐☐ ☐☐☐☐ ☐☐☐☐ ☐☐☐☐ ☐☐☐☐ ■■■■
Ending old relationship(s)
Special care maintaining relationship(s)

Indicate stress level
1 is lowest, 5 is highest
If not applicable leave blank.

Item	Stress past 6 months (1 2 3 4 5)					Stress next 6 months (1 2 3 4 5)				
Not having freedoms and privileges acquaintances enjoy	☐	☐	☐	☐	☐	☐	☐	☐	☐	☐
High popularity	☐	☐	☐	☐	☐	☐	☐	☐	☐	☐
Feelings of superiority towards friends	☐	☐	☐	☐	☐	☐	☐	☐	☐	☐
Feeling inferior to friends and acquaintances	☐	☐	☐	☐	☐	☐	☐	☐	☐	☐
Feeling unwanted and alone	☐	☐	☐	☐	☐	☐	☐	☐	☐	☐
Lack of social stimulation	☐	☐	☐	☐	☐	☐	☐	☐	☐	☐
Death of a close friend	☐	☐	☐	☐	☐	☐	☐	☐	☐	☐
Close friend moves away	☐	☐	☐	☐	☐	☐	☐	☐	☐	☐
Problems with social discrimination	☐	☐	☐	☐	☐	☐	☐	☐	☐	☐
Victim of ethnic, racial, religious or sexual prejudice	☐	☐	☐	☐	☐	☐	☐	☐	☐	☐
Change in social activities	☐	☐	☐	☐	☐	☐	☐	☐	☐	☐

Environment

Item	Stress past 6 months (1 2 3 4 5)					Stress next 6 months (1 2 3 4 5)				
Problems with zoning laws	☐	☐	☐	☐	☐	☐	☐	☐	☐	☐

Noisy or unfriendly neighbors

Construction work in neighborhood

Problems with traffic

Problems with shifts in population

Problems with schools

Local politics or election results

Adjustments to new neighborhood

Neighbors failing to maintain property

Problems with municipal services/utilities

Vandalism/minor crime in neighborhood

Violent crime in neighborhood

Ethnic or racial conflict

Lack of recreational facilities

Crowding

Remodeling in home

Major renovation/construction of home

Financial

Not enough money to pay bills

Loss of income

Increased expenditures

Declining net worth

Indicate stress level
1 is lowest, 5 is highest
If not applicable leave blank.

	Stress past 6 months						Stress next 6 months				
	1	2	3	4	5		1	2	3	4	5
Lack of funds for recreation	☐	☐	☐	☐	☐		☐	☐	☐	☐	☐
Major purchase	☐	☐	☐	☐	☐		☐	☐	☐	☐	☐
Financial loss	☐	☐	☐	☐	☐		☐	☐	☐	☐	☐
Cash flow problems	☐	☐	☐	☐	☐		☐	☐	☐	☐	☐
Loss of credit	☐	☐	☐	☐	☐		☐	☐	☐	☐	☐
Dramatic increase in net worth	☐	☐	☐	☐	☐		☐	☐	☐	☐	☐
Inheritance	☐	☐	☐	☐	☐		☐	☐	☐	☐	☐
Major financial gain	☐	☐	☐	☐	☐		☐	☐	☐	☐	☐
Went on or off welfare	☐	☐	☐	☐	☐		☐	☐	☐	☐	☐
Business readjustment	☐	☐	☐	☐	☐		☐	☐	☐	☐	☐
New mortgage or loan	☐	☐	☐	☐	☐		☐	☐	☐	☐	☐
Foreclosure of mortgage	☐	☐	☐	☐	☐		☐	☐	☐	☐	☐
Work/School											
Beginning new work or school	☐	☐	☐	☐	☐		☐	☐	☐	☐	☐
Poor job description	☐	☐	☐	☐	☐		☐	☐	☐	☐	☐
Ambiguous lines of authority	☐	☐	☐	☐	☐		☐	☐	☐	☐	☐

					Item					
☐					Poorly defined responsibilities at work or school	☐				■
☐	☐	☐			Setting work or school goals	☐	☐	☐		■
☐	☐	☐			Meeting work or school goals	☐	☐	☐		■
☐	☐	☐			Failure to understand or accomplish assignments	☐	☐	☐		■
☐					Lack of necessary skills and abilities to perform adequately at work or school	☐				■
☐	☐	☐	☐	☐	Too tired to get work done	☐	☐	☐	☐	■
☐	☐	☐	☐	☐	Difficulties with career decisions	☐	☐	☐	☐	■
☐	☐	☐	☐	☐	Overwork	☐	☐	☐	☐	■
☐	☐	☐	☐	☐	Pressured deadlines	☐	☐	☐	☐	■
☐	☐	☐	☐	☐	Many emergencies at work	☐	☐	☐	☐	■
☐	☐	☐	☐	☐	Uncooperative co-workers or students	☐	☐	☐	☐	■
☐	☐	☐	☐	☐	Language problems with co-workers or other students	☐	☐	☐	☐	■
☐	☐	☐	☐	☐	Too much responsibility at work	☐	☐	☐	☐	■
☐	☐	☐	☐	☐	Fear of error	☐	☐	☐	☐	■
☐	☐	☐	☐	☐	Fired from job/expelled from school	☐	☐	☐	☐	■
☐	☐	☐	☐	☐	Laid off	☐	☐	☐	☐	■
☐	☐	☐	☐	☐	Work/school hours too long	☐	☐	☐	☐	■

Indicate stress level
1 is lowest, 5 is highest
If not applicable leave blank.

Stress past 6 months 1	2	3	4	5	Item	Stress next 6 months 1	2	3	4	5
☐	☐	☐	☐	☐	Family interfering with work or school	☐	☐	☐	☐	☐
☐	☐	☐	☐	☐	Pressure to do well at work or school	☐	☐	☐	☐	☐
☐	☐	☐	☐	☐	Lack of company/school concern about workers/students	☐	☐	☐	☐	☐
☐	☐	☐	☐	☐	Labor-management/student-school conflict	☐	☐	☐	☐	☐
☐	☐	☐	☐	☐	Out of job or school	☐	☐	☐	☐	☐
☐	☐	☐	☐	☐	Promotion	☐	☐	☐	☐	☐
☐	☐	☐	☐	☐	Outstanding personal achievement at work or school	☐	☐	☐	☐	☐
☐	☐	☐	☐	☐	Change to a different line of work or study	☐	☐	☐	☐	☐
☐	☐	☐	☐	☐	Picking a school, college, or course of study	☐	☐	☐	☐	☐
☐	☐	☐	☐	☐	Equipment malfunctions at work	☐	☐	☐	☐	☐

Company/school interference in personal life ☐ ☐ ☐ ☐ ☐

Insufficient in-service training or supervision ☐ ☐ ☐ ☐ ☐

Boredom with work or school ☐ ☐ ☐ ☐ ☐

Little opportunity for advancement ☐ ☐ ☐ ☐ ☐

Responsibility without authority ☐ ☐ ☐ ☐ ☐

Lack of privacy at work ☐ ☐ ☐ ☐ ☐

Irregular work hours ☐ ☐ ☐ ☐ ☐

Retirement ☐ ☐ ☐ ☐ ☐

Change in responsibilities at work or school ☐ ☐ ☐ ☐ ☐

Trouble with boss ☐ ☐

Change in work hours or conditions ☐ ☐

Muscular System

Tight muscles or muscular aches ☐ ☐ ☐ ☐ ☐

Nervous tics ☐ ☐ ☐ ☐ ☐

Stuttering, voice shaky or strained ☐ ☐ ☐ ☐ ☐

Frowning, wrinkling forehead ☐ ☐ ☐ ☐ ☐

Tension headaches ☐ ☐ ☐ ☐ ☐

Bruxism (grinding or clenching teeth) ☐ ☐ ☐ ☐ ☐

Indicate stress level
1 is lowest, 5 is highest
If not applicable leave blank.

	Stress past 6 months						Stress next 6 months				
	1	2	3	4	5		1	2	3	4	5
Jaw pain or ache											
Pacing, finger- or foot-tapping, difficulty sitting still											
Trembling or shaking											
Back pain											

Parasympathetic Nervous System

	1	2	3	4	5		1	2	3	4	5
Change in appetite											
Nausea											
Gas pains or cramping											
Acid stomach, heartburn											
Problems with urination											
Constipation											
Diarrhea											
Frigidity or impotence											
Dry mouth or throat											
Difficulty swallowing											

Sympathetic Nervous System

- High blood pressure
- Dizziness
- Palpitations
- Sweaty palms, increased perspiration
- Cold hands or feet
- Rapid heartbeat
- Sudden bursts of energy
- Migraine headache
- Chest pain
- Shortness of breath

Emotional

- Feeling things are getting out of control
- Anxiety or panic
- Frustration
- Anger and irritation
- Feeling desperate, hopeless
- Feeling trapped, helpless
- Feeling blue or depressed
- Feeling guilty
- Feeling self-conscious

Indicate stress level
1 is lowest, 5 is highest
If not applicable leave blank.

	Stress past 6 months							Stress next 6 months				
	1	2	3	4	5			1	2	3	4	5
Feeling restless	☐	☐	☐	☐	☐			☐	☐	☐	☐	☐
Cognitive System												
Poor memory	☐	☐	☐	☐	☐			☐	☐	☐	☐	☐
Daydreaming	☐	☐	☐	☐	☐			☐	☐	☐	☐	☐
Indecisiveness	☐	☐	☐	☐	☐			☐	☐	☐	☐	☐
Mental confusion	☐	☐	☐	☐	☐			☐	☐	☐	☐	☐
Racing thoughts	☐	☐	☐	☐	☐			☐	☐	☐	☐	☐
Conviction that everything turns out for the worst	☐	☐	☐	☐	☐			☐	☐	☐	☐	☐
Difficulty falling asleep	☐	☐	☐	☐	☐			☐	☐	☐	☐	☐
Poor judgment	☐	☐	☐	☐	☐			☐	☐	☐	☐	☐
Difficulty concentrating	☐	☐	☐	☐	☐			☐	☐	☐	☐	☐
Preoccupation	☐	☐	☐	☐	☐			☐	☐	☐	☐	☐
Endocrine												
Arthritic joint pain	☐	☐	☐	☐	☐			☐	☐	☐	☐	☐

Menstrual difficulties

Unusual changes in body temperature

Diabetes

Skin rashes or pimples

Fatigue, feeling tired

Infertility

Bloating, water retention

Excessive thirst

Changes in skin color (e.g., gray pallor)

Immune System

Many colds

Frequent bouts of flu

Allergies

Many low-grade infections

Hives

Feeling generally unwell or sick

Sores in mouth

Strep throat

Mononucleosis

Herpes

Indicate your experience from 1 to 5
1 is always, 5 is never

1=always, 5=never				
1	2	3	4	5

Vulnerability to Stress
Please Answer Each Of The Following Items

I eat at least one hot, balanced meal per day.

I get 7–8 hours sleep at least 4 nights per week.

I give and receive affection regularly.

I have one relative within 50 miles on whom I can rely.

I exercise to the point of perspiration at least three times a week.

I limit myself to less than half a pack of cigarettes per day. Fill in 1 if you do not smoke.

I limit myself to fewer than 5 alcoholic drinks per week. Fill in 1 if you do not drink.

I am the appropriate weight for my height.

I have an income adequate to meet basic expenses.

I get strength from my religious beliefs.

I regularly attend club or social events.

I have a network of friends and acquaintances.

- □ □ □ □ ■ I have one or more friends to confide in.
- □ □ □ □ ■ I am in good health (including eyes, hearing, teeth).
- □ □ □ □ ■ I speak openly about my feelings when angry or worried.
- □ □ □ □ ■ I have regular conversations with the people I live with about domestic problems, e.g., chores, money, etc.
- □ □ □ □ ■ I do something fun at least once per week.
- □ □ □ □ ■ I am able to organize my time effectively.
- □ □ □ □ ■ I limit myself to fewer than 3 cups of coffee (or tea or cola drinks) per day.
- □ □ □ □ ■ I take quiet time for myself during the day.

Printed in the United States
By Bookmasters